AF805610

Archimedes

New Studies in the History and Philosophy of Science and Technology

Volume 43

Series Editor
Jed Z. Buchwald
Dreyfuss Professor of History
California Institute of Technology
Pasadena
California
USA

More information about this series at http://www.springer.com/series/5644

Nathan Sivin

Health Care in Eleventh-Century China

Springer

Nathan Sivin
University of Pennsylvania
Philadelphia, PA, USA

ISSN 1385-0180 ISSN 2215-0064 (electronic)
Archimedes
ISBN 978-3-319-20426-0 ISBN 978-3-319-20427-7 (eBook)
DOI 10.1007/978-3-319-20427-7

Library of Congress Control Number: 2015948370

Springer Cham Heidelberg New York Dordrecht London
© Springer International Publishing Switzerland 2015
This work is subject to copyright. All rights are reserved by the Publisher, whether the whole or part of the material is concerned, specifically the rights of translation, reprinting, reuse of illustrations, recitation, broadcasting, reproduction on microfilms or in any other physical way, and transmission or information storage and retrieval, electronic adaptation, computer software, or by similar or dissimilar methodology now known or hereafter developed.
The use of general descriptive names, registered names, trademarks, service marks, etc. in this publication does not imply, even in the absence of a specific statement, that such names are exempt from the relevant protective laws and regulations and therefore free for general use.
The publisher, the authors and the editors are safe to assume that the advice and information in this book are believed to be true and accurate at the date of publication. Neither the publisher nor the authors or the editors give a warranty, express or implied, with respect to the material contained herein or for any errors or omissions that may have been made.

Printed on acid-free paper

Springer International Publishing AG Switzerland is part of Springer Science+Business Media (www.springer.com)

Dedicated to my colleagues at the
China Institute for History of Medicine and Medical Literature,
China Academy of Chinese Medical Sciences,
led for many years by Professor Li Jingwei

Preface

In writing this book I have done my best to say clearly what I have to say for anyone who is simply curious about ancient Chinese health care. I have documented it for historians of medicine, Sinologists, or humanistically inclined physicians.

Don't feel that you are obliged to begin reading this book with the first page and continue to the end. It has three introductory chapters, but if you simply want to know what I have to say about health care in China, you may want to begin with chapter 4, and return to the first three only if something arouses your interest in them. The sequence of the book's remainder, which deals with the varieties of health care, is more or less arbitrary, so read them in an order that fits your own curiosity.

I became curious about science in China because it seemed to me that there were many possibilities for investigating nature and the human body that had never occurred to Western thinkers, and that it might be interesting, rather than simply philosophizing about them, to see if people elsewhere had tried them out. China was the most obvious civilization to explore, since its remarkably rich writings on medicine were freer of Graeco-Roman influence than those of Islam; unlike those of India, they are mostly datable; and its authors were highly articulate about every aspect of human activity.

I did not have the slightest interest in medical history until, not long after I began teaching, a physician studying anthropology named Arthur Kleinman kept reminding me that if I was curious about understanding the human body, medicine was the obvious area to investigate. I was not exactly eager to take this advice, since the early Chinese medical literature is enormous, and to get an idea of it I would have to spend several years reading before I could begin trying to form conclusions. But the prospect was so enticing that before long I began that process. My first attempt to make sense of Chinese medicine was a manuscript that I drafted in 1973 and found quite unsatisfactory. The available analytical tools were too crude, and my understanding was inadequate.

There is practically nothing of that draft left in this book. What prompted me to begin again was the realization (finally!) that, although a fairly large literature has accumulated on classical Chinese medicine, its practitioners were a minority among therapists, and only a small part of the population before modern times had access to their care. At the same time, while reading the medical literature and that of early religion, I had gradually accumulated a rich trove of documents about non-medical therapy. This was obviously the other part of the health care picture, and my task was to make a rough sketch of what it was and how it fit together.

Philadelphia, PA, USA Nathan Sivin

The Contents of This Book

Chapter 2 presents definitions of certain words that play important roles in the book, such as "health care," "medicine," "religion," and "elite." It also sets out my viewpoints on a number of contentious issues, for instance, how to translate early medical terms and what I mean by culture (not just the word, but the disputed concept). The third chapter takes up a question that up to now writers on ancient Chinese medicine have scrupulously avoided: how effective could early health care have been? My answers have shaped this book as a whole.

Chapters 4 through 6 divide the range of therapies that I study historically into four groups: classical medicine, popular curing, elite curing, and a variety of curative rituals carried out by government officials, from the emperor to local magistrates. I take them up in that order, beginning with the classical practice that has been most thoroughly studied by modern scholars.

By classical medicine I mean the practice of physicians before the twentieth century, which was not at all uniform. Physicians in imperial times learned medical doctrines from a cumulative tradition of books as much as two millennia old. They imbibed these classics' view of the body as a microcosm, and of disorders as disturbances of the body's adjustment to seasonal rhythms.

Almost all the historical writing so far about health care in pre-modern China is about classical medicine. I do not see it as the dominant kind of therapy, but rather as a kind of care based on learning, limited to the most articulate minority of the population. Classical medicine kept its vitality by appropriating other kinds of therapy, just as popular, Daoist, and Buddhist curers drew on it.

I will give examples below of the regular interplay of classical and popular therapy. The difference between them was not simply secular vs. religious, but views of health and disease based on cosmic symbolism vs. those based on the bureaucracy of the gods. The cosmos of the physicians accommodated the otherworld, the realm of spirits, which were part of the natural order. There was no supernatural in Chinese thought, at least not before Buddhism. Popular therapists regularly translated dysfunctions of the universe into their own concrete language, and physicians did the inverse.

With that in mind, I take up in chapter 5 therapy as an aspect of popular religion, which has been little explored. Few historians discuss any but the "Three Religions," by which they mean Confucianism, Buddhism, and Daoism. The recent exceptions who discuss popular religion refer to it as folk religion, the common religion, local religion, folk Daoism, popular sects, and so on, and rarely even hint that in early China all these terms refer to a single phenomenon. The result is general confusion.[1]

The few people who are engaged in research on early popular religion tend to see Buddhism and Daoism as elite ritual developments out of common worship.[2] Most learned authors in imperial China ignored popular religion because they believed that emperors and their ministers, not the illiterate peasants who fed and clothed them, had invented all worthwhile techniques and institutions.[3] In the People's Republic of China, until recent decades popular traditions of worship remained unexplored because the government condemns them as superstition. The fact remains that they were the only universally available forms of religious practice. Buddhist and Daoist clerics were distributed across Song China, but beyond the reach of many peasants. Seen from the viewpoints of medical anthropology and history, ritual curing is well worth studying in detail.

The surviving record of popular religion was perforce set down by literate people. It is extremely rich. It is useful if read critically. My sources come partly from the rich Daoist literature, which in adapting the rites of local religious curers (often condemning them at the same time) gives much information about them; partly from medical handbooks, some of which freely adapted folk practices; and to a smaller extent from the collections of jottings about everything under the sun that a number of eleventh-century literati wrote.

Finally I discuss three varieties of religious curing that, unlike the oral traditions of popular practice, depended on writing: those of Buddhism, Daoism, and the state cult. The latter has nothing to do with Confucianism, and would no doubt have outraged the ancient sage. It comprises diverse rituals of worship directed toward gods, carried out by the emperor and his officials as part of their duties.

Poor people seldom saw, and had no direct access to, any official. But all three traditions played important roles in shaping health care. Although the three sharply differ in many obvious ways, in the eleventh century the high status of all three depended on writing and literacy. Not all Buddhist clerics were literate, but those who were not memorized texts. It makes sense to discuss their liturgies as those of elite religions. There was much liturgical borrowing back and forth between the three. Although some movements condemned the practices of popular religion as "excessive cults (*yinsi* 淫祠)," all of them appropriated much from it.

---

[1] Teiser 1995, 378–380, Sivin 2010.

[2] Raz 2012 is a penetrating reconstruction of this process for early Daoist movements.

[3] Csikszentmihalyi 2002, 92, notes that such achievements by legendary emperors depended on their ability "to understand Heaven and the spirit world."

In the conclusion, in addition to drawing together the picture sketched in previous chapters, I suggest that the methods used here may be of some use in evaluating responses to therapy today.

References

Csikszentmihalyi, Mark. 2002. Traditional Taxonomies and Revealed Texts in the Han. In Kohn & Roth 2002, 81–101.
Raz, Gil. 2012. *The Emergence of Daoism. Creation of Tradition.* Routledge Studies in Taoism. London: Routledge.
Sivin, Nathan. 2010. Old and New Daoisms. *Religious Studies Review* 36. 1: 31–50.
Teiser, Stephen F. 1995. Popular Religion. *Journal of Asian Studies* 54. 2: 378–395.

Acknowledgements

One thing that made my current understanding possible was my ambiance, first what is now the Science, Technology and Society program at MIT and then the Department of the History and Sociology of Science at the University of Pennsylvania. A good deal of what may seem brand new with respect to Chinese health care long ago made possible a capacious understanding of how Euro-American health care evolved. Some of the most valuable methods and insights I learned came from, among others, Judith Farquhar at the University of Chicago, Robert Aronowitz and Renée Fox at the University of Pennsylvania, Sir Geoffrey Lloyd at the Needham Research Institute, Giorgio de Santillana and Jerome Y. Lettvin at MIT, and Volker Scheid at Westminster University, London.

I especially wish to acknowledge the help of seven colleagues who have read the complete manuscript and provided me with critical comments, Patricia Buckley Ebrey, Daniel Burton-Rose, Allegra Giovine, Marta Hanson, Volker Scheid, Hilary Smith, and an anonymous reader. I am also indebted to these colleagues who have read and commented on parts of the manuscript: Philip Cho, Theodore Friend, Paul Goldin, Arnold M. Katz, Paul R. Katz, Mujeeb Khan, Lewis Pyenson, Pierce Salguero, and **Zhao** Lu 赵璐.

An earlier draft of chapter 3 appeared three years ago in another book in this same series, *A Master of Science History. Essays in Honor of Charles Coulston Gillispie,* ed. Jed Z. Buchwald, pp. 341–53 (Archimedes, 30. Secaucus: Springer).

Contents

Chapter 1
Health Care, Medicine, and Chinese Society

Abstract This book explores the spectrum of health care available to people in Imperial China, and analyzes important parts of it. It focuses on ideas and methods of therapy in the long eleventh century (960-1127) and their interaction. Historians have concentrated on the high medical tradition, with its rich sources, but its physicians treated few outside the class that governed China and owned most of its wealth. Who, then, cared for the vast majority, illiterate, mostly rural, and largely poor? They depended on the resources available in their own villages—from local herbalists, popular priests, and others—and, for epidemics and other collective crises, from Buddhist and Daoist priests and occasionally from local officials. To most Chinese, curative rites were more familiar than medical prescriptions. The book applies medical anthropology and the sociology of medicine to interpret the rich evidence of ritual therapy in the eleventh century.

Through the two thousand years of imperial China, health care was perpetually in flux.[1] I will explore one period in which change came more quickly than in most. The Northern Song dynasty began in 960 with the reunification of China after a century of growing tumult in multiple regimes that called themselves empires. It ended in 1127 when the Jin Tartars occupied north China. They drove the Song government south of the Yangzi river, where it remained for another century and a half.

The eleventh century was remarkably dynamic in every respect. The center of gravity of society and of wealth had been migrating southeastward to the lower Yangzi river region for a long time; now the shift was definitive, and included the southeastern coast (present Fujian and Guangdong provinces) as well. For the previous three centuries an originally military aristocracy centered in north China wielded power. In the last century of the three, as the population shifted toward the south, the fertile lower Yangzi and Huai river valleys became the most productive and wealthiest part of China.

In the eleventh to thirteenth centuries a main force for change was competition between men from the north, the south, and the southwest (Sichuan had played a

[1] I define "health care" below, chapter 2, p. 9.

© Springer International Publishing Switzerland 2015

N. Sivin, *Health Care in Eleventh-Century China*, Archimedes 43,
DOI 10.1007/978-3-319-20427-7_1

noticeable part for centuries), but by the end of that time southeasterners were predominant.[2]

That was not the only main transition. In early imperial China, commerce was not a source of prestige. As time passed, wealthy merchant families broke through old obstacles, especially in the south, and increasingly attained high social and political status.

In the eleventh century, for the first time, the imperial examination system became a broad avenue of recruitment to civil service posts. It was far from the only such avenue. A large proportion of those appointed had been exempted from the examinations because of family connections to officials.

Marriage could be a matter of mutual benefit. As Robert Hartwell has shown, positions to be filled by examination were limited by quotas for each province, and wealthy local gentry families monopolized some of these quotas for generations. Maintaining such a monopoly demanded that those families regularly produce extremely bright sons devoted to memorizing classical texts. There was an alternative for those who failed. One could marry one's daughter to a very bright young man from an elite lineage already well established in the civil service. Families that could afford to be lavish with dowries were able to compete for sons of families that already had high status. The result after several generations was a trend toward extended families who always had some children in the civil service and others in business.[3] Although by the end of the period the old bias against commerce persisted in some circles, from then on it had less and less to do with social reality.

The result of all these changes was administrations that were more open to change than in the past, even though that change increased imperial power. From then until the present, leadership not only in politics but in society, thought, finance, commerce, science, medicine, art—in almost every field of enterprise—shifted to the southeastern provinces generally, and came from a wider social spectrum than before.

The Diversity of Health Care

When we look beyond the high tradition of medicine, we see a remarkably diverse health care picture, partly on the social periphery of medicine and partly non-medical. This book will explore particularly important parts of the spectrum: medicine, religious curing, and curing by officials.

The literate physicians, probably the smallest group, were the therapists we know most about. They belonged to the educated elite, so they could leave written records. Many of them took up medicine when they failed to qualify for appointment to officialdom. Like literati who prepared for the imperial examinations by

[2] On the transformation of Jiangnan into "the principal arena of continuous social, economic, and cultural development," see Smith 2003.

[3] For the ubiquity of this pattern see Hartwell 1982, 419ff. Hartwell's analysis shows the complexity of regional patterns of social change; I unavoidably simplify his argument.

studying the conventional classics, they learned their trade by memorizing the written classics of their field, and—mostly but not always—learning current methods as disciples or apprentices. They competed with members of hereditary medical families, who passed down proprietary therapies. These retainers remained the majority of therapists to the gentry and others who could afford them. By the Song period, many of that group had learned to read and write, at least well enough to keep records. Some were indistinguishable from the literate physicians.[4]

Since there was no organization to police qualifications, anyone could call himself a doctor *(yisheng* 醫生 or *yi* 醫). Many with scantier educations cultivated a clientèle further down the social scale. Further still down the scale, people with more limited skills tended to present themselves as "therapists *(yishi* 醫士 or *yigong* 醫工)" rather than "physicians." Where the boundary lay was merely a matter for curer and patient to agree on. There was also an indistinct genre of itinerant curers, called "neighborhood therapists *(lüyan yigong* 閭閻醫工)" "doctors of the grassy marshes *(caoze yi* 草澤醫)," "bell-ringing doctors *(lingyi* 鈴醫)," and by other names.[5]

The literati physicians tended to look down on anyone who did not belong to their own group, but had no way to put them out of business. Indeed they were themselves far too few to provide medical care for everyone, and mostly preferred patients who were their social peers or betters.

Since educated doctors (some of them from hereditary medical families) left the records, providing a model for their less learned imitators, my discussion of classical medicine will concentrate on their special world-view and therapeutic methods.[6] I will describe the most important varieties of religious health care separately.

Preventing and curing illness was part of every religion that sought devotees, not only in China but throughout the pre-modern world. Health care was the cutting edge of religious organization. In China, the spirit mediums and others who served as priests of popular religion, as well as the Buddhist and Daoist clerics, had their own curative rituals, which varied with their understandings of the universe and man's place in it. But the neat distinctions between religions that undergraduates are expected to memorize are specious. Freely borrowing back and forth was the norm, partly because all therapists' livelihoods were at stake in their ability to aid the sick, and partly because ordinary people were ready to worship any spirit that they had reason to hope could cure them.

Finally, given the vastness and diversity of China, officials were responsible for governing populations whose cultures often differed from their own. They regularly administered too many people, usually with inadequate resources. They could succeed only if they won the respect of the local gentry. Some of them did so by demonstrating their high-minded contempt for the customs of the poor, popular worship

---

[4] In order to avoid confusion, I use "physicians" for the elite group and "hereditary physicians" for the rest. Members of the latter group often imitated the former, and people commonly called both "physicians."

[5] Yu Gengzhe 于賡哲 2011, 46. *Lüyan* implies poor neighborhoods, and *caoze* remote areas.

[6] For a more detailed discussion see Sivin 1987, 43–199. I use "classical medicine" for what physicians in imperial China practiced; see chapter 4.

among them. Others added to their charisma by practicing religious rituals that the governed would understand. As we will see, many civil servants even learned and practiced rites for controlling demons.

Health Care and Medicine

There is a great difference between health care and medicine. As historians of occidental medicine use the terms, medicine is what physicians do to stop, minimize, and prevent suffering,[7] and health care is what everyone—including physicians—does for the same purposes. "Everyone" begins not with the practitioner, but with the person who feels sick. Most treatment, in ancient times as today, begins with self-therapy. Avoiding confusion between health care and medicine is extremely useful in thinking about the rest of the world, and about the past before physicians were defined by a uniform education.

Speaking of the family, it is a truism that the two largest segments of health care are self-therapy and family therapy. Let me give an example. One summer morning decades ago, when my wife and I were living in Cambridge, England, I woke up, stood up, and promptly fell flat on my face. This seemed odd. As soon as I stood up again the same thing happened. My obvious first response was to ask myself what was wrong. Had it been a headache, I would have diagnosed it and taken an aspirin. It was not a headache. I had no idea what it could be. The only thought that occurred to me was "if this is permanent, it's going to be awfully inconvenient!" It could perfectly well have been permanent.

Since my wife quickly noticed me lying on the floor, the next step after my failed self-diagnosis was indeed family consultation. As a result of it, she telephoned a friend. She found out that the latest quirky virus had rendered several friends horizontal, and that after 48 hours it went away. That information was so satisfactory that neither of us thought of my taking any medicine, much less of troubling a physician. Within a day, as the symptoms began to fade, we were confident that no therapy would be necessary. That was the end of that.

My point is that, except in exceptional circumstances, regardless of time or place the physician is more likely to be the last resort for health care than the first. In the real world even today the norm is a great many varieties of health care besides self-care, family care, and therapy by a physician.

In ancient China the spectrum of therapists was even wider, and the family played a more important role in primary care and in choosing between curers. In the eleventh century there were many patterns of living together, ranging from the nuclear families of the poor to elite households of up to five generations with many resident

[7] This includes both physical and mental suffering, although how far people at a given time and place considered the latter as separate, and as an object of therapy, varied greatly. In practice, eleventh-century Chinese saw mind and body as part of a unitary whole rather than, as in the West, a radical dichotomy.

servants and the servants' families, not to mention the large collective households of some ethnic groups. Family members often disagreed about what a given disorder was, and how to deal with it. They might favor a method passed down in the family: a religious rite, dosage with a medicinal plant that grew nearby, a formula commonly used in the locality, one mentioned in a medical book, adjustments to diet, snake venom or some other panacea offered by a specialist curer, acupuncture or moxibustion, or massage. When they had negotiated what curer to call, still someone often disagreed about the treatment proposed by the therapist.

Today, adults who hurt themselves or fall ill often have some idea of what to do about it. If what they try does not succeed, or if they don't know what is wrong, someone else in the household usually knows, or thinks she knows, how to cope. Only if that fails is it necessary to look for outside help. The first contact outside the family may be a friend with a reputation for medical knowledge, or a pharmacist. If a physician becomes involved, it is usually further down the line, sometimes after a chiropractor or a holistic therapist of some kind. The doctor may come at the end of the line, particularly if he is the most difficult to make an appointment with, and the most expensive, of the available choices.[8]

This pattern familiar from our own experience held as well in eleventh-century China. Wealth and education had a great deal to do with how much choice one had. The great majority of the population had none. That is, laborers and farmers usually had little or no education, and many had no discretionary income at all. Since physicians preferred living in the towns and cities, and most villagers had no opportunity to travel, seeing a doctor was simply not among their options. They or another family member might gather local medicinal plants themselves—botanical drugs were only beginning to be cultivated—or buy them from a neighbor.[9] They might know someone who distributed a family formula as a kind of charity, earning merit for a better rebirth. There might be an itinerant curer of some sort who came through their village from time to time. But the main source of local therapy was the village temple, because the most powerful source of health was its god, or one of them.

A larger village or a town might have more than one popular temple, owned by the community and normally managed by an invoker (*zhu* 祝), who could refer inquirers to a popular, Buddhist, or Daoist ritual master (*fashi* 法師) who was likely to suit their needs. The therapist would perform his ritual at the patient's home or, if more space was needed, at the temple. Everyone involved expected a small gift of money, food, or something else useful, more generous if the rites turned out to be effective.[10] Laborers who earned wages in large towns or cities had more choices than farmers: more temples, more kinds of curers, and more sellers of materia medica who could only attract the poor.

---

[8] If the U.S. patient is poor, without well-informed acquaintances, and the problem urgent, a hospital emergency room may be the first resort outside the family.

[9] How the cultivation of botanicals began and evolved is a practically unexplored topic. See Hu Daojing 1963 and 1981.

[10] Email from Terry Kleeman, 5 September 2013.

City-dwellers who had enough money in their pockets had a great deal of choice not only between drug-sellers and curers with all sorts of special skills, but also among doctors and priests. The government, for part of the century in a few large cities, operated pharmacies that sold at controlled prices medicines recommended in formularies published by the state.

Associated with large temples were diviners, sometimes many of them. Illness was one of the most frequent topics of divination, by consulting an individual if one could afford it, or by drawing fortune-telling lots *(chouqian* 抽籤), available in temples since long before the Song period.[11]

As for physicians, they could be found at every level of society: the old-style doctor whose skills, he was likely to boast, had been passed down for generations as family secrets; the curer who had learned what skills he had by apprenticeship; the new style of literate self-trained doctor, who had learned from manuscripts or printed books, or from a mentor; the retainer to the upper gentry, prominent by his learning and his income; and the imperial physician retired into private practice, accessible to a few, a trophy of high social standing.

Priests, whether popular, Buddhist, or Daoist, were trained in curative rituals. Many of their general ceremonies aimed, among other goals, to treat the sick and maintain health. Their skill at healing was an important facet of their reputations. The approaches of each religion differed, but they borrowed methods back and forth, as we will see in chapters 4 and 5. Many clerics learned secular techniques as well (see, for instance, chapter 6, pp. 138–139).

Goal

The purpose of this book is to begin understanding and thinking about the range of health care available to China's people in the long eleventh century.

This first general exploration of early health care could have studied any period of history. Every era encompassed change, and each had its own style. My choice is not quite arbitrary. In medicine, the Northern Song government became much more active than its predecessors in meeting the health needs of its subjects. The formularies and drugstores it sponsored encouraged self-medication. It attracted young men of elite families to the practice of medicine. The latter move, as it gradually succeeded, encouraged hereditary doctors and others to emulate elite styles of practice. The state's involvement in popular religion, Daoism, and Buddhism encouraged the attention of clerics to curing; a reputation for overcoming illnesses was a strong element in a god's (and a temple's) qualifications for endorsement by the government.

Because there were so many kinds of therapy, my concern for analysis and the paucity of eleventh-century sources on popular curing rule out surveying all of them. I have concentrated on what I believe most needs explanation, and what I understand. In order to comprehend what curers of all kinds did, it is necessary to

[11] On the many varieties of divination in early China see Kalinowski 2003.

use not only sources written in the long eleventh century, but earlier writings that practitioners of the Northern Song dynasty knew. I also use three short accounts written in the century after 1127, simply because they are so rich and colorful, and characters and circumstances like theirs can be found in the century before 1127.

The need to investigate a few exceptionally important themes has kept me from considering in depth others equally interesting but more scantily documented, such as self-medication and therapy by family members; medical divinities and cults; trance healing; local variations in healing practices and beliefs; and the influence of minority (that is, non-Han) peoples on health practices. It would also be good to know more about the practice of medical therapists who did not belong to the literate elite: the hereditary physicians who learned their skills from their fathers or uncles, and the few female physicians whose educations are unknown.[12] There were also many other providers of health care who await investigation: the midwives and other female practitioners; the itinerant curers who provided therapy to poor villagers and townspeople; and the bonesetters, inoculators, veterinarians and others who provided special services.

References

Abbreviations

DZ = Volume number in *Daozang*
ES = *Ersishi shi* 二十四史 of ZS, 1959–1977.
HY = text in Harvard-Yenching Concordance series
j. = *juan* 卷 (chapter)
RW = published by Renmin Weisheng Chubanshe 人民衛生出版社, Beijing
S = Title number in Schipper 1975
SQ = Siku quanshu 四庫全書
SV = Schipper & Verellen 2004
T = *Taishō shinshū Daizōkyō* 大正新修大藏經
UP = University Press
YZ = Yi tong zheng mai quan shu 醫統正脈全書
ZD = Volume, item, *juan,* and page numbers in *Zhonghua daozang* 中华道藏
ZS = published by Zhonghua shuju 中華書局, Beijing
ZZ = Zhongyi zhenben congshu 中醫珍本叢書 ed.

Furth, Charlotte. 1999. *A Flourishing Yin: Gender in China's Medical History, 960–1665.* Berkeley: University of California Press.

Hartwell, Robert M. 1982. Demographic, Political and Social Transformations in China, 750–1550. *Harvard Journal of Asiatic Studies* 42. 2: 365–442.

[12] On female curers see Furth 1999, especially pp. 123–124. Sources on non-elite practitioners in the Song period are scanty, but they are plentiful for Ming and Qing China. See, among others, Unschuld 2010 and Unschuld & Zheng 2012.

Hu Daojing 胡道靜. 1963. Shen Kuo de nongxue zhuzuo *Mengxi wang huai lu* 沈括的農學著作夢溪忘懷錄 (Shen Kuo's agricultural book *Record of Longings Forgotten). Wen shi* 文史, 1963, 3: 221–225.

Hu Daojing. 1981. *Mengxi wang huai lu* gouchen—Shen Cunzhung yizhu gouchen zhi yi 夢溪忘懷錄鈎沉—沈存中佚著鈎沉之一 *(Record of Longings Forgotten* reconstituted. Shen Kuo's lost works reconstituted, 1). *Hangzhou daxue xuebao* 1981, 11. 1: 1–16.

Kalinowski, Marc, ed. 2003. *Divination et société dans la Chine médiévale. Étude des manuscripts de Dunhuang de la Bibliothèque nationale de France et de la British Library.* Paris: Bibliothèque nationale.

Sivin, Nathan. 1987. *Traditional Medicine in Contemporary China.* Science, Medicine, and Technology in East Asia, 2. Ann Arbor: Center for Chinese Studies, University of Michigan.

Smith, Paul Yakov, & Richard von Glahn, eds. 2003. *The Song–Yuan–Ming Transition in Chinese History*. Harvard East Asian Monographs, 221. Harvard UP. On the period 1270–1550.

Smith, Paul Yakov. 2003. Problematizing the Song–Yuan–Ming Transition. In Smith & von Glahn 2003, 1–34.

Unschuld, Paul U. 2010. The Berlin Collections of Chinese Medical Manuscripts: Rural Authors, Rural Contents. Monumenta Serica 58: 281–293.

Unschuld, Paul U., & Zheng Jinsheng. 2012. *Chinese Traditional Healing. The Berlin Collections of Manuscript Volumes from the Sixteenth through the Early Twentieth Century.* Sir Henry Wellcome Asian Series, 10. 3 vols. Leiden: Brill.

Yu Gengzhe 于赓哲. 2011. *Tangdai jibing yiliao shi chu tan* 唐代疾病医疗史初探 (Preliminary historical studies of illness and therapy in the Tang period). Beijing: Zhongguo Shehui Kexue Chubanshe.

Chapter 2
Some Definitions and Viewpoints

Abstract This chapter defines how this book uses such basic terms as "health care" and "medicine." It discusses certain words important in this book such as "elite," "religion," and "ritual." I also set out my positions on a number of contentious issues pertinent to the book, such as how to translate ancient medical terminology, how Chinese medical writings describe the body's contents and metabolic processes, the role of objectivity in historical studies, the meaning of "culture," the value of cultural relativism, and the coinage of technical terminology by historians. The chapter also explains some of the book's conventions, such as the use of "biomedicine" and "formula," and the use of Chinese personal names.

Definitions

Health care

The normal meaning of this term is all of the means that people use, individually and collectively, to maintain and restore health. This is a perfectly satisfactory definition. I emphasize therapy rather than such means of remaining healthy as exercise and entertainment. It would have been good to examine health maintenance—which Chinese discussed as an aspect of "nurturing life (*yangsheng* 養生)"—in relation to minimizing physical suffering, but I have chosen to limit the scope of this book to the many varieties of curing. Part of the fantasy of exotic Cathay is the notion that its inhabitants paid their doctors only so long as they remained healthy. Sensible though that idea may be, I have never seen it expressed in a Chinese source before modern times.

Historians are more likely to call non-medical therapists healers than curers. Experience has led me to prefer the latter word. A good many years ago an eminent authority took me to task for using it to refer to religious therapists, on the ground that, since religious ritual could not possibly cure anything, "curer" is inappropriate. I use it for two reasons. First, a fixed conviction that ritual cannot possibly cure anything is as ignorant as a fixed conviction that it can cure everything. I discuss the efficacy of ritual therapy in chapter 3. I find "healing" implies a passivity that underestimates the power of symbol and meaning that I explore there. Second, therapists

© Springer International Publishing Switzerland 2015

N. Sivin, *Health Care in Eleventh-Century China*, Archimedes 43,
DOI 10.1007/978-3-319-20427-7_2

believed that they were curing disease, and that was how they presented themselves. My concern is to study them, not to correct their language.

Medicine

Medicine may, according to the dictionary, include or exclude self-dosing, surgery, therapy performed by people whose occupation is something else, what folk curers do, what pharmacists recommend, and any number of other activities. Here, like most people who write about medical history, I use the word for what physicians did.

In China a millennium ago, *yi* 醫 meant practitioners who belonged to medical families, scholar-physicians trained in certain medical classics, and a gamut of their imitators. This unorganized occupational group had no clear borders, and no authority to draw its own boundaries and patrol them. It was not unusual for a doctor who considered himself a "literatus-physician *(ruyi* 儒醫)" to be labeled a "mediocrity *(yongyi* 庸醫)" by a competitor. As in the United States before 1920, anyone could set himself up in the business of therapy, and call himself whatever struck his fancy. I will discuss what eleventh-century physicians did in chapter 4.

Medical disorders. The commonest Chinese term for what physicians aimed to cure was *bing* 病, which was a good deal broader in scope than "disease." It included wounds, broken bones, and other traumata, rashes and other skin lesions, disorders of childbirth, and other problems that the patient and doctor faced. Its opposite in this context was *zhi* 治, "curing, cured." The same word in political discussions was the opposite of *luan* 亂, "disorder." *Zhi* is a general term for "order." Thus *bing* is a species of disorder, and is most usefully translated "medical disorder."[1] When doctors wanted to refer narrowly to diseases, they usually used *ji* 疾; and they had a rich terminology for other classes of disorder. There was no clear distinction between syndrome and disease.

Nomenclature for diseases is problematic, largely because therapy is local. China was an enormous and highly diverse country, in which there were innumerable dialects, with a range nearly as wide as that of Western Europe's languages. The names of diseases accordingly varied from one region to another. That largely accounts for their enormous diversity in synoptic handbooks of etiology and symptomatology. One of the things that made such handbooks valuable was that they attempted to separate mere synonyms from terms for different disorders. One could carry such work of disentangling only so far, since it was often impossible to be certain that a disease common in the north was the same as one called by the same name in the deep south that had a dissimilar balance of symptoms.

[1] For details and other pertinent terms see Sivin 1987, 99–100, 106–107.

Elite

In imperial China, there was a juridically defined elite. The people who belonged to this class in the eleventh century were aristocrats and officials, or were closely related to them by birth, or had passed government examinations and were thus eligible for official appointment. Members of the elite and their families were exempt from certain taxes and other obligations, were not ordinarily subjected to judicial torture, and so on. There was no single term for members of the elite. The most common were *shi* 士 and *shidafu* 士大夫, which I translate "scholar-officials" when discussing their roles in governance, and "literati" when thinking of them as practitioners of arts and letters. I use "gentry" to mean *shi* and their relatives and descendants who did not necessarily hold office. The opposite of "elite" was "commoners," *shu* 庶 or *min* 民, widely called *buyi* 布衣, "wearers of cheap cloth." A commoner was someone who was not an examination graduate, and was not closely related to an official. This status affected taxation, periodic labor duty, judicial procedures, and other aspects of life.

The fundamental boundary between classes was literacy. Memorization of certain ancient classics and the ability to write in styles derived from them, not just the ability to read and write basic vocabulary, was the basis of education.

The status and character of the elite changed considerably over time. As Peter Bol has put it, "In the seventh century the *shih* were an elite led by aristocratic great clans of illustrious pedigree; in the tenth and eleventh centuries the *shih* were the civil bureaucrats; and finally in the Southern Sung they were the more numerous but rarely illustrious local elite families who provided bureaucrats and examination candidates."[2]

Religion and its types

The word "religion" has no stable meaning in the English language. For the New England philosopher William James, endeavoring in 1902 to find what underlay the varieties of its experience, religion "is a radically personal matter, a private, subjective, deep experience 'faith-state' … adamantly resistant to the growing claims of the public, the social, and the everyday to be the sole and ultimate dictators of what we may believe." That is how the anthropologist Clifford Geertz sums up James's conclusion, going on to argue that by the end of the twentieth century,

> religious 'experience,' pushed out the door as a radically subjective, individualized 'faith state,' returns through the window as the communal sensibility of a religiously assertive social actor. … in what we are pleased to call the real world, 'meaning,' 'identity,' 'power,' and 'experience' are hopelessly entangled, mutually implicative, and 'religion' can no more

---

[2] Bol 1992, 4. Bol's *shih* are my *shi*.

> be founded upon or reduced to the last, that is, 'experience,' than it can to any of the others. It is not in solitude that faith is made.[3]

Nevertheless, many scholars of comparative religions today define their field in terms of "peak experiences" and see no need for such words as "faith," "divinity," "gods," and "God."

When I take up such matters as religious curing in eleventh-century China, I am talking about something not at all like the make-your-own-choice-if-it-interests-you flux of early twenty-first-century Euro-American faith.[4] In fact, it is equally unlike the flux of quite a different kind that Chinese are now experiencing. The atheism of the second half of the twentieth century, enforced with vigor by Party and state, is being drenched—but not slain—by a vast wave of religious enthusiasm and observance, everything from revived popular religion to Buddhism and Christianity to the latest cults from abroad. But "peak experiences" will not wrap up religion for the year 1050. Nor will any of the other categories Geertz has brandished above. In order to see why this is so, it is necessary to ponder briefly the difference between concepts of identity in modern Euro-America and early China.

Writers on Chinese culture of the last generation often observed that the prevalent sense of identity has little in common with the norm in the U.S., also widespread in Europe. North American identity is based on a notion of unique individuality, which its owner may or may not choose to reveal to others.[5] Whether it is possible to know what lies inside another person, even with her permission, is a problem often discussed but never settled. The more Californian versions of individuality question whether one can even know oneself.

For the generation of people now defining their own individuality and publicizing it with the help of Facebook and other cyber-pseudo-necessities, we are the sum of what we let others know we buy and entertain ourselves with. Despite this shift in identity—to our own particular grab-bag of mass-market brands—the mythologies of modern culture still make it the deeply private property of each person. The Chinese norm since about 1990 has only begun to shift in this consumerist direction.[6]

On the other hand, Chinese a millennium ago often thought of themselves as the sum of all their obligations to others and of all the obligations of others to them. In this view a person is a nexus of social relationships with kin, friends, authority figures, and others. The sense of self pertinent to health care was that of someone

---

[3] James 1902, 418; Geertz 2000b, 169, 178, quotation from p. 184; unpublished discussions over many years at annual meetings of the American Society for the Study of Religions.

[4] I use "Euro-American" to designate the locus of modernism as well as what its proponents call post-modernism—which seems to me odd considering that the level of political comportment in such nations has not advanced far beyond that of the late Neolithic. Some of the poorer states of Europe are in many senses less modern than China.

[5] This is a useful but admittedly weak generalization, given the cultural diversity in nations on both sides of the Atlantic.

[6] See, among many sources, Wang 2001 and 2005.

situated in a stable family and community. This was often the case even when neither was actually stable.

This understanding of identity has survived to a considerable extent in the People's Republic of China and in Chinese communities outside it. Since the 1980's, when the state began encouraging the idea that "to get rich is glorious," it undermined its own expectation that people subordinate themselves to the community. Under the new capitalist form of socialism, more and more Chinese have moved on, not to the partly Enlightenment and partly Romantic ideal of the person as the self-invented independent agent, but to a striving to make their own decisions as consumers and in relationships.[7]

With all of this in mind, when this book takes up eleventh-century religion, it is concerned not with private faith but with the phenomena of worship and the way individuals and collectivities support it. That calls for a break with long scholarly convention, which defines religion in terms of belief, unfathomably diverse though that is. Sinologists used to think in terms of the "Three Religions"—Confucianism, Daoism, and Buddhism—as texts and bodies of doctrine. The research of the last generation, drawing on the tools of anthropology and religious studies, has begun shifting the focus to the actual changing practices of popular religion. Many of us now see the latter as a common backbone out of which the "Three Religions" diverged over the millennia for which we have evidence.

The first derivative phenomena began as the religious rites of princely states, recorded beginning in the mid second millennium B.C. By the end of the first century B.C., when the many states had been digested into a single empire, its liturgy had greatly changed, and was colored—but only colored—by the doctrines of Confucius and many other thinkers. He and his disciples were stating, conservatively and normatively, the usages of their class in a time when social change was fundamentally remaking it. The imperial state as generations of new men shaped it was resolutely opposed in many ways to the faith of Confucius and his main disciples, and diverged even more as time passed.[8] To call the state's changing ideology Confucianism simply muddles this dynamic picture. When I discuss that ideology, I explore the realities of eleventh-century state religion and its involvement in ceremonies for curing.

The Daoist and Buddhist religions, the other main derivatives of popular religion, came on the scene about two thousand years ago. The first superimposed new institutions and rituals atop existing forms of worship. The second combined with practices familiar in China its own set of institutions and rituals based on foreign answers to questions previously of little or no interest to native religious thinkers. An important example is "why be virtuous if bad people are likely to lead as happy lives as good ones?" Confucius' stoicism never satisfied the needs of more than a miniscule part of the upper class.

---

[7] Kleinman et al. 2011, especially 1–77; see also Davis 2005, and Kleinman, Kleinman & Lee 1999 and the studies it introduces.

[8] For a list of these differences see Lloyd & Sivin 2002, 47–48.

Buddhism and Daoism each comprised a number of independent movements with their own structures of authority, none with a controlling center. Movements were frequently transmogrified by the state's patronage, coupled with its attempts to control and regulate them. The two religions were individual and collective Ways: ritual behavior aimed at a better life or at overcoming life's limitations, accompanied by whatever beliefs led each individual to support such behavior.

Robert Ford Campany, in a percipient essay entitled "On the Very Idea of Religions in the Modern West and in Early Medieval China," has pointed out how thinking of Chinese religions as isms engenders basic misunderstandings. Europeans and Americans regularly speak of their religions as holistic entities that grow and flourish like organisms, as agents that accomplish this or that, as essential doctrines that believers accept, and so on. Early Chinese, on the other hand, spoke of Daoism, Buddhism and other kinds of ritual as Ways *(dao* 道), laws or methods *(fa* 法), and teachings *(jiao* 教). But Ways do not act; laws in religion are repertories of practices and understandings, not edicts; and teachings are not personified and do not ordinarily act. *Xin* 信, literally "belief," usually means "not assent to propositions but trust or confidence in a teaching, method, or path." Campany concludes his subtle discussion "when religions are metaphorically imagined as doing things, it becomes harder to see the agents who really and unmetaphorically do things: people."[9] Clarity about agency seems to me an excellent reason to avoid isms —"Daoism," "Buddhism," "Confucianism," etc.—so far as I can, and to stress how actual practitioners followed their Ways. What such terms mean to today's textual and philosophical specialists is equally worthy of analysis, but that is not the subject of this book. As for the names of religions, I use "Daoist"—when it is useful—as an overall label for the various movements that worshiped the ineffable Way; I do not use it at all for the writings of various literary-philosophical figures before the Common Era (which play no part in this book), or in any of the dozen or so other senses that Sinologists freely intermix.[10]

The latter also have been unable to agree on translations for the names of the main movements. For *tianshi* 天師 I use "Heavenly Masters ." For *shangqing* 上清 I use "Highest Purity."[11] As for other movements, I translate *lingbao* 靈寶 "Divine Treasure," *shenxiao* 神宵 "Divine Empyrean," and *quanzhen* 全真 "Complete

---

[9] Campany 2003, quotations from p. 310 and 319. Campany was writing about the second through most of the sixth century A.D., but his analysis, as I summarize it, is applicable to the eleventh.

[10] See Sivin 1978. *Daoren* 道人, commonly but questionably translated "Daoist," was originally used, often without reference to religious organizations, for "someone who has special knowledge and abilities in regard to the spiritual realm," including Buddhists. Only from the Six Dynasties on did outsiders and Daoists *sometimes* use the term for "religious specialists of Taoist organizations" (Kirkland 2009, 342).

[11] "Highest Clarity," the most widely accepted translation, disregards the emphasis on purity in the sources. In scholarship before a decade or so ago, "Supreme Purity" was common. The term refers to what adherents claimed was the highest group of heavens, to which the movement's adepts aspired.

Realization."[12] In view of the terminological anarchy in scholarship on what I call "popular religion," I discuss my reasons for using that term at the beginning of chapter 5.

Ritual

Dictionaries are on the whole not very helpful with the meaning of this word. The *Oxford English Dictionary's* various senses mostly identify its uses with respect to rites. In a sense first documented in 1971, it specifies "repeated actions or patterns of behaviour having significance within a particular social group." How pertinent that is depends on just what "significance" means. Catherine Bell, who most deeply analyzed Chinese ritual, suggested that ritual is "a way of acting," and agreed with the lexicographers that it is better studied that way than as abstract structure. It uses the body of the ritualist or ritualists in alternating movement and stillness, sound and silence, to appropriate and condition experience, displaying a sense of community to which its audience—if there is one—can respond.[13]

That makes sense for religious rites, but my concern is with therapy. Therapy is simply one of the tasks of religion. As I hope to make clear in the course of this book, the curing rites of popular ritual masters, Daoists, and Buddhists are typical of, or adaptations of, those they use for the other benefits they offer worshipers. The classical physician of the eleventh century, like the M.D. of the twenty-first, also depended on ritual (in the *Oxford English Dictionary*'s 1971 sense). The latter's white coat and stethoscope, the equipment in her office, her diplomas and reference works, her authoritative tone, her use of biological language in explanations, the conspicuous value of her time, and the protectiveness of her underlings, help to establish the power of her knowledge in the patient's mind. In the same way, the Song gentry doctor—who usually saw patients on their turf, not his—by dress, by comportment, by a combination of deference and dignity, and by allusions to the conventional classics and those of medicine, demonstrated that he was a gentleman and a master of medical skills. Any therapist, elite or popular, had to convince patients that he knew enough, had enough experience, was respectable, and was personally trustworthy. The significance of therapeutic ritual was to demonstrate that the therapist was not merely a proficient technician—a matter that patients still care about.

[12] The latter title is often given as "Complete Perfection," but that is not translation. *Zhen* does not *mean* "perfection," but rather "true" or "real"; in the name of the religion it seems to have been meant in a dynamic sense, hence "realization."

[13] Bell 1989, 1992, and 2006.

Wizards

Modern scholars have sometimes made their work more difficult than it need be due to a tendency to confuse epithets with names of things. An epithet indicates a characteristic that the speaker or writer is using to describe someone. A common negative example is "lazy" for someone who is not willing to do what the speaker wants in the way he wants, but whose own reasons (the speaker is sure) are not worth knowing about.

Wu 巫 is a negative epithet used by officials and other literati in the eleventh century for several sorts of religious operatives that they looked down upon; I therefore translate it "wizard," which captures the disdain that accompanies use of the term. Most often the word *wu* expresses distaste for ritual masters *(fashi* 法師), popular or Daoist.

Modern scholars of Chinese religion who take what their sources say literally tend to think of *wu* as an actual occupational group, and to translate the word "shaman" or, less often, "spirit medium." In anthropological literature, which introduced and defined both terms, shamans and mediums are more or less opposites. Shamans are political leaders who take spirit journeys to the home of the gods; gods in many cultures enter and control the passive bodies of mediums. Nevertheless most of today's Sinological writing describes *wu* not as ritualists who live and perform liturgy on behalf of a village, town, or city, but as independent wonderworkers who have no regular connection to any collectivity.[14] Since that habit perpetuates the hoary misunderstanding that Chinese religion is nothing more than the sum of Confucianism, Buddhism, and Daoism, I avoid it.

Issues

It will perhaps be helpful if I state my positions on several issues about which people interested in history tend to differ. I will begin with a central problem of translation, and then take up the contents of the body, about which there is no consensus among students of China. Finally I will discuss the questions of objectivity, culture, cultural relativism, and the use of jargon in historical writing. Readers who are not fascinated by these debates need not peruse this section, but may find it useful as they read other parts of the book.

[14] Cedzich 1995, 139, writes of gods with "a following of shamans and mediums," without explaining what she takes to be the difference. Japanese specialists also treat *wu* as a social category, e.g., Nakamura 1978 and 1982. For *wu* associated with town and city temples see Nakamura 1982, 66–67.

Comprehending medical terms

The difficulty of understanding what the words in an old Chinese text are saying is frustrating enough. But there are deeper problems, due to the fact that the meanings of words in any two languages seldom map neatly onto each other, that are impossible to solve completely when producing a translation. One can only urge readers to be aware of the inevitable discrepancies.

As an example, one might easily argue that Chinese before modern times had no bodies. From the biomedical viewpoint, in health and illness, anywhere in the world, one human body is much the same as another. That does not mean that people in other climes or other times experienced health, pain, illness, sensuality and physical vigor in the same way. Early physicians and other curers describe what they saw and reasoned about in terms very different from ours. When we compare two cultures, or the same culture before and after a large transition, the common-sense definition of one time and place may turn out to be absurd in the other. For instance *soma,* which became the classical Greek word for the living body, did not mean that in Homeric Greece. Homer used it only for cadavers.[15] The meaning of *shen* 身, the everyday modern Chinese word for body, is not as close an equivalent as it looks. When Zeng Shen 曾參, a disciple of Confucius, said about 500 B.C. that every day he examined his *shen* three times, his point was not looking at himself in the mirror, or even contemplating his navel. He was asking himself concretely "whether in planning for others I have been trustworthy; whether in give and take with friends I have been unreliable; and whether I have practiced what has been taught to me."[16] His *shen* was a kind of social conscience, but of course not only that.

The modern Chinese equivalent of the English bureaucratic term "identity" is *shenfen* 身分, literally, "*shen* status." For 1500 years *shenfen* meant social origins and standing. It had nothing to do with how tall or strong you are. Other Chinese words that Europeans customarily translate "body" have boundaries that are equally odd from an occidental point of view.[17] *Ti* 體, in addition to the body, can mean personification or the embodiment of some moral quality. An example from one of the commentaries of the *Book of Changes,* of the third or second century B.C. is "When the powers of yin and yang merge, hard and soft have their **embodiments** *(yinyang he de er gangrou you ti* 陰陽合德而剛柔有體)." *Xing* 形 can mean the body as form, or can refer to its characteristics, form, shape, or outline. Scholars therefore often translate this word loosely as "body." But such a translation occasionally misses the point. For instance, from the *Inner Canon of the Yellow Emperor:* "The man with **characteristics** of the Phase Metal … In his conduct … is pure *(Jin xing zhi ren … qi wei ren … shen qing lian* 金形之人 … 其為人 … 身清廉)." A fourth word often translated "body" is *qu* 軀. It can mean the physical body, but in

[15] Snell 1953.

[16] *Lun yu* 論語 (Analects) , 1.4.1. On this translation, see Leys & Nylan 2014, 64, note 1.4.

[17] The examples below come from *Zhou yi* 周易, Xici, B.5; *Huangdi neijing, Ling shu* 黃帝内經靈樞, 64.1.5; and *Mengzi* 孟子, 7B. 29.

other contexts denotes "person" or "life." Here is an instance from the *Mencius:* "He was a man with a little talent who had never heard about the great way of the lordly man; he had just enough [talent] for him to end out his **life** *(Qi wei ren ye, xiao you cai, wei wen junzi zhi da dao ye, ze zu yi sha qi qu eryi yi* 其為人也, 小有才, 未聞君子之大道也, 則足以殺其軀而已矣)." Even in medicine the meanings of *shen, ti, xing,* and *qu* don't draw boundaries between the physical body and various mental, spiritual, and social matters, boundaries that Westerners take for granted. That is too consistent a pattern to ignore.

I am not talking about simple metaphors, like the English one that speaks of a corporate body, but about different ranges of literal meaning. A Chinese a thousand years ago could make it perfectly clear, when he wanted to, that he was talking about a bleeding wound rather than punctured moral pretensions. But in his *shen*, unlike the body that the modern physician sees, skin, vitality, emotion, and ethics were equally important parts of one single thing. If we abide by modern Western common sense, not to mention the concepts of current medicine, what the Chinese words talk about is an entity that is not very concrete and quite miscellaneous—one that is not quite a body. I do not see how it makes sense to take modern or postmodern common sense—or today's medical dictionaries—as a universal standard. This is only one of a good many pertinent examples in which we must understand terms in their original context. I take up in detail another, the translatability of classical Chinese disease names, in chapter 3.

Contents of the body

When discussing classical medicine, I translate *zangfu* (藏府 or 臟腑) as "visceral systems of function" (or "visceral systems" for short) to remind readers that the topic is not usually innards. Chinese medicine's preoccupation with dynamic functions, physiological and pathological, did not generate much interest in exploring the body's physical structures. As ideas of metabolic processes became more and more elaborate, less and less was left for anatomy to explain. Since a physician could get information about inner states from the pulse, there was scant impetus for dissection; only a handful of instances are documented. The organs were not little factories, but rather bureaucratic offices that supervised spontaneous processes.[18] Authors kept repeating early crude, cursory accounts of the physical shapes and locations of the viscera, because they found them adequate to an unimportant topic.

Zangfu is actually an abbreviation of *wuzang liufu* (五脏六府 or 五臟六腑), "the five *zang* and the six *fu.*" The early medical classics variously distinguish between the *zang* and the *fu* in ways that conflict with each other.[19] The only distinction all

[18] Lloyd & Sivin 2002, 218–221.

[19] In the Han period, *zang* and *fu* both literally meant "storehouse" (see *fu* in *Hanyu dacidian* 汉语大词典, 3:1213, sense 1). Some modern scholars translate *fu* "palace," but that meaning (sense 7) came into use after the end of the Han period, and thus postdates the medical classics.

the classics accept is that the former is yin and the latter yang. I therefore render *wuzang liufu* as the "five yin and six yang visceral systems of function."

As Manfred Porkert has shown, anatomy envisions the body as a complex of tissues and organs which may or may not have a function (e.g., the appendix is traditionally vestigial), while classical medicine in China sees the body primarily as a congeries of systems administering vital functions, which may or may not be associated with a physical organ. For instance, medical authorities did not feel the need to agree on whether the Triple *Jiao (sanjiao* 三焦) system corresponded to one organ, three organs, or one or more spaces in the abdomen.[20]

Another technical term that demands attention is *qi* 氣. *Qi* refers to the matter—which may be intangible, liquid, or solid—of which everything is composed. Aristotle's matter was passive stuff on which form must be imposed if it is to become anything. *Qi* is anything but passive. It contains the vitality it needs to maintain its physical form and characteristic activity, and to grow. When you eat, metabolism spontaneously extracts from food and drink their characteristic *qi* and transforms it into your own *qi (zhengqi* 正氣), so that it can keep you alive and support your growth. The visceral systems also excrete the *qi* that you cannot use.

The classical language of the body's processes talks about aspects of the body's *qi,* not about the chemically distinct substances that interest moderns. Thus *qi* and *xue (qixue* 氣血) are not *qi* and blood as separate fluids, but two specific aspects, yang and yin, of the general *qi*. This commonly confuses modern readers. *Qi* and *xue* are yang and yin subtypes of the body's fluid substances, the totality of which also happens to be called *qi*. And *xue*, when it left the body, was just blood. Ancient students of medicine found this aspectual language for what moves in the circulation system clear enough. The constructive and defensive *qi (yingwei* 營衛) are another pair of aspects—of the same *qi*—for another kind of discussion. The constructive *qi (yingqi)* is the contents of the circulation system—its *qi* and *xue*—sustaining life and growth within the body. The defensive *qi (weiqi)* is the *qi* and *xue* that suffuses the body's periphery, protecting it from invasion. These are merely examples of the ways classical authors analyzed *qi* and its functions.[21] Many historians, those who think of their work as documenting the gradual approach of early doctors to correct modern knowledge, prefer to think of the *zangfu* as organs and *xue* as blood, but that approach only encourages further misunderstandings of early medical thought. This disagreement does not amount to a debate; the positivists simply ignore understandings based on critical reading, without attempting to refute them.

Having offered these samples of medical language's flavor, I will now move on to some general issues under debate.

---

[20] See Porkert 1974, 107–108, and Sivin 1987, 124–133. No one has yet proposed a defensible translation of *jiao*, nor can I, so I do not translate the word. The same is true of *qi*.

[21] On this and other technical language for bodily functions see Sivin 1987, 46–53 and 117–171.

Objectivity

Some writers use "objective" merely to announce that they are not easily taken in, or that they try to avoid emotional judgments. By that usage they proclaim that they do not care beyond crude approximation what the words they use mean, encouraging their readers to conclude that they do not necessarily mean what they say.[22]

"Objective" and "objectivity" have for centuries been key terms in epistemology. Thus the *Oxford English Dictionary* defines "objective" as what "is or belongs to what is presented to consciousness, as opposed to the consciousness itself; that is the object of perception or thought, as distinct from the subject; (hence) (more widely) external to or independent of the mind" (sense 3b, from 1648). Since knowledge is objective only if it does not depend on operations of the mind, and by implication is identical for all minds, it must be defined by universal standards.

The only such standards that are truly global today are number and measure.[23] Objectivity is indeed characteristic of conclusions based on quantitative physical, chemical, and biological data—even though their discoverers are likely to feel joy, gloom, etc. Certainty of that kind does not exist, however, for reasoning in the humanities and the non-quantitative social sciences. It is true that a later sense of "objectivity" reduces it to a synonym for "detachment" or "impartiality" (sense 8a, 1838). Even authors who intend only the latter sense often associate their arguments with those of people who claim that they are authorities in the "historical sciences" rather than mere historians—not the best of company, in the minds of many critical readers. Since I do not wish to be taken for a pretender to scientific authority, I avoid the ambiguity of "objectivity," and instead strive—not always successfully, I must admit—for impartiality.

Culture

I use "culture" in a way compatible (so far as that is possible) with the understandings of both Geertzian anthropologists and others who consider them fogies. For Clifford Geertz, culture is "an historically transmitted pattern of meanings embodied in symbols, a system of inherited conceptions expressed in symbolic forms by means of which men communicate, perpetuate and develop their knowledge about and attitudes toward life. Seeing culture as meaning embodied in symbols focuses attention on such phenomena as beliefs, ritual practices, art forms, and ceremonies, and on informal cultural practices such as language, gossip, stories, and rituals of daily life. … Indeed, culture is specifically the set of symbolic vehicles through

[22] Daston & Galison 2007. For definitions and debates in various specialties see Agazzi 2014 for physical science and Megill 1994 for humanities and social sciences.

[23] This doctrine has been challenged by social constructivists and others; their line of attack is to imply that objectivity of every kind is simply a delusion, and that anyone who disagrees is delusionary.

which … sharing and learning take place."[24] Geertzians therefore think in terms of a unified "cultural system."

This understanding fails to take into account the great differences in the values that individuals express, and in their personal responses to any given configuration of symbols. The divergence of those values and responses is why many anthropologists find the Geertzian picture—or the very idea of cultures—too uniform or even (dreaded word!) essentialist. They see persons as situated at the intersections of subcultures or even of cultures, and as responding individually to symbol and meaning generally.

The views of Ann Swidler and Volker Scheid are particularly useful in resolving this standoff. Swidler (on love) sees culture as a repertory of meanings from which, in individual ways, "… people draw disparate ideas, images, and attitudes." Scheid's stance is similar. His topic is narrower than love—he writes about Chinese medicine—but his pluralism is broader and I find it more persuasive. He argues that "it is possible to communicate effectively across apparently incommensurable paradigms, that horizons are essentially open, that plurality is practicable." His work demonstrates effectively that physicians are not at all uniform; they use "plural styles of reasoning, forms of practice, medical gaze, etc."[25] Culture is not a uniform system of any kind, but simply what you might call the vector sum of individual meanings. This is what I mean in this book by culture. I see no need for a more elaborate analysis.

Cultural Relativism

Cultural relativism is an issue that has called down tornadoes of ire on anthropologists and those who draw on their work. To some people it implies that no set of values is better than another, and that truths we hold self-evident are never more than local customs.

It is actually a multifarious and slippery conceit, of which Melford Spiro has given the most helpful analysis. He distinguishes several varieties[26]:

Contextual relativism is simply the belief that the significance of action or thought varies depending on its context. That is hardly a contentious notion, since it does not imply that such significances are universal.

Descriptive relativism, which animated nineteenth-century anthropology, was the insight that variations in social and psychological patterns reflected—or, as I see it, were part of—a larger pattern of variations in culture.

---

[24] Geertz 1973b, 89. There is much to be said for the minimal definition of "culture" from the sociologist Howard Becker: "the shared understandings that people use to coordinate their activities" (1986, 15). Note Becker's emphasis on action rather than knowledge and attitudes.

[25] Swidler 2001, 43; Scheid 2002, 158, 163.

[26] Spiro 1986; compare the different stance in Spiro 1978.

The **normative relativism** that shaped anthropology in the early twentieth century saw all judgments of merit or worth as derived from the particular cultures in which they occur. It originated much earlier, as witness Montaigne's (1685) "… every one gives the Title of Barbarity to every Thing that is not in use in his own Country: As Indeed we have no other Level of Truth and Reason, than the Example and Idea of the Opinions and Customs of the Place wherein we live."[27] By 1950, anthropologists no longer insisted on an uncrossable boundary between savages, the object of their study, and ourselves, who did the studying or learned from its outcome. Some over the next decades even created ethnographies of English communities.[28]

There survived no generally accepted basis for any universal moral standard, any invariant human nature or mind. Although nostalgic guardians of public morality have often excoriated relativists for trashing conventional standards, those standards had lost their power to compel by the time the progeny of Franz Boas pronounced them ethnocentric.

Finally, **epistemological relativism** resulted from the flowering of symbolic anthropology in the 1960s. Many practitioners believed that symbolism shaped social reality. The worlds it shaped varied so greatly in the minds of individuals that a single culture could not subsume all the people of France, its Rhone department, its city of Lyons, or the sausage-makers of that city. Some denied that the cultural patterns seen by any two people coincide, and found culture a useless or merely distracting essence. The best one could hope to do was interpret symbolic structures one by one.

The arguments still continue, and there is no sign that they will come to an end. In polemics over normative relativism, anthropologists who believe civilization requires fixed moral standards persist in identifying examples of universal values, e.g., Melford Spiro's taboo against parent–child incest, avoidance of pain, and so on. Those who find that stance merely nostalgic can usually cite a group somewhere who happen not to find the taboos deviant.

As for epistemological relativism, the notion that the culture of a group of individuals does not add up to anything larger, and that in view of local cultures one cannot speak of national ones, is hard to take seriously. In affirming that there is much of which I do not partake in the culture of Philadelphia, I imply that it exists; one cannot have it both ways. A number of social scientists a generation ago spoke forcefully against the idea of culture, but what matters is that they offered nothing better.

Finally, it is hard to take solemnly the notion that today's anthropologists and their readers, questioning fixed beliefs, are unable to form their own convictions about what makes life worth living. As Geertz has put it, "What looks like a debate about the broader implications of anthropological research is really a debate about how to live with them." That, it seems to me, nobly echoes Bertrand Russell's defi-

[27] Montaigne 1685/1711, 1:287.

[28] See in particular the work of Mary Douglas and her students.

nition of philosophy: "how to live without paralysis in a world that knows no certainty."[29] My own belief, then, is that normative relativism, applied not to all judgments of merit or worth but to some of them, is an essential tool of historical inquiry. It in no sense threatens my own values, which have never presupposed that in life anything qualitative can be certain.

Technical Terminology

One frequently glimpses in medical anthropology (and history that draws on it) a tendency to turn from ordinary language, not to technical terminology, but to jargon. By technical terminology I mean language that makes it possible to lucidly and systematically think through matters too complicated for everyday language to express adequately; by jargon I mean the use of words that (whatever the author's announced intent) make the expression of thought less rather than more clear. An example is "discourse." This word had some novel uses in the analytic technique of the same name (a generation ago), but enthusiasts before long smudged it into a vague grab-bag that might denote speech, discussion, debate, concept, writing, narration, or a half-dozen other notions.

In some instances (mostly but not always in dissertations) an author tries to demonstrate that he is at the cutting edge by quoting trademark usages of authors greatly in fashion—usually at least a decade earlier. Among people interested in the history of medicine, Michel Foucault is most often cited with reverence, much as, in Chinese books that appeared during the Great Proletarian Cultural Revolution, writers felt obliged to quote Chairman Mao or Friedrich Engels. Other historians are partial to what I think of as yesteryear's Seven B's, namely Bachelard, Bakhtin, Barthes, Baudrillard, Benjamin, Bhabha, and Bourdieu. I have learned from most of these, but, oddly enough, what I have learned I can always somehow express in plain English.

In other cases, critical students of medicine, out of the desire to establish clear distinctions, invent jargon instead. As a half-century-old instance of the latter, I will remark on attempts to turn the synonyms "disease," "illness," and "sickness" into words of art.

What underlies this effort is a faith that objective scientific knowledge is the only kind that can comprehend disease. This implies that the clinician's authoritative understanding (by this definition, of disease) differs decisively from the patient's mere subjective experience (of illness) which, the conventional wisdom assures us, is more likely to get in the way of therapy than to be useful. Ritual, magic, persuasion, psychology, charisma, can affect illness—what the patient experiences—but

[29] That is how Russell's definition stuck in my mind since, ca. 1955, I read his *History of Western Philosophy*. His original formulation is less concise: "To teach how to live without certainty, and yet without being paralyzed by hesitation, is perhaps the chief thing that philosophy in our age can still do for those who study it" (1945, xiv). See Geertz 2000c, 45–46.

only correct diagnosis and specific bio-physico-chemical therapy can end the disease—a biological entity validated by methodical research. So goes the distinction.[30]

Avoiding confusion is always desirable, but the outcome is sometimes other kinds of confusion. Regardless of where and when the treatment takes place, the disease-illness distinction implies that correct diagnosis of and therapy for disease can come only from a graduate of an accredited medical school. That is, only an M.D. who has mastered the current state of clinical knowledge can determine whether what the traditional physician, herbalist, or wizard did a thousand years ago could have been effective.[31] Since the ancient curer was not an up-to-date physician, his own experience must be irrelevant. His effectiveness, if any, must have been unconscious, and his convictions about how he attained it deluded. Non-biomedical therapists can at best instinctively support the body's ability to heal itself, but the up-to-date doctor who calls upon objective science can not only cure but comprehend the ability of others to do so. Eleventh-century practitioners were obviously wrongheaded because they aimed to cure, and did not consider curing and healing mutually exclusive.

The obvious problem with the disease-illness dichotomy is that in China eleven centuries ago there were no M.D.'s. Even in 1950, of the very few Chinese trained in biomedicine, none was acquainted with today's state of the art, and all were therefore doomed to medical unreliability. The actual medieval therapist, whether classical physician, herbalist or priest, does not figure in the dichotomy at all, except as an ignorant person blindly playing a part.

I find it impossible to agree that most traditional practitioners who saw their patients repeatedly were not intelligent enough to judge whether they got better or worse. Still, the disease-illness model assumes that since the therapist was not trained in science he had no way to tell whether he had cured the patient's disease (by having done unknowingly what the M.D. retrospectively approves) or merely eased the symptoms while the patient recovered on her own.

The fallacy is elementary. Such an analysis of therapeutic interaction is based on the recorded experience of only one of the two people actually involved—the putatively irrelevant therapist. In every eleventh-century instance when we have details, it was the practitioner who left the record. It was he who set down what information we have about the person he treated. The few records by patients of therapy are so much scantier and less detailed that it is not possible to compare adequate accounts of the same patient's "disease" and "illness."[32]

---

[30] See Eisenberg 1977.

[31] This American prejudice overlooks the parochiality of the rule that physicians must have doctoral degrees. The norm in many countries of the world, some where the quality of medical care is generally higher than the United States, is the degree of M.B.B.S. (Bachelor of Medicine, Bachelor of Surgery).

[32] In the only detailed accounts of therapeutic interactions between patients and their physicians, in the Palace Medical Archive of the Qing period (1644–1911), we have minute reports by the traditional practitioners, and responses to them by royal patients. For a study that shows the possibilities

On the other hand, many expect today's biomedical physician, as arbiter of past practice, to diagnose and assess a program of therapy without full details about the patient, a physical or verbal examination, or laboratory test results—that is, without the data that make responsible evaluation possible. No competent M.D. would diagnose in these circumstances.[33]

There is no point in following the dichotomy further. It typifies the mental confusions that spring from assuming modern medicine provides adequate understanding of data from every time and place.

One might define other special language to express the two *pertinent* types of past experience, those of the patient (about which we lack details) and of the actual practitioner.[34] But new technical terms sometimes launch their inventors into flights of fancy that transform them into jargon. Having reflected on the flaws in these attempts to turn ordinary language into technical terminology, I will depend throughout this book on generally accepted nomenclature and ordinary English usage, which are more likely than jargon to reveal sloppy thinking.

Conventions

Biomedicine

People call the medical theory and practice now conventional in Western Europe, the United States, and a number of other countries by many different names. Some consider it the only real "medicine"; others prefer "allopathy," "biomedicine," or "cosmopolitan medicine." In a study of this kind, "medicine" in the Euro-American sense is merely parochial. "Allopathy" is the English version of a term that German homeopaths originated to distinguish traditional practice from their own. "Cosmopolitan," which implies practice in diverse countries, is equally true of the medicine that originated in China, now practiced in as many countries as that of

and limits of these sources for the studies of medical encounters, see Chang Che-chia 1998. Materials from the archive appear in Chen Keji 1990 and his other publications.

[33] That has not kept a number of technically reputable medical authors from reducing historical studies to a kind of parlor game. See, among others, Dale 1952, Lerner 2006, Als et al. 2002, and Colp 1977.

[34] Kleinman & Sung 1979, in a valuable study of efficacy in Taiwan, use "disease" in different contexts to refer to the M.D.'s and the spirit medium's understanding (p. 22). The result is confusion, since they consider the M.D.'s evaluation, unlike that of the popular curer, "objective" (p. 19). Kleinman & Seeman 2000, 231, provide a definition of "disease" broad enough to encompass the varieties of health care: "the practitioner's construction of patient complaints in the technical terminology of a particular healing system." But other medical anthropologists do not use the word in this relativistic way; and how many physicians are willing to admit that a spirit medium's definition of a given disease is apposite and their own, if it conflicts, may be irrelevant? See the early but thorough critical discussion in Young 1982. Young also points out attempts—which clash with each other—to enlarge this set of distinctions by adding "sickness" (p. 265 and elsewhere).

Europe and America. The only term that does not take sides, so to speak, is "biomedicine," which first appeared in print in 1923 for "clinical medicine based on the principles of physiology and biochemistry." One definition is "the ethnomedicine in which physicians are trained."[35] The word was adopted as the title of a medical journal in 1973, and most anthropologists use it. So do I.

Formula

In writing on Chinese medicine there has been a fair bit of confusion about the meaning of *fang* 方, which specialists often translate "prescription."[36] A prescription is "A doctor's instruction, usually in writing, for the composition and use of a medicine" (*Oxford English Dictionary*, sense 5a). A *fang*, on the other hand, is a "formula," a standard method that a physician learns from a book or a teacher, which may involve drugs or some other therapy. He then adapts it to the case at hand, producing his own prescription *(jiajianfang* 加減方).[37] Primary sources sometimes refer to the latter informally as a *fang* as well. It seems to me worth while in this book to maintain the distinction.

Names

It was usual for educated Chinese to have over a lifetime, in addition to a formal name *(ming* 名, sometimes called the "taboo name *(hui* 諱)"), a variety of given names, including but not limited to courtesy names *(zi* 字) and alternative names *(hao* 號) chosen by themselves *(zihao* 自號, *shiming* 室名, etc.) or by others *(biehao* 別號). Two or three names were usual for literati, and a dozen not unusual.

There was an elaborate etiquette for using them.[38] Some medical authors were, and still are, better known by alternative names than by their formal names, which during their lifetimes it was polite to avoid in most circumstances. For instance, Chinese authors, ancient and modern, call the man who wrote the *Treatise on Cold Damage Disorders* Zhang Zhongjing 張仲景, his courtesy name, more often than Zhang Ji 張機, his formal name. I consistently give the formal name, since it is standard in reference books and thus most useful in further research.

---

[35] Rubel & Haas 1996, 116.

[36] Some scholars translate *fang* "recipe," an obsolete usage outside of cooking.

[37] See the analysis with respect to TCM in Farquhar 1994, 175–190. *Jiajianfang* literally means "formula to which something has been added or from which it has been subtracted."

[38] Wilkinson 2013, 112–145, provides a detailed summary of names and their uses.

Miscellaneous

The form 1123–1125 refers to the three consecutive years; 1123/1125 means a date at some unknown time in this interval.

I use Pinyin transcription for Chinese. I give book titles and authors' names in old-style or simplified characters depending on how they were originally published.

I cite old-style Chinese books in the form *m: n–n*, where *m* is the *juan* (roughly, chapter) number and *n* is pages.

For official titles, I rely on Hucker 1985, the standard reference work.

Now let me consider a question that necessarily takes priority: how can we fruitfully comprehend the efficacy of health care?

References

Abbreviations

DZ = Volume number in *Daozang*
ES = *Ersishi shi* 二十四史 of ZS, 1959–1977.
HY = text in Harvard-Yenching Concordance series
j. = *juan* 卷 (chapter)
RW = published by Renmin Weisheng Chubanshe 人民衛生出版社, Beijing
S = Title number in Schipper 1975
SQ = Siku quanshu 四庫全書
SV = Schipper & Verellen 2004
T = *Taishō shinshū Daizōkyō* 大正新修大藏經
UP = University Press
YZ = Yi tong zheng mai quan shu 醫統正脈全書
ZD = Volume, item, *juan,* and page numbers in *Zhonghua daozang* 中华道藏
ZS = published by Zhonghua shuju 中華書局, Beijing
ZZ = Zhongyi zhenben congshu 中醫珍本叢書 ed.

Classical Chinese Sources

Huangdi neijing ling shu 黃帝內經靈樞 (Inner canon of the Yellow Emperor: Divine pivot). Anonymous. First century B.C. or first century A.D. In *Ling shu jiao shi* 靈樞校釋 (2 vols.; RW, 1982).

Huangdi neijing su wen 黃帝內經素問 (Inner canon of the Yellow Emperor: Basic questions). Anonymous. First century B.C. or first century A.D. Taipei: Xuanfeng Chubanshe, 1973.

Huangdi neijing tai su 黃帝內徑太素 (Inner canon of the Yellow Emperor: Grand basis). Yang Shangshan 楊上善. 666/683. In *Tōyō igaku zempon sōsho* 東洋醫學善本叢書 (Collected rare books on Oriental medicine). Osaka: Tōyō igaku kenkyūkai.

Huangdi neijing. See *Huangdi neijing su wen, Huangdi neijing ling shu,* and *Huangdi neijing tai su.*

Lun yu 論語 (Analects). Successors of Confucius. 479/249. HY. Translation and notes in Leys & Nylan 2014. For tentative dating, see Brooks & Brooks 1998.
Mengzi 孟子 (Mencius). Anonymous. Chapters written between ca. 320 and the first century B.C. HY.
Shanghan lun 傷寒論. See *Shanghan zabing lun*. In YZ.
Shanghan zabing lun 傷寒雜病論 (Treatise on Cold Damage and miscellaneous disorders). Attributed to Zhang Ji 張機. 198–220. Divided into *Shanghan lun* (q.v.) and *Jin gui yao lue* 金櫃要略 by 1057.

Other Sources

Agazzi, Evandro. 2014. *Scientific Objectivity and its Contexts*. Cham: Springer.
Albrecht, Gary L., Ray Fitzpatrick, & Susan Scrimshaw, eds. 2000. *Handbook of Social Studies in Health and Medicine*. London: Sage Publications.
Als, C., et al. 2002. Visible Signs of Illness from the 14th to the 20th Century. Systematic Review of Portraits. *British Medical Journal* 325: 1499–1502.
Becker, Howard S. 1986. Culture: A Sociological View. In Becker, *Doing Things Together: Selected Papers*. Evanston: Northwestern UP.
Bell, Catherine. 1989. Religion and Chinese Culture: Toward an Assessment of 'Popular Religion,' *History of Religions* 29: 35–57.
Bell, Catherine. 1992. *Ritual Theory, Ritual Practice*. New York: Oxford UP.
Bell, Catherine. 2006. Paradigms Behind (and Before) the Modern Concept of Religion. *History and Theory: Studies in the Philosophy of History* 45. 4: 27–46.
Cedzich, Ursula-Angelika. 1995. The Cult of the Wu-t'ung/Wu-hsien in History and Fiction. The Roots of the *Journey to the South*. In David Johnson 1995, 137–218.
Bol, Peter K. 1992. *"This Culture of Ours." Intellectual Transitions in T'ang and Sung China*. Stanford UP.
Brooks, E. Bruce, & A. Taeko Brooks. 1998. *The Original Analects. Sayings of Confucius and his Successors*. Translations from the Asian Classics. New York: Columbia UP.
Campany, Robert Ford. 2003. On the Very Idea of Religions (in the Modern West and in Early Medieval China). *History of Religions* 42. 4: 287–319.
Chang, Che-chia. 1998. The Therapeutic Tug of War. The Imperial Physician-Patient Relationship in the Era of Empress Dowager Cixi (1874–1908). Ph.D. dissertation, Asian and Middle Eastern Studies, University of Pennsylvania.
Chen Keji 陳可冀 et al. 1990. *Qing gong yian yanjiu* 清宮醫案研究 (A study of the Qing medical archives). Beijing: Zhongyi Guji Chubanshe.
Colp, Ralph, Jr. 1977. *To Be an Invalid: The Illness of Charles Darwin*. University of Chicago Press.
Dale, Philip Marshall. 1952. *Medical Biographies: The Ailments of Thirty-three Famous Persons*. Norman: University of Oklahoma Press.
Daston, Lorraine, & Peter Galison. 2007. *Objectivity*. New York: Zone Books.
Davis, Deborah. 2005. Urban Consumer Culture. *The China Quarterly* 183: 692–709.
Douglas, Mary, ed. 1982. *Essays in the Sociology of Perception*. London: Routledge & Kegan Paul.
Douglas, Mary. 1966. *Purity and Danger*. London: Routledge & Kegan Paul.
Douglas, Mary. 1970. *Natural Symbols*. New York: Vintage.
Eisenberg, Leon. 1977. Disease and illness. Distinctions between professional and popular ideas of sickness. *Culture, Medicine, and Psychiatry* 1. 1: 9–23.
Farquhar, Judith. 1994. *Knowing Practice. The Clinical Encounter of Chinese Medicine*. Studies in the Ethnographic Imagination, 4. Boulder: Westview Press.
Geertz, Clifford. 1966/1973b. Religion as a Cultural System. In Geertz 1973a, 87–125.

Geertz, Clifford. 1973a. *The Interpretation of Cultures. Selected Essays*. New York: Basic Books, 1973.
Geertz, Clifford. 2000a. *Available Light. Anthropological Reflections on Philosophical Topics*. Princeton UP.
Geertz, Clifford. 2000b. The Pinch of Destiny: Religion as Experience, Meaning, Identity, Power. In Geertz 2000a, 167–186.
Geertz, Clifford. 2000c. Anti Anti-Relativism. In Geertz 2000a, 42–67.
Hucker, Charles O. 1985. *A Dictionary of Official Titles in Imperial China*. Stanford UP.
James, William. 1902/1929. *The Varieties of Human Experience. A Study in Human Nature*. New York: Modern Library.
Johnson, David, ed. 1995. *Ritual and Scripture in Chinese Popular Religion. Five Studies*. China Popular Culture Project, 3. Berkeley: The Project.
Kirkland, Russell. 2009. The Taoist Priest *(Daoshi)* in Comparative Historical Perspective: A Critical Analysis. *Pacific World: Journal of the Institute of Buddhist Studies*, series 3, 11: 307–349.
Kleinman, Arthur, & Lilias H. Sung. 1979. Why Do Indigenous Practitioners Successfully Heal? *Social Science and Medicine* 13B: 7–26.
Kleinman, Arthur, & Don Seeman. 2000. Personal Experience of Illness. In Albrecht et al. 2000, 230–242.
Kleinman, Arthur, et al. 2011. *Deep China. The Moral Life of the Person. What Anthropology and Psychiatry Tell Us about China Today*. Berkeley: University of California Press.
Kleinman, Arthur, Joan Kleinman, & Sing Lee. 1999. Introduction to the Transformation of Social Experience in Chinese Society: Anthropological, Psychiatric, and Social Medicine Perspectives. *Culture, Medicine, and Psychiatry* 23: 1–6. Overview of special issue from 1996 conference.
Lerner, Barron H. 2006. *When Illness Goes Public. Celebrity Patients and How We Look at Medicine*. Baltimore: The Johns Hopkins UP.
Leys, Simon, & Michael Nylan, translators. 2014. *Confucius. The Analects*. Norton Critical Editions. New York: W. W. Norton.
Lloyd, G. E. R., & Nathan Sivin. 2002. *The Way and the Word. Science and Medicine in Early China and Greece*. New Haven: Yale UP.
Megill, Allan, ed. 1994. *Rethinking Objectivity*. Durham: Duke UP.
Montaigne, Michel de. 1685/1711. *Essays of Michael Seigneur de Montaigne*. 4th ed., 3 vols. London: Daniel Brown et al.
Nakamura Jihei 中村治兵衛. 1978. KitaSōchō to fu 北宋朝と巫 (The Northern Song dynasty and wizards). *Chūo Daigaku Bungakubu kiyo. Shigaku ka* 中央大學文學部紀要. 史學科 23: 63–78.
Nakamura Jihei. 1982. Sōdai no fu no tokuchō 宋代の巫の特徵 (Special characteristics of wizards in the Song period). *Chūo Daigaku Bungakubu kiyo* 104: 51–75.
Porkert, Manfred. 1974. *The Theoretical Foundations of Chinese Medicine: Systems of Correspondence*. MIT East Asian Science Series, 3. Cambridge: The MIT Press.
Rubel, Arthur J., & Michael R. Haas. 1996. Ethnomedicine. In Sargent & Johnson 1996, 113–130.
Russell, Bertrand. 1945. *A History of Western Philosophy, and its Connection with Political and Social Circumstances from the Earliest Times to the Present Day*. New York: Simon and Schuster.
Sargent, Carolyn F., & Thomas M. Johnson, eds. 1996. *Medical Anthropology: Contemporary Theory and Method*. Rev. ed. Westport, CT: Praeger.
Scheid, Volker. 2002. *Chinese Medicine in Contemporary China: Plurality and Synthesis*. Durham: Duke UP.
Sivin, Nathan. 1978. On the Word Taoism as a Source of Perplexity. With Special Reference to the Relations of Science and Religion in Traditional China. *History of Religions* 17: 303–330.
Sivin, Nathan. 1987. *Traditional Medicine in Contemporary China*. Science, Medicine, and Technology in East Asia, 2. Ann Arbor: Center for Chinese Studies, University of Michigan.

Snell, Bruno. 1953. *The Discovery of the Mind.* Oxford: Blackwell.
Spiro, Howard. 1986. *Doctors, Patients, and Placebos.* Yale UP.
Spiro, Howard. 1997. Clinical Reflections on the Placebo Phenomenon. In Harrington 1997, 37–55.
Spiro, Melford E. 1978. Culture and Human Nature. In Spindler 1978, 331–60.
Spiro, Melford E. 1986. Cultural Relativism and the Future of Anthropology. *Cultural Anthropology* 1. 3: 259–286.
Spindler, George Dearborn, John Wesley, & Mayhew Whiting. 1978. The Making of Psychological Anthropology. Berkeley: University of California Press.
Swidler, Ann. 2001. *Talk of Love. How Culture Matters.* University of Chicago Press.
Wang, Jing. 2001. Culture as Leisure and Culture as Capital. *Positions* 9. 1: 69–104.
Wang, Jing. 2005. Bourgeois Bohemians in China? Neo-Tribes and the Urban Imaginary. *The China Quarterly* 183: 532–548.
Wilkinson, Endymion. 2013. *Chinese History: A New Manual.* Third, revised printing. Cambridge: Harvard UP. This edition originally published 2012.
Young, Allan. 1982. The Anthropologies of Illness and Sickness. *Annual Review of Anthropology* 11: 257–285.

Chapter 3
The Question of Efficacy

Abstract Historians have tended either to avoid asking whether the therapies described in their ancient sources had any curative value, or to assume that they were effective to the extent that modern biomedicine can validate them. But today's knowledge is not the only reliable criterion. This chapter, on the basis of recent studies in medical anthropology and sociology, observes that the success of therapy in every culture depends on three kinds of response by patients: the autonomous response (the tendency of the body heal itself), the meaning response ("the biological consequences of knowledge, symbol, and meaning"), and the specific response to biological, chemical, or physical intervention. The book's analyses of therapeutic instances look for the first two responses (the third played only a small role in pre-modern therapy). It also notes that the medical disorders and even the symptoms of ancient China were different from those of biomedicine. Recorded judgments of the efficacy of care in the eleventh century came as regularly from members of patients' families as from physicians. Examples suggest that in order to use biomedical knowledge productively, it is essential first to understand the sources on their own terms.

Some scholars of ancient medicine trustfully accept the judgments of physicians—Western or Eastern, ancient or modern. Others dismiss reports of cures except for the few instances, mostly of drugs, in which biomedical research has validated the specific therapy. Physicians generally agree with the doubters, shrugging off the rich literature of medical case records as mere anecdotes, by which they mean that none of it is worth thinking about. The utility of religious or other popular curing does not come up.

Surely one has to understand differently therapy that powerfully affects suffering and treatments that cannot significantly change it. Personal inclination, whether that of the true believer or the inveterate skeptic, is not a productive basis for thinking critically about that difference. Clarifying what makes therapy effective can correct some common misunderstandings about health care before modern times—or, for that matter, at any time.

Yes, at any time, emphatically including our own. If we want to find a reasonable way to approach the problem of efficacy, we cannot put the most quantitatively rigorous contemporary biomedical knowledge in one category and everything else in another. Anthropologists sensibly demand that any general principle, if it is true

© Springer International Publishing Switzerland 2015

N. Sivin, *Health Care in Eleventh-Century China*, Archimedes 43,
DOI 10.1007/978-3-319-20427-7_3

of one culture, be true for all. If it is true of every culture but the one that invented academic anthropology, it isn't general.

Concentrating on principles that hold for not only popular but scientific medicine, for not only ancient but modern medicine, seems to me a good way to avoid self-delusion. In exploring the meaning of efficacy, therefore, I will mention examples from both the modern United States and ancient China. My concern in this chapter is not to determine whether the therapeutic means of a given time and place are generally effective or not—a question too vague to be answerable—but to see in what ways the issue of efficacy can be productive in studying the past, recent or distant. This seems to me essential before taking up what the kinds of health care were. The central question of this chapter, then, is who decided what is efficacious in a given case in eleventh-century China, and on what grounds?

What Does Efficacy Mean?

In most conversations, "efficacy" is what happens when competent physicians prescribe drugs or do something else that gets rid of, or lessens the seriousness of, patients' diseases or symptoms. In thinking about drugs, the word usually applies to the verified and published results of double- or triple-blind testing on a statistically representative sample, preferably large, of patients. Such tests compare the drug's effects with those of a biomedically inert substance, a placebo, given to part of the sample. The difference between the two results becomes a numerical measure of efficacy.

This "gold standard" is useless in studying health care in the past—and in considerable parts of today's world where people consider it unethical to give patients who need care an inert substance. In records from China (and elsewhere) in the eleventh century, we have only fragmentary information, and no statistics at all. Many therapies do not even involve medicines. We need a less narrow approach.

A more productive approach needs to set aside some of the mythology of present-day medicine. There are several sources of confusion that get in the way of rational discussion. First, the term "placebo effect" is woefully confused. It originally referred to the use of a pharmacologically inert substance (placebo) as a drug, but medical writers now routinely use it for the sum of verified effects that medicine cannot explain.[1] "Placebo effect" is used so carelessly in discussions of medical efficacy that we are better off without it. Second, modern convictions about the power of medicine tend to rest on success with acute infectious and other epidemic disorders and with traumata; it is to the point that much (but not all) of the power of ancient drug therapy had to do with chronic disorders (see p. 40). Third, the assumption that records of other times can be unambiguously translated into modern diagnoses is mere wishful thinking.

[1] See Spiro 1997, 40–41.

I will therefore set aside much of the conventional wisdom that pervades medical discussions of history, and begin with what anthropologists have learned from empirical studies of a wide range of cultures, including some in the past.

The sophisticated analysis in Daniel Moerman's *The Meaning Response*, based on his field experience and his survey of a large literature in medicine and the social sciences, is an excellent starting point.[2] Moerman, a medical anthropologist and expert on ethnopharmacy, makes it clear that efficacy in health care—the response of the patient to therapy—includes several distinct things.

What Moerman calls the **autonomous response** is the patient's ability to recover spontaneously. As Moerman puts it, abnormal conditions of the body tend to regress to the mean.[3] The distress due to a peak in blood pressure will ordinarily, before long, subside as the pressure becomes lower. He notes as well the general tendency of organic systems toward homeostasis, the tendency to maintain a fairly constant internal state despite changes in conditions outside it. The patient's will to recover can speed its work. This response, for all of the primary-care physicians with whom I have discussed their work, makes patience and encouragement the most effective resources for the self-limiting majority of clinical problems—colds, flus, muscular aches and pains, and common digestive problems.

Second is the patient's **specific response** to biological, chemical, or physical intervention. It is this sort of response on which public spokesmen for medicine base their claim that it is an applied science. The central role of the specific response in modern medical research is responsible for the primacy of the gold standard, which aims to exclude the effects of *everything* but specific agents.

Evidence-based medicine provides clinicians with summaries of research on the specific response alone, and leaves it to them to decide what else they need to think about in order to treat an individual patient. Since medical schools devote little time to the systematic study of other kinds of knowledge, and since practicing clinicians are expected to keep schooling themselves only in new positive developments, the specific response is the only one that the average practitioner is prepared to recognize and evaluate. Some recognize its inadequacy as the sole guide to diagnosing the people who come to them for help, but most see no alternative.

This high-minded narrowness also motivates physicians to dismiss most of the Chinese medical armamentarium. Clinicians often insist that if a drug has not been proven specific, any therapeutic success can be due only to the placebo effect.[4] The biologically active ingredients of thousands of Chinese drugs have been scientifically

---

[2] Moerman 2002, 16–21. For an example of its use by anthropologists see Whyte et al. 2002, 29.

[3] An important clarification is Lock 2000, which emphasizes that normality is not a universal category. The mean depends on ethnic, social, cultural, and political circumstances which medicine usually ignores, often at some cost to the quality of treatment.

[4] E.g., Shapiro & Shapiro 1997, 13–19, which on this basis claims that almost all the results of medical care everywhere before the mid 20th century were due to the placebo effect—a perfect example of misusing the term. On the vagueness of the distinction between specific and general action, see Csordas & Kleinman 1996.

studied.[5] By the standards of multinational drug corporations, which now spend something close to a **billion** dollars on synthesis—so that it can be patented—and clinical testing of a single drug, this is only a small first step. But early Chinese physicians had ample means to affect symptoms and, in many cases, control disease.

Finally, the **meaning response** resonates with Clifford Geertz's celebrated definition of "culture" as a symbolic system, given above (p. 20). Symbols are not the only carrier of meaning. Moerman included "meaningful events—involving relationship, discourse, form, belief, knowledge, commitment, history." We also have to comprehend how the patient's body feels in health and sickness, as well as other esthetic dimensions.[6] The individual's meaning response—the curative power of meaning—encompasses "the biological consequences of knowledge, symbol, and meaning." That is, it includes everything outside of specific therapy and spontaneous healing: the physician's persuading the patient that the problem is curable, the moral support of people around the patient, the color of the prescribed pills.[7] Among its many advantages, it ignores the mind-body split that has caused so much mischief in European thought.

This way of looking at it challenges the quasi-religious faith of medical hardliners that such matters may affect the patient's subjective illness, but can have no effect whatever on biological realities. This unwillingness to confront anything but the physical aspects of disease traps narrowly trained physicians in what Ann Harrington has called an "existential deficiency." It leaves them powerless to help patients with any but the biological components of suffering.[8]

The analytic power of medical anthropology and sociology comes from their systematic examination of ailment and cure in a very wide variety of cultures distributed in space and—increasingly—in time. This broad perspective reveals the fallacies in much of the conventional wisdom. Studies of these kinds find greatly varied patterns of response to meaning among patients and practitioners. Patients' medical experience has never been uniquely medical, but is one with their experience of life as a whole. They respond to therapists, whether cardiologists or mediums in trance, in ways that are part of their responses to other people in general, and in particular to people with powerful knowledge or people whose status differs notably from theirs. These are social dimensions of the meaning response.

This approach implies that physicians engaged in therapy, however they may present themselves, are not scientists manipulating laboratory animals, but human beings interacting in complex ways with other human beings who are suffering and who have gone to them for help. For common ailments, doctors' medicaments often

---

[5] See Liu Shoushan 刘寿山 1963 and subsequent volumes in the series.

[6] Moerman 2000, 56. Feeling is a main aspect in Desjarlais 1992. In ancient Chinese documents sources that reflect patients' perceptions rather than those of doctors are rare, mainly to be found in poetry. See, for instance, the poem cited in chapter 6, p. 146.

[7] Moerman 2002, 4. This formulation is analogous to, but more clearly thought out than, the analysis of doctor-patient relations into "technology, caring, and values" in Payer 1988, 9.

[8] Harrington 2008, 17.

matter less than their social, moral, or spiritual influence.[9] In any system of health care, a practitioner who knows how to facilitate more than the specific response is more likely to help patients than one who cannot.

As a corollary, those trained narrowly in current medical fashions, defensive doctoring, and reliance on tests rather than attention to the patient's signs and symptoms and empathetic listening, are likely to be least successful except in acute emergencies for which specific therapy is known. As Kleinman & Sung put it,

> …the physician is trained to systematically ignore illness [i.e., the patient's experience]. This represents a profound distortion of clinical work which is built into the training of physicians. It pays off on the application of biomedical technology to the control of disease, a less common but crucial clinical function, while it founders on the psychosocial and cultural treatment of illness, which is a much more common clinical function. Failure to heal illness is not articulated in the health professional's system of evaluating the efficacy of healing, but it is articulated in patient non-compliance and dissatisfaction, use of alternative health care facilities, poor and inadequate care, and medical-legal suits.[10]

Once physicians enter practice, most of them, willy-nilly, cultivate their ability to listen attentively to their patients. But increasingly, medical-school curricula ingrain attitudes that many are too rushed in their clinical practices to overcome, above all a reductive mindset that is useful in laboratory research but impedes care of patients.

What Role Does the Placebo Effect Play?

Before proceeding further, let us look at efficacy in the long-term evolution of biomedicine. As a historian of medical professionalism has put it, "the peculiar history of physicians in Eurocentric societies provided a focus for understanding the role of the healer who was found in all cultures of which we have knowledge."[11] Peculiar though that history was, in most instances positivism has been the only focus that non-social-scientists have used. But the history of diseases, and of the placebo effect, does not fit this model. Let us first consider the use of placebo in studies of efficacy, which is by no means a recent innovation.

Blind assessment combined with placebo (substances known not to affect the body) or other sham controls go back to 1784, and were used frequently from then on.[12] Out of this development, about 1955, randomized controlled trials evaluated by statistical tests of significance became the hallmark of clinical research that claimed to be objective. Those who carried out such trials have assumed that all therapy, no matter whether with effective drugs or inactive pills, incorporated "a

[9] See the overview in Waldram 2000.

[10] Kleinman & Sung 1979, 24. On the cost of this dissatisfaction, see Eisenberg et al. 1993.

[11] Burnham 1996, 23.

[12] This paragraph is based on the reconstruction in Kaptchuk 1998a and 1998b. The quotation is from 1998b, 1724.

monolithic effect which was present to the same degree and same direction in both the treatment and dummy arms … one could simply subtract the amount of the placebo effect to determine the presence (or absence) of specific drug effect." But no one has ever rigorously tested this not at all obvious assumption. Few clinical experiments have investigated the placebo effect itself. For ethical reasons, almost no trials have incorporated a group of patients who receive no treatment at all to determine how the results differ from those of patients who receive placebo. T. J. Kaptchuk has recently published an experimental study of placebo, which also pioneered making such a trial with informed consent.[13]

What most researchers without further thought call the placebo effect is (in Kaptchuk's words) a hodge-podge of "nature taking its course; regression to the mean; routine medical and nursing care; regimens such as rest, diet, exercise, and relaxation; easing of anxiety by diagnosis and treatment; the patient-doctor relationship; classic conditioning and learnt behaviours; the expectation of relief and the imagination; and the will and belief of both patient and practitioner." It also includes the circumstances of research itself: "the method of recruiting patients, manner of giving informed consent, procedures for blinding, vehicle of delivery (colour of pills, pills vs injection), provider characteristics, provider verbal attitudes, and physical setting of the environment."[14]

It is not hard to see why Moerman's "meaning response" is a better label than "placebo effect" for what results from this hodgepodge. In fact, endless confusion has arisen because the placebo itself—an inert substance, from the pharmacodynamic point of view that rigorous experimentalists insist upon—obviously cannot be what causes the physiological changes.[15] Such changes cannot be its specific effects. What causes them, in Kaptchuk's first few instances in the last paragraph, is the body's autonomous processes, and in the others, the personal meaning of the circumstances to the patient.

The thoughtless usage of the term "placebo effect"— ignoring these distinctions within the clinical encounter, in research circumstances, and in individual healing processes —results from the collective irrationality of diligently rational medical researchers. As David B. Morris has put it, "for over two hundred years the best scientific minds have steadfastly denied the bond between what we think and how we feel." That has changed gradually as the evidence against the complete separation of conscious and unconscious mental processes has become undeniable. But many are still committed to the strict dichotomies of the eighteenth century. Some consider placebo "a kind of gratifying fraud, pleasant but useless"; some assume it does not work for any purpose except those already proven one by one in clinical

---

[13] Kaptchuk et al. 2010; Kaptchuk 2013, esp. p. 331.

[14] Kaptchuk 1998a, 1998b, all quotations from 1998b, 1724–1725. Pellegrino 1976 writes of the placebo effect as "closely related to the aura which surrounds ingestion of any chemical substance properly invested with healing powers by the ritual of prescribing" (p. 628).

[15] Moerman 2002, 94.

tests. For others less narrow-minded, the question is not "whether placebos work but rather … how they work."[16]

Some of the scanty clinical studies of the meaning response have separated patients who improve after treatment with inert substances from those who do not, and have tested them for differences in individual personality. They find no significant correlation between personality traits and response. Moerman reports that the patient's response to placebo has "no significant impact on the character and quality of meaning effects." Other investigations reveal strong effects due to the *therapist's* "nature, character, personality, behavior, and style," especially empathy with patients and the ability to persuade them "that things will turn out well."[17] In some studies, enthusiastic physicians have registered considerably higher therapeutic effectiveness than inattentive ones. Studies of other kinds indicate that old medications commonly become statistically less effective after new ones appear, due to physicians' growing enthusiasm for the latter. This linkage has proven manifest even when the doctors are not consciously aware of their changed preference.

Studies of placebo, although few, have shown variations in effectiveness depending on the color of the inert pills, their size, their reputed price, the number taken per day, and whether the medicine was taken by mouth or injected. Sham surgery works even better than injection, and "high-powered machines with snappy names … may be at the top of the heap."[18]

The reasons postulated for these patterns have consistently had to do with meaning. For instance, blue placebo pills generally have been more effective as sedatives than as stimulants. But this was not true in studies of Italy in the 1970's. Blue substitutes for sleeping pills worked nicely for women, who tended to associate blue with the robes of the protective Virgin Mary, but not for men, who connected the color with the uniforms of the national soccer team, Azzurri, and thus with dynamic movement and excitement.[19]

Because ways of experiencing the world differ from one gender and one culture to another, the effect of the meaning response on recognized patterns of medical disorder varies greatly. For instance, although U.S. medical manuals assume that menopause is common to all women, is purely biological in origin, and often needs medication, in Japan and other countries its symptoms are rare or absent.[20]

The very frequent diagnosis of Attention Deficit Hyperactivity Disorder (ADHD) in the school systems of many American states—and the resulting use of psychotropic drugs, commonly without examination by licensed physicians—divides the United States from much of the world. The most pertinent difference is the expectation of

---

[16] Morris 1997, 188, 195, represents this third stance; for examples of the first and second in the same volume see, respectively, Shapiro & Shapiro and Price & Fields.

[17] See, for instance, Kaptchuk et al. 2009, 388. Howard Spiro 1986, 227–228, calls the crucial characteristic loyalty to the patient.

[18] Moerman 2002, 66.

[19] For references and interpretation, Moerman 2002, 35–49; for responses to colors of pills in southeast India, Nichter 1980, 231.

[20] See the extensive study in Lock 2005.

many U. S. schools that young children sit still for long periods and otherwise exhibit considerable self-discipline. This demand is often at odds with the early training of the same children by their parents. Some couples encourage freedom and creativity (whatever that may mean to them) over predictable behavior, and others simply make little effort to teach self-control. Circa 1980, U.S. medical manuals attributed ADHD to minimal brain dysfunction, but neurological examination so rarely played a role in diagnosis and dosing that this reductive etiology is now rarely mentioned.[21]

Moerman's survey of drug experiments for ulcers and hypertension show great national differences between the U.S., Germany, and Brazil, for both drug and placebo. The variation in placebo effectiveness, as always, "carries over to the drug healing rate."[22]

These are only examples of what we can infer so far about the meaning response in disease and therapy. The biomedical view of the body as a complex of purely biological, chemical, and physical systems has discouraged inquiry into its non-material aspects. Few clinical researchers challenge the conventional wisdom that dichotomizes mind and body, the psychological and the somatic, pain sensation and pain affect, and so on.[23]

Psychosomatic medicine, the enterprise that aimed to overcome this either-or approach to mind and body, is now only a distant memory. Research in it flourished from ca. 1930 to the 1950's, and it even gained a modest role in educating medical students, but from that decade on it disappeared from curricula —and with it much of the flexibility that might have integrated Moerman's varieties of response. It was a casualty of the drive to recast medicine into the mold of physical science.[24] This successful campaign transformed what it discarded into mere psychological factors or cultural peculiarities, and (in the words of Robert Aronowitz) relegated them to "illness but not disease, to therapy but not etiology, to symptoms but not pathology, and finally to the course of the disease but not to its cause."[25]

The picture I have just sketched indicates that an adequate account of therapeutic efficacy depends on three kinds of bodily response to medical disorder: the body's

---

[21] The classic study is Rubinstein & Brown 1984. Lock & Scheper-Hughes 1996, 67, discuss ADHD as an instance of recasting social frictions and miseries as "individual pathologies rather than as socially significant signs." On NIH doctrine re ADHD, see National Institutes of Health 2012. For diagnosis rates in some other countries approaching those of the U.S., see Hinshaw & Scheffeler 2014.

Payer 1988 gives other examples of important discrepancies in diagnosis and therapy between the U.S. and Western European countries. This exceptionally useful book does not reflect current practice, but no one has done a comprehensive study since. Ikels 1998 compares the experience of dementia in China and the U.S.

[22] Moerman 2002, 72–83.

[23] See, for instance, Price & Fields 1997, which even takes the last dichotomy seriously (pp. 133–134).

[24] Renée Fox further correlates the decline of psychosomatics with that of psychoanalysis and the supplanting of pathophysiology by molecular biology (personal communication, 31 August 2011).

[25] Aronowitz 1998, 51–52, in a historical analysis of ulcerative colitis. He lists several reasons for the demise of psychosomatic medicine.

autonomous ability to recover normal functioning, its specific response to biological, chemical, and physical agents, and the response of the individual to interaction with other people, which depends on the quality and meaning of that interaction. The combination of these three responses is useful in understanding any therapy in any time and place. This is true for China ca. 1000.

An obvious rejoinder to this proposition is that symbolic curing, which uses religious or ritual means, is simply an early form of psychotherapy. That claim is so close to the conventional wisdom that it calls for careful examination. I will look at it closely later (chapter 5, p. 122).

What Was Efficacy in Ancient Health Care?

Anthropological findings suggest a general viewpoint on therapy in culture that I have found useful in comparing early Chinese therapeutic approaches with each other and with other varieties of health care.[26]

What laymen and most practitioners today consider significant therapy tends to concentrate on only part of the spectrum of possibilities. In the modern societies that can afford to make biomedicine the norm, people evaluate the power of therapy according to what it can do for acute—particularly exotic—disease and serious physical trauma, and pay much less attention to its shortcomings with respect to chronic disorders. In traditional societies, I will argue, the situation is very different. What biomedicine classes as chronic rather than acute disorders, as well as epidemic febrile disorders, provide the criteria. This difference is so fundamental that ignoring it causes much mutual misunderstanding.

Look at it this way: every culture—or subculture in a society as complex and regularly changing as China's—commands many diverse techniques and strategies for the care of health. What has mattered in past evaluations of the art is relieving the suffering of patients. The value of a technique is not a fixed quantity, but depends on how it is used, how the therapist and patient understand it, and how the two (and other people present) interact. In any culture, roles, attitudes, rituals[27] and techniques interact through normal social processes to make available the fullest provision of health that lies within the means of its people.

---

[26] The first sophisticated studies of these issues, still useful in many respects, are Kleinman & Sung 1979, Kleinman 1980, and Kleinman & Gale 1982.

Some theoreticians condemn the use of the word "traditional" on the ground that it implies lack of change and thus of dynamism. I use the word simply as an antonym of "modern" when discussing patterns of practice. As this book makes clear, I believe Chinese society, and health care as part of it, was constantly changing in unpredictable directions.

[27] See, for instance, the discussion of ritual in prognosis in Christakis 1999, 163–178.

This tendency toward greatest feasible efficacy within given limits is bound to be imperfect. Before modern times the certainty of diagnosis[28] and the power of therapy were greatly limited. No society attained—nor has one yet attained—an integrated consciousness of all the dimensions of disease and health. What people observed to be the most effective means tended to play a disproportionate part in forming medicine, and in coloring the conceptions of health care in general.

I have already mentioned the conventional modern distinction between acute and chronic disorders. The usual dictionary definitions, which state that the first kind move quickly from onset to crisis and the second linger or recur, can hardly do justice to their significance either for the patient or for society.

In acute illnesses, time is of the essence. Patients commonly experience the illness as an attack, which curers must repel within the short time it is developing. Otherwise the patient can only withdraw into herself and survive as best she can by dint of her own vitality and will.

The experiential hallmark of today's chronic disorders is simply that one learns not to expect recovery. Some (for instance, Crohn's disease) comprise a succession of crises. Through habit the crucial period loses some of its vividness, though rarely its pain and dysfunction. Some such disorders (e.g., senility) limit activity without crises. Others, such as diabetes, escalate and sometimes kill, but they are not typical.[29] The paradigmatic chronic disease is old age, the irreversible loss of capacities until none is left. The medical problem in chronic ailments is not curing, but making it possible for the patient to live with disability, to resume some approximation to a normal life. That makes social support as essential as—and generally more effective than—chemical and physical therapy.

No pre-modern society had powerful means to control most acute disease. A certain number of people were struck one at a time or in an epidemic, and a certain proportion survived. The death toll from cholera, smallpox, or diphtheria was often very high. Preventive quarantine, an array of drugs with which to manipulate vital processes, quinine for malaria, and smallpox variolation or vaccination: these were widespread in the major civilizations well before 1900, but those who became ill with most diseases were still largely thrown back upon their own resources and the encouragement of others. Only after another half-century did antibiotics make it possible to broadly eradicate microorganisms.

One of the most dramatic changes in European and American medicine during the twentieth century was the specialization of its institutions to prevent and cure one acute illness after another—or to control serious trauma with safe surgery—through means uncovered by scientific research. Most diseases that meant a private encounter with death a century ago now mean, at worst, an agonizing but temporary withdrawal from full activity. This remarkable victory, which has greatly changed the world's demographics, is built upon more than wonder drugs. It has called into

[28] I do not mean that doctors generally lacked confidence in their findings, but that their diagnoses of the same patient were more likely than today to disagree. The limits in their ability to cure also made them more attentive to prognosis than M.D.'s are today. On this topic see Christakis 1999.

[29] For an eloquent discussion, see Kleinman 1988, 44–49.

being a medical system which isolates the patient, controls his immediate environment, and provides clinicians with rapid access to emergency technologies.

As the capacity to cope with acute diseases and emergencies evolved, the roles of the doctor and patient gradually adapted to the new institutions. The interaction was increasingly shaped by the convictions of doctors and their organizations about the need to base health care solidly on technical research (and in the process to give physicians the status they needed to reach these professional goals, as well as their personal ones).

The balance tipped away from general practice toward specialization, away from the physician treating the patient at home and toward examination in a clinic or an emergency room. The physician came to resemble the scientist manipulating an experimental object which had to be kept immobile and passive so as not to hinder operations measured to the millimeter and timed to the second.

This association of the clinic with the biological laboratory spread even in circumstances where it was irrelevant and distracting. The patient's biochemistry and physiology became crucial, his signs and symptoms rendered less relevant to diagnosis by laboratory tests, and his feelings beside the point. The examples of their mentors encouraged medical students to see the patient's experience as a mere obstacle to decisions best made unilaterally by the therapist on technical grounds. The life-or-death decisions, although a small minority, justified the rest. Once the patient entered the hospital, the people he lived with were no longer involved in caring for him.[30] This new complex of practice and attitude justified itself by bringing under control one acute infectious disorder and surgical emergency after another—at least in societies that could afford the technology, in cases that reached the hospitals, and in patients who could afford the expense.

A consensus has developed among public health physicians in the United States that this specialization of institutions has led to a disastrous imbalance. The direction of greatest development has been almost diametrically opposed to what meets the needs of chronic patients. Prevention of serious dysfunction, the most powerful means, is under-funded and, despite a consensus about its importance, is not a priority of hospitals, planners, or medical practices. Most practitioners attentive to prevention pay more attention to statistical risk factors—which hold only for large populations—than to the personal situations of their clients. As a well-informed recent U. S. survey of progress in chronic disease control puts it, "at present less than 3% of health funding is directed to prevention efforts. The bias against prevention is so pervasive, so embedded, so intractable, that many people, including policy makers, fail to recognize that the development of most chronic illnesses is almost entirely outside the purview of clinical care. Chronic disease control today is similar to where the nation was a century ago with regard to basic sanitation."[31]

It is not normal for a doctor to be available whenever the patient needs understanding, support, and unhurried explanation. It is exceptional in modern middle-class

[30] In much of China and elsewhere in East Asia, members of all except wealthy families still tend to stay in the hospital to feed and care for the patient, as European families used to do.

[31] National Association of Chronic Disease Directors 2007, 8.

American society for doctors to know their patients well enough to encourage in them—leaving aside the occasional one-minute lecture or printed handout—a minimally impaired style of life. It is practically unheard of for doctors to enter the patient's home and form an independent impression of personal or family circumstances that affect physical well-being.

Many patients—the uninsured middle class, the poor, and the elderly, among others—cannot adapt to the highly routine, stressful procedures of municipal clinics that will accept them. They cannot avoid disorientation when treated impersonally by a succession of unknown doctors whose time is rationed.

Physicians have largely given up the role of social mediator, despite the large role of the patient's setting in recovery. Society has changed in ways that make mediation almost impossible. The wasting away of communal bonds and common values has meant that in large sectors of modern societies there is seldom a circle of relatives, friends, and neighbors to encourage what a chronically ill person has to contribute, and to support his efforts toward a useful life. Many old people ("senior citizens") with degenerative diseases, barely subsisting on social security in a city, have no relative or friend with whom they can regularly keep in touch.

In summary, the transformation of modern medicine—of which I have mentioned only a few manifestations—has been part of, and has been made possible by, replacing the values and forms that defined earlier societies. The result has been a differently unbalanced ability to deal with the spectrum of suffering. There has been no significant evolution toward better balanced institutions and roles. In fact, in the wealthier societies and those whose wealth is increasing, rising life expectancy and growing inequality of income have increased the pressure that skews medical institutions.

The situation I have just described is so striking that it immediately suggests contrasts with that of China before the dislocations of the twentieth century. The limitations of classical medicine notably differed from those just described. Its doctrines guided the deployment of an enormous variety of therapeutic measures, including thousands of physiologically active drugs. Physicians used these mostly to produce changes in the balance of body processes. Few such remedies were specific in the biomedical sense. Elite culture established ritual forms for the relation of doctor and patient, and adapted from the culture of the commoners other forms useful in that relationship. All this happened in a society where the physician had access to the patient's social milieu. The curer could easily learn, in an unhurried way, what his patient believed, how he saw the world, what his inner experience of illness was, who in his family tended to lessen his distress, and who to increase it.[32] Some practitioners were perfunctory in diagnosis and inflexible in therapy, but the norms encouraged responsiveness. The settings of health care for the majority, who had no access to classical medicine, were extremely varied.

[32] The situation was often different from the fourteenth century on with women and children, since other family members often presented their ailments for diagnosis, but this was not normally the case for women ca. 1050.

It is impossible to compare in detail the strengths and limitations of classical Chinese therapy in the eleventh century with those of modern biomedicine. They have too little in common. We could reduce the absurdity if we were to compare Chinese and European medicine at the same time, ca. 1000. The most conspicuous strengths of both lay in the provision of what we now call chronic care. Even so, the great variation in medical practice in different parts of Europe and in the different levels of its society would limit the value of any vague Sino-European comparison. So long as the history of medical ritual remains unstudied, we have no way to adequately comprehend care for chronic suffering. And given the negligible role of the high medical traditions in health care at both ends of Eurasia then, an impartial comparison of religious curing, that of local curers of every kind, and the work of illiterate and semi-literate herbalists, would be much more to the point—but about such matters we are abysmally ignorant.[33] This book, at least, aims to encourage it by working out a first rough idea of the spectrum of Chinese health care. Keeping this pattern in mind will prepare us to appreciate the power of Chinese health care, classical and popular, and the importance of rituals in both kinds.

Efficacy for Which Disorders?

It is natural to assume that what curers in other times and places contended with were the same diseases that physicians diagnose today. If we believe that biomedicine provides infallible knowledge of every time and place, that is an obvious corollary. But both this article of faith and the assumption based on it are wrong.

Medical therapy treats human beings in societies. Comprehending it depends on our understanding—still all too fallible—of culture, of thought and feeling, of the ways people interact, and of how the varieties of human suffering are related to one another.

It is no news that diseases vary according to place, change over time, and come into being and pass away. Typhus and typhoid are now rare enough that American general practitioners[34] are seldom able to diagnose them. Paralytic polio is no longer a constituent of U.S. health statistics. I have already mentioned the precipitous rise of Attention Deficit Hyperactivity Disorder in those statistics. Habitual drunkenness, once a "despised although tolerated moral condition" (and a crime in many localities), within living memory became the medical disorder alcoholism.[35] Even

[33] There are a few useful monographic studies of popular therapy in Europe and the United States up to the nineteenth century, e.g., Beier 1987, Ramsey 1988, Brockliss & Jones 1997, Green 1994, MacDonald 1981, Pelling 1998, Porter 1985 and 1989, and Ulrich 1990. For an overview see Gentilcore 2004. Important more recent publications are Lindemann 2010 and Rankin 2013.

[34] I realize that this term is no longer respectable, but it is less stiff than the bureaucrats' "primary health care provider." I was involved in a medical case in which it took a team of hospital physicians two weeks to learn that a case that they could not identify was typhoid.

[35] Stein 1973, quoting p. 367.

more recently, senile dementia has metamorphosed into Alzheimer's disease. These instances are all the more remarkable because medicine cannot explain how any of these newish diseases originate, prevent them, or cure them. New organic diseases, such as Ebola hemorrhagic fever, Lyme disease, and HIV AIDS, appear with some regularity.

When we look some distance into the past, the picture becomes even more obviously discrepant. Fever today is elevated body temperature, a mere symptom that the patient may or may not feel, but that the physician measures to a tenth of a degree. In the U.S. in the late nineteenth century, fever was a disease with many symptoms, including cold sensations and elevated pulse rate. In a diagnostic handbook very widely used in the early twentieth century, it included even more symptoms. Although the well-trained, experienced biomedical physician of 1930 likely felt that his knowledge and habits of reasoning held for all time, as we look back from the present day his limitations are all too obvious.[36]

The same is true when we look at other cultures. The definition of *re* 熱 in dictionaries of modern Chinese is "fever." Indeed that is what it means to Chinese M.D.'s. Most practitioners of Traditional Chinese Medicine, trained since the 1950's using textbooks that aimed to impose science on old ideas, also now understand it as fever. But in classical medicine its meaning was quite different. From early medical writings on, authors paired *re* with *han* 寒 as antonyms. *Han* meant "chills," cold feelings within the body—a symptom that the patient reported, not a physical sign—and *re* meant hot sensations of exactly the same kind; the combination *hanre* 寒熱 meant alternating hot and cold sensations. In some sources before modern times a different word, *fare* 發熱, meant the dynamic manifestation of heat at the periphery of the body—which is not the same thing as elevated temperature there or within the body. The ancient roster of diseases, and even of symptoms, not only differed greatly from the constituents of modern nosology, but changed regularly.

Let me give an example. Hilary Smith has studied in considerable detail the repeated metamorphoses of the medical disorder *jiaoqi* 腳氣 through Chinese history. Dictionaries of the modern language list its meaning unambiguously as "beriberi," and that is how most historians of medicine have understood it. But that definition held true only for a limited time in the late nineteenth and the twentieth century. *Jiaoqi* began by about A.D. 500 as an often fatal disease and in time became a group of diseases, repeatedly changing its great range of symptoms. In modern times, for biomedical physicians, it became beriberi, but it now increasingly refers to athlete's foot! To practitioners of classical medicine over the centuries, even as its manifestations changed, it remained—like fever in early modern Europe—one disease.[37]

Most competent modern-day physicians are sensibly reluctant to diagnose diseases in people they have not examined. Andrew Cunningham, in a recent study that questions "the continuous identity of past diseases with modern diseases," has looked closely at the pitfalls. In England, as he demonstrates for several points over

[36] Dunglison 1874, 416; Savill 1930, 498; more extensive discussion in Sivin 1987, 107–109.

[37] Smith 2008.

the past four hundred years, the categories used for reporting causes of death differed fundamentally from those that physicians today are qualified to choose between. The law for much of this time designated bystanders with no medical education to decide for the record what disease killed someone. In 1672 the requirement was "two ancient Matrons" appointed as Searchers; in the act of 1836 it was "some person present at death, or in attendance at the last illness." It was the sum of such reports that entered official records and statistics. Looking closely at "how diagnosis happens," Cunningham argues that "the identity of any disease is made up of a compound of elements, of which the biological or medical is only one, and sometimes the least important." With due attention to the social dimension, he demonstrates that human decisions regularly change disease entities. The notion that reality lies elsewhere than in how witnesses identified these entities in the language of a given time and place may be unimpeachable as mystical faith, but has no value for historical study.[38]

To take the example of *jiaoqi*, someone familiar with modern nosology may well notice that several of its symptoms in the sixteenth century resemble those of modern gout, but to say that *jiaoqi* at the time was gout is an elementary error. It is easily corrected by citing its other defining symptoms that had nothing to do with gout.[39] And sixteenth-century gout, unlike that of 2010, was not defined by the deposition of crystals from sodium urate in a joint. To understand how the two differ is, as Cunningham puts it, a matter of studying historically the social process of diagnosing them. His point extends perfectly to eleventh-century China. The diseases were those that a wide variety of curers and laymen could name. The family of the deceased, more often than a therapist or a functionary, determined the cause of death for records we can consult, namely funeral inscriptions and official biographies derived from information that the family provided.

Instead of beginning with a biomedical disorder, let us take the case of someone ca. 1000 whom a classical physician diagnosed with Pulmonary Abscess Disorder *(feiyong* 肺癰). The standard reference for nosology was still the 400-year-old *Origins and Symptoms of Medical Disorders* (611).[40] The descriptions in that book provide a common denominator for cases where, as usual, we know nothing about the doctor's own classification of disease. According to *Origins and Symptoms,* this ailment is due to damage to the lung functions caused by wind and cold factors in conditions of *qi* 氣 depletion. The cold pathogens from outside the body, contending with its yin vitalities *(xue* 血), congeal them to form a hidden abscess and, if hot factors are also involved, the result is likely to be purulent, bloody sputum often accompanied by trembling.

[38] Cunningham 2002, citing pp. 13 and 16 (the second quotation is italicized in the original). On searchers see Munkhoff 1999. For an analogous study, see MacDonald 1989. For significant differences between medical practice in Germany, France, England, and the U. S. in the late twentieth century see Payer 1988, 25.

[39] Smith 2008, 183–186.

[40] *Zhu bing yuan hou lun* 諸病源候論, 33: 177b–178a. This book was superseded only by *San yin ji yi bing yuan lun cui* 三因極一病源論粹, ca. 1174.

The M.D. without a body to examine but willing to diagnose words will perhaps conclude that the patient is ill with pulmonary tuberculosis, some anemic or neurasthenic syndrome, or another ailment characterized by hemoptysis. But it is not that simple. Instead of merely scanning a list of symptoms, as Cunningham reminds us, we need to ask about the process of diagnosis. Were there other options? If so, who chose, and how?

There were in fact a great many alternatives, even for classical physicians. Any doctor might also have considered the large class of Depletion Exhaustion Disorders *(xulao* 虛勞). Among the seventy-five disorders that it comprises are several obvious prospects, for instance Depletion Exhaustion with Hot Sensations *(xulao re* 虛勞熱), Depletion Exhaustion with Alternating Cold and Hot Sensations *(xulao hanre* 虛勞寒熱), Depletion Exhaustion with Bone Steaming *(xulao guzheng* 虛勞骨蒸), Depletion Exhaustion with Upset and Inner Tension *(xulao fanmen* 虛勞煩悶), Depletion Exhaustion with Vomiting due to Reversed Flow of Yin *Qi* and with Spitting Blood *(xulao ouni tuoxue* 虛勞嘔逆唾血), Depletion Exhaustion with Vomiting Blood *(xulao ouxue* 虛勞嘔血), which vary not only by symptoms but by the etiologies that some of their names reflect.[41]

Other likely disorders occur among the thirty-four consumptive disorders in the class of Infusion (that is, possession) Disorders *(zhu* 注, 疰), also due to *qi* depletion and exhaustion, as well as to possession by the *qi* of ghosts, which can be transmitted from a dying patient to a bystander.[42]

Every one of these more than a hundred distinct pathological entities has its own list of symptoms and indications, often as long as that of Pulmonary Abscess Disorder. An M.D. willing to accept some symptoms and blankly ignore others may decide that all are simply names for pulmonary tuberculosis or some other modern entity, but that is too high-handed a procedure and too inattentive a method for anything but a parlor game. A physician who insists on understanding past experience is likely to agree with the historian in taking all of the sources—and their nosology—seriously.

In fact, modern medical knowledge, if combined with careful attention to exactly what the original records say rather than substituted for the original concepts, can be indispensable in study of distant times and places. An excellent instance is the long-debated death of the nineteen-year-old Tongzhi Emperor on 12 January 1875. Generations of scholars have argued about whether it was due to smallpox or syphilis, or whether the monarch was poisoned. They freely ignored the recorded cause of death, *zouma yagan* 走馬牙疳 (literally, "galloping gum ulcerations"). A recent study has reconstructed from the extremely detailed contemporary accounts of the emperor's medical care a remarkable denouement. It has done so by paying attention to the substance of discussions by the physicians involved, without at that stage letting modern diagnostic entities obscure them.

---

[41] For *xulao* see *Zhu bing yuan hou lun*, 3: 17a–4: 27b; *xulao re*, 3: 19b; *xulao hanre*, 3: 22b; *xulao guzheng*, 4: 23a–23b; *xulao fanmen*, 4: 23b; *xulao ouni tuoxue* and *xulao ouxue*, 4: 24a.

[42] *Zhu bing yuan hou lun*, 24: 130a–134b.

On 9 December 1874, the emperor was indeed diagnosed with *douzhen* 痘疹, a disease that at the time overlapped with symptoms of what English calls smallpox. Within a week his condition had stabilized, and in less than two his doctors announced that recovery was well under way. He decided unilaterally to stay in bed for a hundred days to ensure complete recovery. But by 23 December he had developed large purulent sores about his waist, and these spread over his back and arms until by 7 January 1875 his face and gums swelled and he developed grave infections in his mouth and gums. As they worsened, he died five days later.

The historians could never settle their long-running debates. Nevertheless, with the publication of the palace medical archives in 1990, it became clear that there had been no symptoms of syphilis, and that the emperor was indeed recovering quickly from *douzhen.* Finally in 1998 Chang Che-chia plausibly explained for the first time what the archives and other important sources revealed. "Galloping gum ulcerations" were indeed what killed the young ruler. What led to them were symptoms well known in Europe, but to which Chinese physicians at the time did not give a distinct place in their nosology, namely bedsores. It took the whim of a youthful emperor to lie abed for many weeks, a circumstance that so far as Chang knows did not otherwise occur under the eyes of imperial physicians, to allow the infection to become systemic. His several outstanding doctors, with no experience of bedsores out of control, were flummoxed—and he died.[43] Modern knowledge can be most helpful in sorting out the ambiguity of ancient records, but only when they are exceptionally detailed and after exactly what they say is well understood.

Who Decided What is Efficacious?

The results of self-care or care by a family member were evaluated within the family (depending on its constellation of authority or informal power). The family also decided, when it was necessary to consult an outsider, whom to see. Its members—the patient not necessarily participating—eventually reached consensus about whether the treatment was satisfactory. They might well disagree on whether the patient was recovering. As often happened in families that could afford it, they might try someone else. The medical case records of physicians over the past five hundred years often speak of their protagonist as the last of several assorted therapists called. Their authors often complain that family members present in the sickroom upset the patient, disagreed with the doctor's judgment, or found fault with him in favor of some other curer.[44] If we had case records left by earlier physicians or other types of curers, we would no doubt be left with an even more complicated impression of the family's role. The decisions about efficacy that mattered, like other decisions, were usually those of the people around the patient.

---

[43] Chang Che-chia 1998, 85–120. For the archives, see Chen Keji 1990.

[44] See, for example, Grant 2003, chapter 3, and, on case records, Furth et al. 2007, especially part 2.

That does not quite answer the question of what process led to judgments about diagnosis and therapy, since in almost every instance the only record we have is that by the therapist. They did tend to see patients frequently. The literature indicates, however, that ancient practitioners of various kinds made judgments of success or failure in much the same way as biomedical physicians still do. That is, once the treatment was concluded to their satisfaction, they did not follow up systematically but, unless they heard otherwise, assumed that the patient recovered. They tacitly agreed with the patient that, even in obviously self-limiting disorders, the therapist is entitled to the credit.

Thus the failure of the patient to reappear, or of anyone to complain, was what usually closed the case. Sometimes the physician's—or someone else's—decision that the patient needed no more care, or would be better off with care from someone else, led to the end of the therapeutic relationship. But the judgment of all concerned about whether the patient had recovered was commonly based on habitual assumptions rather than investigation. It makes sense to conclude that the assessment of therapy resulted from often complex interactions between the patient, the family, and the various curers involved. If there were several therapists, it is perfectly possible that they all numbered the same case among their successes.

Conclusions

Any historical investigation of curing, no matter where or when, may benefit if the inquirer knows biology, chemistry, physics, and clinical practice. But translating traditional accounts of disease directly into biomedical language usually leads to grossly inadequate understanding. We have seen that therapy depends as greatly on the body's tendency toward homeostasis, and on the patient's response to symbolic and personal interaction, as it does on technology—and often more so. This implies that the present-day physician's personal cultivation, sensibility, and empathy may play as large a role as her mastery of pathology. To put it the other way round, Americans often explain their resort to an acupuncturist by the fact that their primary care physician spent more time looking at his computer monitor than at them.

We have also seen that there is no consensus within the medical profession about the meaning of "the placebo effect," which all too often lumps together an ill-assorted gaggle of phenomena. Some medical spokesmen use that term to dismiss all scientifically unexplainable curing; others take it seriously as due to a biochemically inert substance, but are mystified by it. A mere handful of researchers has thrown odd but revealing glimmers of light on it. Fewer are inclined to undertake research directed toward understanding it. In short, the concept of placebo is too vague to be useful in an investigation such as this. A more productive method is to leave it to the clinical researchers, and follow Moerman in pondering the role of the meaning response in every sort of therapy.

We can deduce from the discussions above several aids useful in exploring the varieties of curing in China ca. 1000:

- Although every kind of health care is unique, we can take as a working hypothesis that, in a given time and place, all are likely to share some notions of the causes and character of disease, even as they disagree about the rest. To assume that, say, religious curing has nothing in common with the classical medicine of the scholarly doctors is counterproductive. What in a given instance they have in common is an empirical question worth asking.
- The way curers and patients evaluated the strengths and weaknesses of medical care in their time and place can vary greatly, and always calls for attention. The criteria of modern medicine (for instance, the ability to deal with acute emergencies and serious traumata) are likely to be irrelevant. Major surgery was extremely rare and dangerous, and there is little evidence that early physicians could do more than bolster the body's own ability to recover from serious disease. Again what criteria are pertinent is an empirical question.
- Every culture slices up the spectrum of suffering in its own way. It can be seriously misleading to assume that the diseases, or even the symptoms, that people experienced long ago or in a different culture are the same as those of the U.S. or China today.
- The records of medical disorders that this book will study were shaped by their own culture and subculture, and have to be seen in their light. To evaluate (or dismiss) accounts as though they were modern case histories is to lose the opportunity to learn from them.

What we learn can throw light not only on the medical experience of many times and places, but on current assumptions about how to improve health care and facilitate wellness. With these principles and cautions in mind, let us explore the world of early Chinese health care.

References

Abbreviations

DZ = Volume number in *Daozang*
ES = *Ersishi shi* 二十四史 of ZS, 1959–1977.
HY = text in Harvard-Yenching Concordance series
j. = *juan* 卷 (chapter)
RW = published by Renmin Weisheng Chubanshe 人民衛生出版社, Beijing
S = Title number in Schipper 1975
SQ = Siku quanshu 四庫全書
SV = Schipper & Verellen 2004
T = *Taishō shinshū Daizōkyō* 大正新修大藏經
UP = University Press
YZ = Yi tong zheng mai quan shu 醫統正脈全書
ZD = Volume, item, *juan,* and page numbers in *Zhonghua daozang* 中华道藏
ZS = published by Zhonghua shuju 中華書局, Beijing
ZZ = Zhongyi zhenben congshu 中醫珍本叢書 ed.

Classical Chinese Sources

San yin ji yi bing yuan lun cui 三因極一病源論粹 (The three causes epitomized and unified: the quintessence of doctrine on the origins of medical disorders). Chen Yan 陳言. 1174 or shortly after. Beijing, 1957 ed., under the title *San yin ji yi ping zheng fang lun* 三因極一病證方論. Commonly referred to as *San yin fang* 三因方.

Zhu bing yuan hou lun 諸病源候論 (Origins and symptoms of medical disorders). Chao Yuanfang 巢元方. Completed 610. RW, 1955.

Other Sources

Albrecht, Gary L., Ray Fitzpatrick, & Susan Scrimshaw, eds. 2000. *Handbook of Social Studies in Health and Medicine*. London: Sage Publications.

Aronowitz, Robert A. 1998. *Making Sense of Illness. Science, Society, and Disease*. Cambridge History of Medicine. Cambridge UP.

Beier, Lucinda McCray. 2008. *For Their Own Good: The Transformation of English Working-Class Health Culture, 1880–1970*. Columbus: Ohio State UP.

Brockliss, Laurence, & Colin Jones. 1997. *The Medical World of Early Modern France*. Oxford UP.

Burnham, John C. 1996. Garrison Lecture: How the Concept of Profession Evolved in the Work of Historians of Medicine. *Bulletin of the History of Medicine* 70. 1: 1–24.

Chang, Che-chia. 1998. The Therapeutic Tug of War. The Imperial Physician-Patient Relationship in the Era of Empress Dowager Cixi (1874–1908). Ph.D. dissertation, Asian and Middle Eastern Studies, University of Pennsylvania.

Chen Keji 陳可冀 et al. 1990. *Qing gong yian yanjiu* 清宮醫案研究 (A study of the Qing medical archives). Beijing: Zhongyi Guji Chubanshe.

Christakis, Nicholas A. 1999. *Death Foretold. Prophecy and Prognosis in Medical Care*. University of Chicago Press.

Csordas, Thomas J., & Arthur Kleinman. 1996. The Therapeutic Process. In Sargent & Johnson 1996, 3–20.

Cunningham, Andrew. 2002. Identifying Disease in the Past: Cutting the Gordian Knot. *Asclepio* 54, 1: 13–34.

Desjarlais, Robert R. 1992. *Body and Emotion. The Aesthetics of Illness and Healing in the Nepal Himalayas*. Series in Contemporary Ethnology, 2. Philadelphia: University of Pennsylvania Press.

Dunglison, Robley. 1839/1874. *Medical Lexicon: A Dictionary of Medical Science: Containing a Concise Explanation of the Various Subjects and Terms*. Revised ed. Philadelphia: Henry C. Lea.

Eisenberg, David M., Ronald C. Kessler, Cindy Foster, et al. 1993. Unconventional Medicine in the United States—Prevalence, Costs, and Patterns of Use. *New England Journal of Medicine* 328: 246–252.

Furth, Charlotte, Judith T. Zeitlin, & Ping-chen Hsiung, eds. 2007. *Thinking with Cases. Specialist Knowledge in Chinese Cultural History*. Honolulu: University of Hawai'i Press. Cases in law, medicine, religion and philosophy.

Gentilcore, David. 2004. Was There a 'Popular Medicine' in Early Modern Europe? *Folklore* 115: 151–166.

Grant, Joanna. 2003. *A Chinese Physician. Wang Ji and the 'Stone Mountain Medical Case Histories.'* Needham Research Institute Series, 2. London: RoutledgeCurzon.

Green, Monica H. 1994. Documenting Medieval Women's Medical Practice. In *Practical Medicine from Salerno to the Black Death*, ed. Luis Garcia Ballester, 322–352. Cambridge UP.

Harrington, Anne, ed. 1997. *The Placebo Effect. An Interdisciplinary Exploration.* Harvard UP. Nine papers from a 1994 conference.

Hinshaw, Stephen P., & Richard M. Scheffeler. 2014. *The ADHD Explosion. Myths, Medication, and Today's Push for Performance.* New York: Oxford UP.

Ikels, Charlotte. 1998. The Experience of Dementia in China. *Culture, Medicine and Psychiatry* 22: 257–283.

Kaptchuk, Ted J. 1998a. Intentional Ignorance: A History of Blind Assessment and Placebo Controls in Medicine. *Bulletin of the History of Medicine* 72. 3: 389–433.

Kaptchuk, Ted J. 1998b. Powerful Placebo: The Dark Side of the Randomised Controlled Trial. *The Lancet* 351: 1722–1725.

Kaptchuk, Ted J. 2013. Placebo-controlled Randomized Trials and Chinese Medicine. In Hinrichs & Barnes 2013, 329–331.

Kaptchuk, Ted J., et al. 2009. 'Maybe I Made Up the Whole Thing': Placebos and Patients' Experiences in a Randomized Controlled Trial. *Culture, Medicine and Psychiatry* 33: 382–411.

Kaptchuk, Ted J., et al. 2010. Placebos without Deception: A Randomized Controlled Trial in Irritable Bowel Syndrome. *Plos ONE* 5. 12: 1–7 (e15591).

Kleinman, Arthur. 1980. *Patients and Healers in the Context of Culture: An Exploration of the Borderland between Anthropology, Medicine, and Psychiatry.* Comparative Studies of Health Systems and Medical Care, 3. Berkeley: University of California Press.

Kleinman, Arthur. 1988. *The Illness Narratives. Suffering, Healing, and the Human Condition.* New York: Basic Books.

Kleinman, Arthur, & James M. Gale. 1982. Patients Treated by Physicians and Folk Healers: A Comparative Study in Taiwan. *Culture, Medicine and Psychiatry,* 6: 405–423.

Kleinman, Arthur, & Lilias H. Sung. 1979. Why Do Indigenous Practitioners Successfully Heal? *Social Science and Medicine* 13B: 7–26.

Lindemann, Mary. 2010. *Health and Healing in Early Modern Europe.* Rev. ed. Cambridge University Press.

Liu Shoushan 刘寿山, ed. in chief. 1963– . *Zhongyao yanjiu wenxian zhaiyao* 中药研究文献摘要 (Abstracts of research publications on Chinese drugs). Beijing: Kexue Chubanshe. Ongoing; the first volume covers research published between 1820 and 1961.

Lock, Margaret. 2000. Accounting for Disease and Distress: Morals of the Normal and Abnormal. In Albrecht et al. 2000, 259–276.

Lock, Margaret. 2005. Symptom Reporting at the End of Menstruation: Biological Variation and Cultural Difference. In *Controversies in Science and Technologies: From Maize to Menopause,* ed. D.L. Kleinman, A.J. Kinchy, & J. Handelsman. Madison: University of Wisconsin Press, 236–253.

Lock, Margaret, & Nancy Scheper-Hughes. 1996. A Critical-Interpretive Approach in Medical Anthropology: Rituals and Routines of Discipline and Dissent. In Sargent & Johnson 1986, 41–70.

MacDonald, Michael. 1981. *Medical Bedlam. Madness, Anxiety, and Healing in Seventeenth-century England.* Cambridge UP.

Moerman, Daniel. 2000. Cultural Variations in the Placebo Effect: Ulcers, Anxiety, and Blood Pressure. *Medical Anthropology Quarterly* 14. 1: 1–22.

Moerman, Daniel. 2002. *Meaning, Medicine and the Placebo Effect.* Cambridge Studies in Medical Anthropology. Cambridge UP.

Morris, David B. 1997. Placebo, Pain, and Belief: A Biocultural Model. In Harrington 1997, 187–207.

Munkhoff, Rachelle. 1999. Searchers of the Dead: Authority, Marginality, and the Interpretation of Plague in England, 1574–1665. *Gender and History* 11: 1–29.

National Association of Chronic Disease Directors. 2007. *Public Health Advances through Chronic Disease Prevention: 1986–2006.* Atlanta: The Association.

National Institutes of Health. 2012. 'Attention Deficit Hyperactivity Disorder.' NIH Publication 12–3572. http://www.nimh.nih.gov/health/publications/attention-deficit-hyperactivity-disorder/index.shtml (accessed 2015.3.2).
Nichter, Mark. 1980. The Layperson's Perception of Medicine as Perspective into the Utilization of Multiple Therapy Systems in the Indian Context. *Social Science and Medicine* 148: 225–233.
Payer, Lynn. 1988. *Medicine & Culture: Varieties of Treatment in the United States, England, West Germany, and France*. New York: Henry Holt.
Pellegrino, Edmund D. 1976. Prescribing and Drug Ingestion: Symbols and Substances. *Drug Intelligence and Clinical Pharmacy* 10: 624–630.
Pelling, Margaret. 1998. *The Common Lot: Sickness, Medical Occupations and the Urban Poor in Early Modern England*. London: Longman.
Porter, Roy, ed. 1985. *Patients and Practitioners. Lay Perceptions of Medicine in Pre-industrial Society*. Cambridge History of Medicine, 9. Cambridge UP.
Porter, Roy. 1989. *Health for Sale. Quackery in England 1660–1850*. Manchester UP.
Price, Donald D., & Howard L. Fields. 1997. The Contribution of Desire and Expectation to Placebo Analgesia: Implications for New Research Strategies. In Harrington 1997, 116–137.
Ramsey, Matthew. 1988. *Professional and Popular Medicine in France, 1770–1830: The Social World of Medical Practice*. Cambridge History of Medicine. Cambridge UP.
Rankin, Alisha. 2013. *Panaceia's Daughters: Noblewomen as Healers in Early Modern Germany*. Synthesis. University of Chicago Press.
Rubinstein, Robert A., & Ronald T. Brown. 1984. An Evaluation of the Validity of the Diagnostic Category of Attention Deficit Disorder. *American Journal of Orthopsychiatry* 543: 398–414.
Sargent, Carolyn F., & Thomas M. Johnson, eds. 1996. *Medical Anthropology: Contemporary Theory and Method*. Rev. ed. Westport, CT: Praeger.
Savill, Thomas Dixon. 1930. *A System of Clinical Medicine: Dealing with the Diagnosis, Prognosis, and Treatment of Disease: For Students and Practitioners*. 8th ed. New York: William Wood. First ed., 2 vols., London, 1903–1905.
Shapiro, Arthur K., & Elaine Shapiro. 1997. The Placebo: Is It Much Ado about Nothing? In Harrington 1997, 12–36. Medical reductionists' view.
Sivin, Nathan. 1987. *Traditional Medicine in Contemporary China*. Science, Medicine, and Technology in East Asia, 2. Ann Arbor: Center for Chinese Studies, University of Michigan.
Smith, Hilary. 2008. Foot Qi: History of a Chinese Medical Disorder. Ph.D. dissertation, History and Sociology of Science, University of Pennsylvania.
Stein, Howard F. 1973. Ethanol and its Discontents: Paradoxes of Inebriation and Sobriety in American Culture. *Journal of Psychoanalytic Anthropology* 5. 4: 355–377.
Ulrich, Laurel Thatcher. 1990. *A Midwife's Tale. The Life of Martha Ballard, Based on her Diary, 1785–1812*. New York: Alfred A. Knopf.
Waldram, James B. 2000. The Efficacy of Traditional Medicine: Current Theoretical and Methodological Issues. *Medical Anthropology Quarterly* 14. 4: 603–625.
Whyte, Susan Reynolds, Sjaak van der Geest, & Anita Harden. 2002. *Social Lives of Medicines*. Cambridge Studies in Medical Anthropology. Cambridge UP.

Chapter 4
Classical Medicine

Abstract The medicine of the classical physician was based on a integral understanding of the universe, society, and the human body. The long eleventh century marked an important transition in medical care. In certain reigns, the imperial government, responding to a series of epidemics and other needs, deeply involved itself in medicine. It collected ancient classics, edited, and printed them, to furnish a corpus on which education could be uniformly based. It founded a medical school to prepare the sons of elite families for therapeutic careers. It opened pharmacies to minimize inflation in the prices of drugs. It attempted to sponsor medical education and medical care in the provinces. The political infighting of the time limited the success of these initiatives. Classical therapy saw health as a dynamic balance of metabolic and circulatory processes adjusted to the body's physical environment, and disease as the result of either inner imbalance or invasion by pathogens. The eleventh century was the first time in a millennium that doctors and other scholars were able to synthesize disparate earlier approaches to diagnosis and therapy. They enriched these methods with others adapted from popular, Buddhist, and Daoist health care. This chapter explains basic concepts and their application, and provides some examples of doctor-patient relationships and of the applications of doctrine in medical care.

The high tradition, what I call classical medicine, was based on a special way of seeing the body, as well as of thinking about the cosmos and society, and of contemplating the possibility of change in all three.[1] Unlike other kinds of medicine, and health care generally, it was based primarily on the study of books, on memorizing classical texts. More than ten thousand medical books survive from imperial China.[2] They were mostly written by the minority of physicians who belonged to the tiny educated elite bred to govern the empire. Physicians before the eleventh century had been almost entirely hereditary practitioners or itinerant curers. The exceptions were literati who took up medicine for personal reasons, often because when they

[1] What most writers now call "Traditional Chinese Medicine" or simply "TCM" has appropriated so much from biomedicine, and has been so reshaped by social transformation since 1911, that it differs greatly from classical medicine; see Scheid 2002 and 2007, Taylor 2004, and Sivin 1987.

[2] Xue Qinglu 薛清录 1991, a union catalogue of medical books in Chinese libraries, lists well over ten thousand titles from before 1911.

© Springer International Publishing Switzerland 2015

N. Sivin, *Health Care in Eleventh-Century China*, Archimedes 43,
DOI 10.1007/978-3-319-20427-7_4

were growing up they or a parent had been seriously ill. A few others were trained in the imperial palace to serve in its medical bureaucracy. It was not until ca. 1100, in fact, that the government set out to create a large class of doctors at the top of the social scale (see p. 64).

The eleventh-century medical books that we can read today give a very different impression: that the care of health lay entirely in the hands of highly literate physicians. Their authors acknowledge the existence of other kinds of therapist mainly when scoffing at the incompetence of practitioners unlike themselves. Although most historians have let themselves be guided by this view, it is myopic, confusing medicine and health care.

Historians of medicine have consistently assumed that, despite the importance of religion in the ritual curing of the poor, classical medicine for the gentry was consistently secular in its therapy. As Joseph Needham put it in 1966, writing about talismans, incantations, and prayers to deities, "they were quite peripheral to the practice of medicine as such, kept far indeed from the centre of the stage, and it can confidently be asserted that, from the beginning, Chinese medicine was rational through and through."[3]

This was not true of the beginning of classical medicine, where religious ritual played an important part. It was not true for the eleventh century; scholar-officials—even those who despised popular curers—believed that the society of gods, ghosts, and ancestors interpenetrated human society. But for classical physicians, both societies were part of a larger order, the cosmic order with which the healthy body maintained harmony.

Those who practiced medicine recognized that success depended on supporting the patient's ability to recover. The physician aimed to reinforce the healing power of nature when he and his patient believed it was inadequate. The early doctor could not determine beyond doubt how far he, and how far nature, succeeded—nor can we. As important as his knowledge of therapy was his mastery of symbols and meanings that could overcome the disorder by guiding and encouraging the patient in habits of thought and of life that furthered recovery.

At the same time, to both physicians and patients, the world of gods and ghosts was real, so religious ritual was one department of therapy. For instance, the handbook of etiology and symptomatology that was authoritative in the eleventh century explained causation of disease by ghosts in three of its chapters.[4] The great materia medica collection of 1108, compiled by officials, includes many examples of religious rites to be used when taking medicines.[5] The *General Record of Sagely Benefaction*, an enormous imperial formulary of 1117,[6] devoted three chapters

---

[3] Needham et al. 1954–, 6, part 6:44.

[4] *Zhu bing yuan hou lun* 諸病源候論 (Origins and symptoms of medical disorders), written 611 but still standard in the N. Song period. On this topic, and especially on changes in medical understanding of exorcism from the sixteenth century on, see Cho 2006.

[5] *Jing shi zheng lei Daguan bencao* 經史正類大觀本草; see, for instance, those for cinnabar in 3: 3a–3b.

[6] *Sheng ji zong lu* 聖濟總錄, j. 195–197.

(195–97) to therapy by "talismans and exorcism." The Imperial Medical Service included Erudites for Exorcism (Shu jin boshi 書禁博士) who trained exorcists for service in the palace. I will return to the role of religious curing in health care in later chapters. In this one I will concentrate on explaining the ideas behind the classical doctrines current in the eleventh century.

What Was Classical Medicine?

The traditional physician's willingness to integrate any kind of remedy that experience taught him was effective is not a sign of primitive mentality or deficient acumen. Chinese doctors, like their Western contemporaries, formed doctrines for their utility in diagnosis and therapy, not for their formal philosophic rigor.[7] Their purpose was to integrate and make coherent a vast body of recorded observation and experience. Authors aimed to provide a guide among possibilities that the physician could master over years of experience.[8] As I argued in the last chapter, physicians were able to draw on several kinds of effectiveness, and to recognize—within limits—when their treatments helped patients to recover.

The documents of Chinese medical therapy before the eleventh century are by far the world's richest. The classical tradition uninterruptedly recorded the medical experience of a large clientele.

In order to understand how classical medicine worked, we will need to reflect on several of its dimensions. First, the eleventh century was a period of transition in medicine. It is essential to understand what those changes were as well as why and how they took place then. Second, we will need to comprehend in what sense the medicine of the time was classical: its assumptions and concepts, the traditions on which it was based, what practitioners disagreed about, and its social milieu. Neither a purely intellectual nor a purely social analysis can make its character clear. Third, we will need to examine its practice of healing, and the relationships of physicians and patients in that practice. Fourth, we will need to look at the persona of the doctor as cosmologist, and how it could evoke the meaning response in patients.

First, let me explain what I mean by "classical medicine." I use that term to make it clear that medicine in the eleventh century was fundamentally different from what English speakers today call "Traditional Chinese Medicine."

The latter is actually a hybrid of modern biomedicine with practices and doctrines that originated in earlier China. The result differs in every physician.[9] Its teachers stress its continuity with earlier medicine, but the impact of modern knowledge has changed it greatly. The Chinese word for it, *Zhongyi* 中医, means simply "Chinese medicine." Nothing in that term implies tradition. Since most people outside of East

---

[7] As a reminder of this difference, in referring to China I usually speak of doctrine underlying practice rather than of theory, which for many historians is distinct from action.

[8] Farquhar 1994 establishes this point by ethnographic and historic study.

[9] Scheid 2002, especially chapter 8, gives examples.

Asia think of today's medicine as exotic, with a savor of ancient wisdom, government spokesmen have added "traditional" to the official English label to make it more consumer-friendly. After all, the use of native herbal drugs (often packaged in new value-added forms) and other medical commodities abroad is a great source of income to the state and to Chinese industry. And the cultural prestige of TCM, as it is called, is considerable.

The medicine practiced by elite physicians *(yi* 醫) before 1911 was classical in that its basic doctrines, like the ideology of the state and the gentry, were based on the conviction that the most ideal state of affairs existed in the archaic past. This implied that among the most fundamental activities were preserving what survived in written form of ancient knowledge, and retrieving, so far as was possible, what had been lost. This ideal had been attenuated for several centuries before the year 1000, because most of the early classics no longer widely circulated. It revived with great impact in 1057 after a new government bureau began recovering, selecting, editing, printing, and distributing what it advertised as the medical canon. We find a wide variety of practices in the Northern Song period, but with increasing emphasis at the top of the social scale on the Yellow Emperor texts, the *Divine Farmer's Materia Medica*, and the newly classic *Treatise on Cold Damage and Miscellaneous Disorders*.[10]

Medicine, like most other aspects of high culture, began changing into new forms during the long eleventh century. The government created a new ideal of medicine. It sought to attract gentlemen educated to fill positions in the imperial civil service but unable to qualify for generalist official careers. I will explain what sort of transition it was, and how medicine came to be an attractive alternative.

Through the eleventh century, the physicians remained too few for the competition to be intense, so there was little visible friction. It was changes at the end of the Northern Song period that sharpened the division between hereditary doctors and literati physicians. Emperor Huizong's efforts to raise the status of the latter, although short-lived, made medicine attractive to more elite men.[11]

From the Song on, the gentry, high and low, played a large part in medicine, and a small but noticeable part in health care as a whole. After the eleventh century, large numbers of elite men entered therapeutic careers, frequently occupying positions of prestige and shaping new doctrines and patterns of practice. As their numbers increased, the rivalry for patients became sharper, and we find more and more diatribes against doctors called inadequate because they lacked a firm foundation in the classics.[12]

That leads naturally to the questions of what classical health care was, and what it meant to elite practitioners and the gentry patients who preferred them. As

---

[10] *Huangdi neijing* 黄帝內經, *Huangdi bashiyi nan jing* 皇帝八十一難經, *Huangdi jiayi jing* 黃帝甲乙經, *Shennong bencao* 神農本草, and two books extracted from *Shanghan za bing lun* 傷寒雜病論, namely *Shanghan lun* and *Jin gui yao lue* 金匱要略 (Essentials in the golden casket).

[11] See Zhang Haipeng 張海鵬 2014 on how praise for hereditary physicians and those trained by apprenticeship shifted to elite physicians.

[12] Leung 2003 has nicely documented this point.

I will show, the long eleventh century was the period in which classical medicine, with its emphasis on man as a microcosm and disease as due to imbalances in bodily function, became the standard for patients who wanted their treatment to be up-to-date and could afford it. It was also the time when its ideas and practices began to exert a large influence on popular curing; earlier the impetus tended strongly the other way.[13]

The Early Norm

If we look at known medical practitioners over the centuries up to the Song period, the pattern is fairly consistent. They are either sage rulers of antiquity credited with medical innovations, legendary figures recalled in anecdotes, or authors. The first group is prominent because literati believed that rulers and those around them discovered or invented every important aspect of culture, the second because everyone knew stories about cures by wise, spiritually advanced figures, and the third because the literature was very large, and the literati were avid readers. The tendency to identify great physicians by their authorship of important books—sometimes (as in the Hippocratic case) their putative authorship—was as habitual in China as in Greece. Of the three groups, over the twelve hundred years of the empire before the eleventh century, the first stopped expanding, the second became smaller except in accounts of religious healing, and the third grew larger. All of the doctors of the seventh through ninth centuries that orthodox historians identified as outstanding were historical figures whose writings were available.

The early classics mention physicians as artisans. For instance, the *Record of Rites (Li ji* 禮記, early second century A.D.) notes that "all those—exorcists, clerks, archers, carriage-drivers, doctors, and diviners—who profess an art in the service of their superiors" are not permitted to abandon their calling, and warns "if he is not the third generation in medicine, don't take his prescriptions." This, like the other ritual classics, asserts what the authors believed ought to be the case in a time when distinctions were breaking down. But that breakdown had not progressed to completion even in the Tang period, when we are assured that "astronomers, diviners, physiognomists, doctors, and ingenious artisans are all craftsmen"—that is, mere craftsmen.[14] But when we look at the individual doctors who were immortalized in the histories, they are clearly gentlemen.

Table 4.1 lists twenty-four of the most prominent physicians between the beginning of the Tang period (627) and that of the Song (960). All except one of the

[13] A number of influential authors drew freely on popular therapy. The best known of these are Ge Hong 葛洪, author of *Zhouhou jiu zu fang* 肘後救卒方(ca. A.D. 340), and Sun Simiao 孫思邈, (also pronounced Simo), whose medical books include *Beiji qianjin yao fang* 備急千金要方 (650/659) and *Qianjin yi fang* 千金翼方 (late seventh century).

[14] *Li ji,* 5/42 and 2/18, contexts in Legge 1885, pt. 3, 235 and 114; *Xin Tang shu* 新唐書, 204: 5797. On historical interpretations of the *Li ji's* second dictum see Chao Yuan-ling 2000.

Table 4.1 Physicians of 620–960

Name	Dates	Home	Position	Involvement	Source
Zhen Quan 甄權	ca. 541-643	Henan	official	acupuncture, pulse, exceptional cures	J305-6
Zhen Liyan 甄立言	545-627/649	Henan	official	formulary, acupuncture; materia medica, brother of Zhen Quan	J306
Yang Shangshan 楊上善	ca. 575-670		medical, general official	classics, acupuncture, pulse, etc.	J306
Su Jing 蘇敬	599-674		palace official	materia medica, monograph	J308
Cui Zhiti 崔知悌	b. ca. 620		high official	formulary, moxibustion, monograph	J308-9
Zhang Wenzhong 張文仲	ca. 620-700	Henan	medical official	monograph, formulary	J309
Meng Shen 孟詵	621-713	Henan	palace official	dietetics, formulary	J309
Wei Xun 韋訊 (Cizang 慈藏)	644-741	Shaanxi	medical, general official	no special field or books	J309
Wang Tao 王燾	ca. 670-755	Shaanxi	palace official	formulary	J310
Jianzhen 鑒真	688-764	Jiangsu	Buddhist teacher	introduced Chinese medicine to Japan	J310
Wang Bing王冰	ca. 710-805		palace official	classics, phase energetics	J312
Sun Simiao (Simo) 孫思邈	fl. 673	Shaanxi	client of emperor	formulary, etc.	J307
Chen Cangqi 陳藏器	ca. 685-757	Zhejiang	local official	materia medica	J310
Zheng Qian 鄭虔	d. 760?		palace official, painter, poet	materia medica of border region	X5766
Jia Dan 賈耽	730-805		palace official, geographer	formulary, veterinary medicine	X5083
Cui Xuanliang 崔玄亮	ca. 761-833		palace official, physician	formulary	X613
Liu Yuxi 劉禹錫	772-842	Jiangsu	palace official, polymath	formulary	J313
Zan Yin 昝殷	ca. 797-859	Sichuan	local medical official	dietetics, obstetrics	J313-14
Gan Bozong 甘伯宗	fl. ca. 700		unknown	medical biography	J314
Yang Sunzhi 楊損之	fl. after 742		medical official	edited materia medica	X3:38
Li Xuan 李暄	fl. before 907		unknown	monographs	X1:317
Li Xun 李珣	fl. 925	Sichuan	poet, foreign descent	foreign drugs	J314

(continued)

Table 4.1 (continued)

Name	Dates	Home	Position	Involvement	Source
Hou Ningji 侯寧極	fl. 925		high examination rank	materia medica	X2:142
Han Baosheng 韓保生	fl. 934/965	Sichuan	official in Shu court	materia medica	J314

Note: Where dates of birth and death are unavailable, I have given a *floruit,* often the date of a book. "Monograph" refers to a book on a single disorder or group of disorders.

Sources: J=*Jiu Tang shu* 舊唐書; X=*Xin Tang shu* 新唐書

group, Wei Xun (better known as Wei Cizang), were authors. Wei's medical ability approached the legendary, like that of the great Sun Simiao; both were among the several physicians later worshipped in popular temples as the divine Medicine King (Yaowang 藥王).[15]

There is no simple pattern. We have no data about the careers of two of those listed. A third was the Buddhist monk who carried religion and medicine to Japan. The last three people on the list lived in the confused but short period of political fragmentation from 907 to 960, when careers tended to be unstable. All the rest were either imperial officials, or supported by the personal patronage of emperors. Only six of those were medical officials. Although generally appointees in the various medical bureaus were hereditary physicians, the sources do not so identify any of the six. In other words, the medical celebrities were socially as well as technically exceptional. As Table 4.2 shows, the social situation in the Northern Song period was not greatly different. But expertise in Cold Damage, and the increased role of material medica, make the importance of the government's involvement in defining and publishing a standard canon clear.

In writing on what physicians ought to be, medicine was never disconnected from values. The emphasis on the doctor as perfected human being rather than mere technical expert was a matter of express intention.

Sun Simiao 孫思邈 remarked that for one of his medicinal wines to be effective the patient "must be honest and straightforward in his dealings, and may be deficient neither in filial devotion nor in his sense of what is right." Sun expected even more of the physician than of the patient:

> In the great physician's therapeutic practice, he must make his spirits serene and his will firm, so that he desires nothing and seeks nothing. First he resolves to attain a compassionate and concerned frame of mind, and vows to relieve the suffering of all sentient beings. If someone endangered by sickness comes and asks him for help, he is not concerned whether the patient is noble or humble, poor or rich, old or young, beautiful or ugly, enemy or intimate, acquaintance or friend, Chinese or foreign, foolish or wise. He treats all equally, and thinks of all as though they were his nearest kin. Looking neither forward nor backward, he

[15] Lee T'ao 1940 discusses Medicine Kings and the state worship of physicians. On Sun Simiao, see Zhang Zuoji & Zhang Ruixian 1995. For antiquity to ca. 550, see the table in Lloyd & Sivin 2002, 24.

Table 4.2 Physicians of 960-1127

Name	Dates	Home	Position	Involvement	Source
Liu Han 劉翰	919-990	Hebei	high medical official	therapy, materia medica	T385
Wang Weiyi 王惟一	ca. 987-1067		medical official	acupuncture	187
Zhang Yuxi 掌禹錫	992-1068	Henan	high official	materia medica	T387
Su Song 蘇頌	1020-1101	Fujian	high official	materia medica	T390
Qian Yi 錢乙	ca. 1032-1113	Shandong	medical official	pediatrics	1426
Pang Anshi 龐按時	ca. 1042-1099	Hubei	physician	broad range	1105
Tang Shenwei 唐慎微	ca. 1056-1093	Sichuan	hereditary physician	materia medica	1464
Xu Shuwei 許叔微	1079-1154	Jiangsu	official	Cold Damage, formulary	T393
Wang Huaiyin 王懷隱	fl. 978-992	Henan	medical official	formulary	185
Sun Yonghe 孫用和	fl. 1020	Henan	high medical official	therapy, formulary	T386
Xu Xi 許希	fl. 1034	Henan	high medical official	acumoxa	T387
Zhu Gong 朱肱	fl. 1088-1118	Zhejiang	official	Cold Damage	619
Chen Cheng 陳承	fl. 1092-1110	Sichuan	official	materia medica , formulary	T388
Dong Ji 董汲	fl. 1093	Shandong	physician	pediatrics, *jiaoqi* 腳氣	1677
Yang Jie 楊介	fl. 1102/1106	Anhui	physician	anatomy	809
Chen Shiwen 陳師文	fl. 1107	Zhejiang	official	formulary	959
Kou Zongshi 寇宗奭	fl. 1116		minor official	critical study of materia medica	1659

does not worry about what is propitious for himself, or begrudge his own life. When he sees the suffering of others, it is as if it were his own. With this concern deep in his heart, he does not avoid personal risk. Night and day, despite heat and cold, hunger, thirst, and fatigue, with concentrated mind he sets out to save them. He does not permit himself a frame of mind that lets him waste time and engage in social niceties. In this way he may be a great doctor to all mankind; otherwise he will be a great thief among sentient beings.[16]

Sun's model for behavior, the best-known of all in China, inspired many who chose careers in medicine. Of course there were other ideals; some saw medicine as

[16] *Qian jin yi fang* 千金翼方, 21: 16b (p. 252); *Bei ji qian jin yao fang* 備急千金要方, 1: 1b (p. 1). The translation of this passage is continued in chapter 6, p. 140.

a kind of warfare against disease.[17] Other doctors at any given time varied as much in their ethical ideals as present-day doctors of medicine do.

The Eleventh-century Mutation

Occasional emperors of earlier dynasties patronized medicine, and rulers of the Tang period, from the eighth century on, paid some attention to public health. A government order of 710 issued materia medica books and a collection of therapeutic formulas, along with other books, to provincial headquarters. But these were still manuscripts, which had to be copied. There is no hint that access by the public was encouraged. One medical Erudite and an assistant were assigned to each province to train physicians, collect drugs, and treat the population, especially in epidemics. But with the populations of provinces in the millions, the effect of such a policy—when it was carried out—was wholly negligible. Edicts of the mid eighth and the early ninth century mandated posting important formulas from government compilations in prefectural and district capitals, and in villages and along important roads. Since these were written on a kind of outdoor blackboard, they would not have remained legible for long. Text engraved on stone tablets was durable but rarer, and still would have been of no use to the vast illiterate majority.[18] These measures showed that high officials considered public health important, but had not begun thinking about what would effectively promote its spread.

Innovations

The rulers of the eleventh century were much more involved, and gradually evolved less quixotic, although not always pragmatic, policies.[19] The Song dynasty's founder (r. 960–976) was a warlord, but among his other interests he avidly collected information about therapy, and practiced it. The three rulers who followed him, altogether reigning for nearly a century (976–1063), were also interested in medicine, thoughtful about the needs of public health, and eager to improve its quality. Their successors continued their diverse initiatives until 1127, the end of the Northern Song period, and beyond. Huizong 徽宗 (r. 1100–1126), that dynasty's last ruler, accomplished the most of all, but most of his innovations ended with his reign. The civil service, as it changed, responded to these new imperial enthusiasms to bring about empire-wide changes. The consistent aims were to make medicine compre-

[17] For the 18th-century physician Xu Dachun 徐大椿's entertaining essay on the topic "Using medicines is like deploying troops," see *Yixue yuanliu lun* 醫學源流論, 1: 185–186, tr. Unschuld 1989, 183–185.

[18] The account of Tang activities in Liu Shufen 2008b, 162–172, notes their limitations.

[19] What follows is partly based on Goldschmidt 2009, especially chapter 1.

hensive, enhance its practice in a way that would meet the needs of public health, and standardize its teaching to reflect state policy.

Recovering and improving on the lost medical doctrines of antiquity were not a simple matter of looking up classics in the palace libraries. Over the three hundred years before the Song period, war and political turbulence had severely depleted the state's holdings of medical books, and the imperial collections would not have been neatly catalogued. For centuries, few physicians had had access to the early classics. Most depended on a few formularies that offered little in the way of doctrinal foundations. Almost all handbooks up to and beyond 1100 depended for etiology and symptomatology on a manual compiled in 610.[20]

To provide an authoritative corpus of classics that would meet the need for textbooks, in 971 and 981 the government not only scoured its own collections but solicited rare manuscripts on a large scale from private owners, offering generous rewards. It also sought them in Korea and Japan. On the basis of these finds, officials assembled and published massive collections of formulas.

Official agencies had begun to print non-medical classics before the Song period. Its government now used woodblock printing—which had matured technically and esthetically—to issue large standard sets of authoritative texts. The earliest was a series of new commentaries on twelve Confucian classics in 988–996. The state also began to publish texts in special fields, not only medicine but mathematics. In 1026–1027, the palace issued three important medical classics out of the many that had not been widely available. In 1057 the emperor Renzong 仁宗 (r. 1023–1063) set up an Office for Revising Medical Texts that gathered other scarce writings, prepared eleven careful new critical editions, and before 1070 printed them for distribution to district offices—not to the public—throughout the realm.[21]

In Renzong's long reign, the emphasis shifted from formularies and their therapy to the early classics and the doctrines they contained. It once again became feasible to study the doctrinal perspectives of the *Inner Canon of the Yellow Emperor (Huangdi neijing* 黃帝內經), of the late first century B.C. or a little later (but considered millennia older). This was originally a compilation of short books that differed in their concepts and their use of terminology, so it was hard to understand, particularly for readers who believed that as a classic it was bound to be an archaic source of infallible—and therefore consistent—wisdom. Eleventh-century readers therefore also studied three books written in the second and third centuries A.D. by authors who had tried to reconstruct what they believed was the inner unity of the *Inner Canon.* The three were, to use the early forms of their names, *Huangdi bashiyi nan jing* 黃帝八十一難經 (Canon of eighty-one Problems in the Inner Canon of the Yellow Emperor, probably second century A.D.), *Huang di jiayi jing* 黃帝甲乙經 (A–B Canon of the Yellow Emperor, 256/282), and *Mai jing* 脈經 (Canon of the

[20] This was *Zhu bing yuan hou lun* 諸病源候論; see the appendix, p. 163.

[21] The products included important materia medica collections, formularies, and early classics. See Meng Yongliang 孟永亮 & Yang Yongxuan 梁永宣 2014 and Goldschmidt 2009, 87–95, for details on the Office and its publication program.

pulse, 280). Mastery of these classics, like those of the Confucians, usually meant memorizing them, preferably under the guidance of a master.

Physicians of the Song period also noted the therapies on which these classics were based, acupuncture and moxibustion rather than drugs. For centuries, many elite physicians preferred moxa to needling, and some shunned the latter. In the hands of poorly-trained practitioners it often caused harm.[22] Furthermore, the written sources had been far from unanimous about where needles should be inserted and moxa burnt. In 1023 (Renzong's inaugural year) an official was assigned to prepare an illustrated textbook of loci[23] to serve as a single standard. Over the next four years he not only produced this manual but manufactured a life-size hollow bronze figure of a human body with circulation tracts and loci inscribed on its surface, and with openings for what he designated as the standard places to insert needles. This figure, when coated with wax and filled with liquid, was used to test students in the palace medical school; a spurt of water indicated immediately and unarguably when they had inserted the needle in the right place.[24]

These changes depended on more than imperial exuberance. High officials were aware that between 1040 and 1057 there had been eight serious epidemics in various parts of the empire, a very high rate. One major classic of antiquity long out of circulation, the *Treatise on Cold Damage and Miscellaneous Disorders (Shanghan zabing lun* 傷寒雜病論), was a drug formulary particularly concerned with epidemic febrile diseases. Works already available mentioned or summarized parts of its contents, but Cold Damage disorders remained marginal, one topic among many. The Office edited and printed the *Treatise* in 1065–1066. That edition was too luxurious to spread far beyond various government headquarters, but after a more affordable small-character text appeared in 1088 it gradually moved to the center of attention. In the interval between the two versions, only scholar-officials discussed the book in their writings. Their response made it clear that medicine was a respectable subject of elite interest.

As physicians gained access to the book (increasingly from copies by commercial printers) they tried to combine its contents with contemporary therapy. They gradually integrated acupuncture, moxibustion, and a wide range of drug therapy, based on such doctrines of the early classics as yin-yang and the five phases *(wuxing* 五行). This process, which reunified doctrine and practice, continued well after the end of the Northern Song period.

The purpose of all this new activity was not simply to disseminate important books, but to provide a basic curriculum for the education of official physicians

[22] These two therapies were largely performed by popular curers, so learned treatises on them often fail to reflect their typical use. See Goldschmidt 2009, 28–37 and, for details, Yu Gengzhe 于賡哲 2011, 154–170. On dangerous acupuncture loci see Grant & Ma 2013.

[23] Therapists and historians often call them acupuncture points, but this word neither translates *xue* 穴 (literally, "pit") nor accurately conveys its meaning. The *xue* are not dimensionless points, but spots of quite perceptible width.

[24] Exact locations actually vary according to the proportions of the patient's body parts, but students learned how to compensate.

analogous to the classical education that had long been normal for generalist civil servants.

The reforms of 1043–1045 established the Imperial Medical Service *(Taiyiju* 太一局) to train doctors for the imperial family and capital functionaries.[25] Because of its small enrollment and policy of open admission, it had little effect in the capital city. There is no reliable evidence that it had any impact beyond it. From then on, incremental steps somewhat raised the prestige of the central school and its graduates. In 1076, the reformer Wang Anshi made it independent.

In 1103, Huizong established a Medical School *(Yixue* 醫學) designed to match the National University *(Taixue* 太學) in status. He aimed to recruit sons of elite families into medicine by creating and publicizing the ideal of what he called the "literatus physician *(ruyi* 儒醫)," a doctor who was also a scholarly gentleman. This innovation succeeded in inspiring sons of the gentry to learn the rudiments of classical medicine, and gradually to enter medical practice. Applying for entrance to the Medical School was not normally a personal decision, since it was usually parents rather than sons who decided what occupations would accrue honor to the ancestral line. The emperor also made the posts in the palace more attractive to graduates. These were the boldest of many gestures to raise the social status of medicine and its practitioners. Despite the vicissitudes of reform in the long eleventh century, highly placed gentry families were beginning—but only beginning—to accept the notion that medicine, as a variety of classical learning, was a fit career for the well-born.[26]

Other forces were coming into play at the same time. The large state-sponsored formularies of the early Song period, like earlier private compilations, extolled the physician's desire to help everyone, not just his family or clan. This ethical principle, combined with the spread of printing, encouraged literati—some of them civil servants—to compile short, simple formularies using widely available simples, for the express purpose of encouraging others to study medicine without a teacher. A typical example is the official Wang Gun 王袞. It was the incompetent medical treatment of his father, and the many illnesses of his mother over a long period, that prompted his studies.

> In the time I could spare from my official duties, I devoted myself to the skills of medicine. Over twenty years I widely collected secret formulas, amassing more then seven thousand formulas and discussions of them. They had been passed down in family records, or I received them from relatives and friends. Those that I had not heard from someone or that were not transmitted to me by word of mouth, I tried out. Thus I chose from among them the most important, those most reliable for therapy, that were certain to prove themselves in

[25] Wang Zhenguo 王振国 2006 studies Song medical education and testing in detail.

[26] Shinno 2007, 93, argues that in the Yuan period medical practice became "a more accessible and attractive option than it had been in the Song." Zhang Haipeng 張海鵬 2014 documents the shift in medical ideals from hereditary physicians or those trained by apprenticeship to those who learned by studying books. After the Mongol invasion (in the 1240s in the north and the 1270s in the south), when the examinations stopped and official posts became rarer, medicine became attractive to men who earlier would have had excellent generalist official careers. Study without a teacher became even more prevalent, as Hymes 1987 and Wu Yiyi 1993–1994 have shown.

> a formulary. The result was five hundred formulas. … This is all in the hope that someone untrained in medicine can, by reading with due care, master it, and that someone practiced in medicine can, with deliberation, use [these formulas] flexibly. …
>
> I have felt that when someone has an illness, it is as if your own parents have it; you urgently want them to get better. Thus I have used all my energy to compile this collection and put it in the hands of the curious. This is one approach to helping everyone …[27]

Books of this kind, reflecting similar sentiments, became a large genre for the first time in the long eleventh century.[28] They attracted printers and booksellers. Their readership was the many young men who had not passed the imperial examinations and were looking for a respectable and remunerative career.

Two other dimensions of medical practice, hospitals and pharmacies, were also important.

Although for a millennium imperial governments had routinely claimed responsibility for popular welfare, attention to it in the palace did not normally go beyond fitful, limited responses to large-scale disasters. The norm was that extended families took care of those for whom nuclear families were unable to care. Those who had no families might or might not receive help from clerics or officials personally devoted to the relief of suffering. The reforms of the 1040's began—on a very small scale—with state institutions for the old, the sick, the abandoned, and the indigent.

At the beginning of the twelfth century, Huizong's government founded a series of charitable institutions, including hospitals. Unlike most innovations, they were initially established in the provinces. This was in part because earlier ones had been local, the charities of Buddhist monasteries or the benefactions of local officials. Like pre-modern European hospitals, they were not primarily medical institutions, but sick-houses for people too poor to recover or die at home. Nevertheless, some drug therapy was available. These hospitals did not long survive the end of the Northern Song period.[29]

The "New Policies *(xin fa* 新法*)*" of the 1070's associated with the activist premier Wang Anshi 王安石 put in place a system of state economic enterprises to end the manipulation of commodity prices by large-scale merchants—and to bring income to the state to pay for the additional responsibilities it was taking on, and for its expanding military ambitions. One of these new initiatives was an Imperial Pharmacy (1076) meant to buy up drugs when costs were low and sell them cheaply when prices went up. It was designed to maintain a higher standard of quality than was the norm in the drug trade. It also was expected to store large supplies of drugs and distribute them free when they were needed to deal with epidemics. Branches were established in many prefectural and some district cities, especially after the end of the Northern Song period. Some even survived into the seventeenth century.[30]

---

[27] Preface to *Boji fang* 博濟方 (1047).

[28] Yan Ruixue 閻瑞雪 2009.

[29] Goldschmidt 2009, 63–65 and 132; Liang Jun 1995, 102–103.

[30] On the Imperial Pharmacy, Goldschmidt 2009, 123–136, and Liang Jun 1995, 78–86. Both take up the later history of the Pharmacy.

These pharmacies initially sold simple drugs so that they could fill doctors' prescriptions. About 1108, they shifted to selling packaged formulations as listed in a manual that the Pharmacy published—another government innovation. This book, the *Formulas of the Imperial Medical Service (Taiyi ju fang* 太醫局方), which originated in the 1080's, was revised up to the mid thirteenth century. In versions from 1108 on its diagnoses were based on lists of symptoms. In principle any literate person, without medical training, could buy and take—or administer—the right formula. This meant doing without an essential step in classical therapy, namely the skilled physician's adjustment of a standard formula *(fang* 方) to the case at hand, producing a prescription *(jiajianfang* 加減方).

The result was, predictably, indignation on the parts of doctors.[31] The eminent blamed the new system for lowering the quality of care. The marginal understood that they would lose patients. Modern historians have speculated that the introduction of the *Formulary* was a government attempt to drive physicians out of business. That conspicuously misses the point.

Given the miniscule number of physicians by comparison with the population, they were never capable of meeting the needs of health care—even that of all gentry families. On the other hand, many scholar-officials were unhappy about abandoning the needs of the poor to herbalists, religious curers and others that the poor might afford. What the *Formulary* accomplished was to provide a cheap and simple form of conventional therapy to large numbers of city-dwellers with cash to spend who otherwise would have had no medical treatment. I doubt that most peasants even heard about it. If the therapy it offered was not up to the standard of the most eminent physicians, its recommendations were cheap, and as good as many rank and file doctors delivered.

Outcomes

What was the net outcome of all these innovations? We do not have a great deal of data, but we can crudely estimate their effectiveness. My opinion is that, although they went far beyond any previous attempt at building a public health system, the benefit was slight in a few cities and negligible everywhere else. This was predictable so long as the government insisted on basing its policies on medical therapy that was not highly available, and a number of officials did everything they could to suppress popular health care (see chapter 5, p. 96).

The only medical school was that for palace functionaries, but the government repeatedly tried to establish similar schools in the provinces. No one says outright that these efforts fizzled, but then the state neither encouraged nor rewarded reports that its initiatives had failed. Be that as it may, the frequency of complaints and the

[31] This was perhaps akin to the complaints from U.S. medical organizations when Medicaid, Medicare, and other government initiatives began, but there were no counterparts to these organizations in China.

repetitiveness of the edicts suggest that provincial medical training and health care had little effect in most places. *Formulas of the Imperial Medical Service* obviously accomplished more than the Medical School did in making conventional therapy available to a somewhat wider public than earlier. As for how much wider, we have yet to find data that can answer that question.

Medical schools and other initiatives that originated in the palace had wider, if less tangible, consequences. They reinforced the idea, long soundly entrenched, that the best training for a medical career (as for other civil-service careers) was the study and memorization of classical texts. This, more than the therapeutic apprenticeship that was the norm among socially inferior doctors, fit the inclinations of students from the gentry.

The government offered an approved canon of medical writings for this purpose. The growth of private printing—which, early on, tended to copy state publications—ensured the eventual centrality of this canon in the educations of physicians everywhere.[32] It encouraged the neglect, and in many cases the loss, of books not included.

This initiative dovetailed with other innovations—particularly during the political reforms of 1043–1045 and the 1070's—that gave medicine unprecedented prestige. Most important was the expansion and enhanced importance of education and examination in recruiting for the medical service.[33] Massive innovation would have been essential for this initiative. The ideal of physicians well-qualified by elite standards treating the whole population could have been met only by enormously increasing the number of qualified practitioners, and by the government paying them to doctor the poor. They eventually would have had to replace the popular curers of all types who actually delivered health care to most of the population. Given the limited effectiveness of the centralized government, and its ignorance about popular health care, all of this was infeasible.

Despite these limitations, as we have seen, the Song ordered medical care extended to localities. This initiative, too, came late and varied in quantity and quality. Assignment of medical officials to prefectures began between 1056 and 1063 (that is, after a century of the Song), closing a great gap after Tang measures had ceased to be effective in the mid eighth century. By 1077, physicians were also to be assigned to districts at a rate of one per ten thousand families, up to a maximum of five. There were so few official doctors, in other words, that they could have accomplished little but treating a number of officials and people of high standing in the district capitals, and—if so inclined—some teaching. Memorials to the court complained that, in the prefectures their authors had visited, there were no medical officials and no teaching facilities.[34] In some, medicine was merely a nominal extra duty of an administrative official. In the districts there was no teaching and, despite

---

[32] Weerdt 2006 gives evidence that private printing grew more quickly in the Song period than most historians have acknowledged.

[33] Wang Zhenguo 2006 documents this process in detail, but does not examine its effectiveness.

[34] Goldschmidt 2009, 49.

the quota, competent classical physicians were rare.[35] In the capital there were hundreds of unassigned medical officials, who did all they could to avoid provincial assignments. It was not until 1122 (five years before the end of the dynasty) that an emperor (Huizong), ordered such officials fired.[36]

The Northern Song government was not only the first but the last seriously to attempt such ambitious programs before the twentieth century. The Medical School, which trained palace physicians, lasted only twenty years. As I have already noted, there is no evidence that several attempts to found provincial schools of the same sort succeeded in any significant way. Nor has anyone shown that a substantial number of graduates practiced outside the palace bureaucracy.

From the mammoth *Divine Physician's Formulary for Universal Relief* (*Shen yi pu jiu fang* 神醫普救方) of 986 on, the government compiled and distributed large formularies. In 992, the merely massive *Imperial Grace Formulary of the Great Peace and Prosperous State Era (Taiping sheng hui fang* 太平聖惠方*)* was sent to prefectures, with a qualified doctor to teach it, and copying authorized.[37] But in practice such imperial compilations were usually locked up, not necessarily accessible even to rank and file officials. Some officials publicized a few of the formulas by posting them in public places or engraving them on steles. In 1088 and 1094, the state had small-character editions of books useful to doctors printed for general sale (see p. 63), but provided only ten copies for each Defense Command (a very large unit) and five for each prefecture.[38] Many such books did not survive, even in the largest collections of rare books. The main utility of these mega-compilations, then, would have been as reference books for palace and prefectural medical officials. The pedagogical usefulness of a collection of more than ten thousand formulas is questionable, all the more so in a society where introductory study depended on memorizing texts. The main utility of the *Imperial Grace Formulary*, not surprisingly, was as a source of abridged collections small enough to learn by heart.

The organization to gather, edit, and print medical books began with a clear view of what was needed for a basic curriculum: early classics that had long been out of circulation, a couple of formularies of manageable size, collections on materia medica, and a few specialized works such as a manual of ophthalmology.[39] In order to bring the materia medica up to date, emperor Renzong in 1058 ordered every district to gather data on local botanicals, as well as on imported drugs (by interviewing passengers on ships, traveling merchants, and others). By that time a succession of empire-wide campaigns to collect medical books had greatly

---

[35] On the frequency of corruption in education see Levine 2009, 577–588 (and in other government initiatives, 598–599).

[36] Liu Shufen 2008a, 177–179.

[37] The number of formulas in the first work, which comprised 1000 chapters, is unknown. The second, in a tenth as many chapters, included 16,000 formulas. The lengths of chapters in Chinese books varied considerably.

[38] Liu, pp. 184–186.

[39] Goldschmidt 2009, 37–39, 53–54.

strengthened the holdings of the imperial library.[40] The government did not plan to distribute its editions beyond local offices, but private commercial publishers, as they began to proliferate, soon reproduced them to meet the demand. That initiative, in the long run, succeeded in making the state's choice of textbooks nearly universal.

How about the other celebrated innovation of the Northern Song period, the Imperial Pharmacy? As with medical schools, the number of drugstores that edicts ordered greatly surpassed how many actually opened and survived. Many of those decreed for prefectural capitals did not appear until after 1127.[41] There were a number of them in the imperial capital and a very few other metropolises, and none in other important cities.

In the beginning, at least, the pharmacies turned out to be very profitable. They became popular because they sold at reasonable prices drugs of higher quality than one could count on from their private competitors. Like other profitable civil service enterprises, they were liable to corruption. Eventually, civil servants and other powerful people went directly to the head of the proverbial line when buying their stock. Officials and medical students got into the habit of stealing the drugstores' high-quality drugs, substituting inferior kinds. Thus in Hangzhou, capital of the Southern Song dynasty, the official names became sources for jokes. People called them not Bureaus for Benefiting the People *(Hui min ju* 惠民局) but Bureaus for Benefiting Officials (*Hui Guan ju* 惠官局), and the factories not Bureaus for Compounding Medicine *(He ji ju* 合劑局) but Bureaus for Harmonizing Bureaucrats (*He li ju* 和吏局).[42]

To sum up, the state, especially during the periods of reform in the eleventh century, tried out many innovative approaches to health care. A second stage of change at the beginning of the twelfth century under Huizong took stock of them, and responded by abandoning some initiatives and rethinking others. This to some extent increased the success of the government's efforts and, perhaps most important, increased the social prestige of medical practice, attracting better-educated and more classically inclined students. Nevertheless, many of the most promising policies lasted less than a quarter-century before the debacle of the Northern Song in 1127.

Liang Jun 梁峻 has pointed out that the greatest flaw in the entire Song dynasty's health care innovations was their fitfulness. The reformers of the Northern Song period began late; the changes were concentrated in short periods, and at other times suffered at the hands of people opposed to direct use of state power. The political battles over fiscal and other reforms that began in the 1040's and became Pyrrhic in the 1070's discouraged long-term planning. As a result, governmental concern and

---

40 Liang Jun 1995, 81–85.

41 Liu Shufen 2008a, 188, gives evidence that they were ordered to be established in prefectures only in 1151.

42 Liu 2008a, 194–195.

responsibility for health care tended to shift abruptly, adding to the instability of new institutions and the repeated failure of new policies.[43]

Despite the government's good intentions, thinking about how to maximize health care for everyone never became realistic. As officials spread central administration to many areas of the south for the first time, some of them, with the approval of the central government, relentlessly persecuted the practitioners of popular religion who provided much of the health care available to ordinary people.[44] In other words, while they were creating a new classical medicine that could treat more patients of the highest social classes, they righteously endeavored to destroy a major component of health care for the majority of the population. I will discuss this situation in chapter 5 (p. 96).

Classical Therapy

The obvious next step is asking what classical physicians did, before we look into the even more interesting question of why they did it. First, they determined what the abnormality was, and whether it was treatable. The canons listed four basic methods of diagnosis: (1) visually examining (the fully clad body, except for external disorders); (2) asking questions to elicit information; (3) listening (in other words, hearing what the patient—or a surrogate—said as well as the sound of the patient's voice, and smelling abnormal aromas),[45] and (4) palpating the pulse and any unusual body forms or textures. Some doctors used all four methods, and some ostentatiously depended on reading the patient's radial pulse (which, they believed, indicated the states of body functions).

Two conventions of diagnosis drew on these findings. The millennium-old Yellow Emperor tradition was in some ways parallel to the Hippocratic approach. Its preferred therapies, as I have mentioned, were acupuncture and moxibustion. But these were not central to the doctor's work. His first resort was discovering what in the patient's style of life was responsible for the dysfunction, and changing it. He focused on supporting the patient's ability to recover.

The Cold Damage tradition, which set the pattern for drug formularies, emphasized organizing symptoms to identify a disease or syndrome—which ancient medicine did not sharply distinguish—and treating it with compounded medicines. The *Treatise on Cold Damage Disorders*, in fact, named its disorders after the chief drugs used to treat them. In it one need not concentrate on a dysfunction of the body as a whole. What mattered was what pathogenic *qi* had invaded the body, and in what circumstances, matters that analyzing the symptoms and other characteristics could determine.

An important accomplishment of the Northern Song period was creating a synthesis of the Yellow Emperor and Cold Damage approaches.[46] The two had

[43] Liang 1995, 105–106.

[44] Hinrichs 2003.

[45] The word *wen* 聞 means either to listen or to smell, depending on the context.

[46] On this synthesis see Goldschmidt 2009, 178–197.

not previously conflicted in the practice of individual physicians, since few had the opportunity to master both types of source. Both were compatible with the fundamental idea that health was a dynamic balance of somatic processes, those of metabolism that produced life-maintaining *qi* 氣, and those that governed its circulation. Disease was an imbalance, and therapy was a matter of restoring the lost equilibrium.

From the eleventh century on, therapists used a varied repertory of tools to overcome dysfunctions in the body's processes. The most familiar are drugs and—only in certain periods and lineages—acupuncture and moxibustion. Many doctors regulated the patient's diet or exercise; some used massage or other physical manipulation, and some used meditation or other spiritual exercises. Medical doctrines, as we will see, represented all of these as ways of regulating the flow of *qi*.[47]

These methods go back to late antiquity or even further. Curers other than physicians used them to varying extents, although—as we will see in later chapters—their understanding of health, illness, and therapy differed considerably.

Little research has been done on changes in therapy among classical physicians.[48] It is clear that there was a gradual increase in the number of drug ingredients recorded in formularies and books on materia medica. By 500, the best-known handbook of pharmacognosy included 730 substances, vegetable, animal, and mineral; the *Tang Materia Medica* of 659 increased that number to 850; by 1116, the number had more than doubled in the officially published *Materia Medica of the Regnant Harmony Era*.[49] The expansion in the cosmopolitan Tang period resulted largely from empire-wide and international trade. The further growth in the Song was due in part to tighter incorporation of southern and western products in commerce, and in part to the proliferation of medical writings, which drew more fully on existing knowledge.

Underlying Assumptions

The classical art was the medicine of the governing elite, defined partly by birth, to some extent by landed property, and above all by education. These three criteria meant that the experts were almost exclusively men. Because upper-class women were occasionally educated, there were a few significant exceptions in medicine, as in other fields.[50] What marked off classical medicine from popular curing was the

---

[47] One can also find therapists, unbeknownst to the patient, inducing emotions to overcome unbalanced emotion of an opposite kind. This method for restoring *qi* balance was rare until the Northern Song period. See below, p. 136.

[48] The outstanding exception is the series of four articles (1976–1980) by, Miyasita, which first revealed changes in the customary use of drugs for a range of ailments in the Northern Song period.

[49] *Zhenghe xin xiu jing shi zheng lei bei yong bencao* 政和新修經史證類備用本草. The compilation of ca. 500 was *Bencao jing ji zhu* 本草經集注.

[50] Furth 1999, 68, 284–298.

ideas and beliefs that shaped the encounter between therapist and patient while they left diagnosis flexible and the choice of therapeutic measures open.

Writing on classical medicine was cumulative. Authors began new writings by critically reflecting on what was already known. They tended to recapitulate earlier knowledge, but they reconciled their own clinical experience with it, frequently producing new understandings. Unlike modern scientists, they did not presume that their own work had made received knowledge obsolete, and mentally toss old books into the discard heap of merely historical sources. In fact, they tended to see the oldest writings—the classics—as most authoritative, and often most pertinent to their therapeutic decision-making.

Medical authors responded to therapeutic success of all kinds. Many of them accepted religious and other ritual therapies, some of which originated among the illiterate majority, reinterpreting and revising them to fit their own cosmology and their own rituals. Some of the innovations of classical physicians came from just such adaptations.

The kernel of classical medicine is the conceptions of diagnosis and therapy worked out in the *Inner Canon* and other writings in which doctors were educated, especially from the eleventh century on. These classics and the commentaries needed to explain them made up only a miniscule part of the medical literature, but they above all others formed the doctor's conception of himself and his work. Doctors near the top of the social scale were deeply versed in the doctrines of these classics, which they regularly memorized. They used them constantly in thinking out diagnoses and therapies—so constantly, in fact, that they did not need to make their assumptions implicit in their accounts of cases. They could be certain that their peers understood them.

Physicians' responses to the popular ideas that found their way into the large therapeutic literature varied greatly with the individual, the lineage of masters in which he was educated, and the circumstances of his career. Knowledge of the classics guided the educated in diagnosis and therapy, gave them prestige, and attracted the gentry patients who could afford their care. Socially marginal practitioners usually knew the classics less deeply. They had less use for the abstract ideas in them, which they sometimes ignored but more often interpreted in the light of their own more concrete universe of meaning.

Basic concepts

Disease was a disorder in the finely balanced, rhythmic inner workings of the body, in its delicate adjustment to its physical environment (especially to the regular variations of the seasons and unpredictable vicissitudes of the weather), or in the relation between the bodily functions and the emotions. People expected the emotions to be appropriate in both quality and intensity not only to the situation but to the character of the moment in its relation to the daily and seasonal cycles of nature. The view of medical disorder as a disturbance of these rhythms was highly dynamic. Disease was a process, not a state. Practitioners of the medical art organized its body of practice and its underlying doctrine in terms of the abstract concepts universal in natural philosophy, above all yin-yang, the five phases, and *qi*.[51]

In the period when classical philosophic, political, and medical thought took shape (roughly the last four centuries B.C.), a considerable range of meanings evolved for these terms. By the time an enduring style had taken shape in medical discourse, and a series of classical syntheses had embodied it (between the 1st century B.C. and the 3rd century A.D.), their thought patterns reflected the conviction that the body, like society, was a microcosm.[52] As was true of Chinese speculative thought as a whole, these concepts were strongly functional, concerned much more with what things do and how things change than with what they inherently are. I will review a few of their main medical senses.[53]

"Qi" in early thought had many meanings—mists, fogs, and cloud forms, life-giving air or anything carried by it (emanations, vapors, aromas, and so on), and the vitality that depends on breathing it. In addition, it is the basic stuff of every material substance, solid, liquid, or gaseous. In sum, the word is untranslatable.[54]

In all thought about nature, it was the vitality of *qi* that made configurations, phenomena, and processes coherent, kept them what they were instead of randomly changing into something else. When the appropriate point in the cycle for metamorphosis arrived, it was *qi* that made the outcome of change orderly and rhythmic. *Qi* was always a qualitative conception, unlike contemporary science's purely quantitative concept of energy. One could have more or less of a given type of *qi* than the norm, but never a measured amount.[55] It was a question of what kind rather than how much, defined by what it did rather than by its composition.

In medical writing, yin-yang and the five phases were normally ways of specifying *qi* function. That is to say, these concepts stand for the sets of two or five phases of *qi*, distinct in quality, into which one may analyze any complete process (in time) or configuration (in space). Just as important, one could use them to understand two or five aspects of any integrated whole. If one thinks of a temporal process as composed of two opposed but complementary phases, for instance, the one character-

[51] The only work of analytical depth on these concepts published in any Western language is Porkert 1974, limited by its narrow range of sources. For an extremely detailed exegetical discussion of them in the *Huangdi neijing su wen* 黃帝內經素問 (hereafter *Su wen)* see Unschuld 2003, 83–124. Sivin 1987, 43–94, explains less technically the relationships and uses of concepts in classical medicine.

[52] Lloyd & Sivin 2002, 214–226, discuss the various correspondences involved.

[53] For a detailed explication of what follows see Sivin 1987, 147–164.

[54] Some Sinologists have made valiant efforts to translate it nonetheless, but their attempts to use a single English equivalent ("pneuma, vapor, influence," etc.) have inevitably led to less clarity rather than more.

[55] There are several passages in *Huangdi neijing* that speak of more or less *qi* or *xue* than normal (not more or less than each other, as *duo qi duo xue* 多氣多血, "more *qi,* more *xue,"* shows), but none specifies a quantity; see *Suwen,* 24.1, *Huangdi neijing ling shu* 黃帝內經靈樞 4.3.1, 12.2, 14.6, 49.6, 59.3 (hereafter *Ling shu),* and *Huangdi neijing taisu,* 10–16.

ized by latency is called the yin, while its active opposite is labeled the yang. Thus the cycle of the day is due to the interaction of yin dark and yang light.

The five phases *(wuxing)*, named Wood, Fire, Earth, Metal, and Water, provide a finer division of characteristic activity. For instance, Wood always denotes the phase of growth, quickening, and increase, and Earth the momentary point of balance between opposed tendencies. This pattern of thought was usual in thought about nature over the past two thousand years. Modern scholars have sometimes misleadingly described yin and yang as forces, and *wuxing* as five elements. These misunderstandings derive from archaic senses that by the eleventh century played no significant part in the language of medicine.[56]

In the course of adapting yin-yang and other universal concepts to medical phenomena, physicians refined and reinterpreted them. They supplemented them with many special notions in order to describe the relations of the body, physical and mental activity as an aspect of it, the body's physical surroundings, and the cosmos. (These developments of specialized doctrine were like those developed in other disciplines such as alchemy and astronomy.) Such entities as the Six Warps *(liujing* 六經)[57] gave clinical experience a sturdier framework of abstract concepts. By "abstract" I do not mean that medical thought cast out subjectivity—that cannot be said of clinical reasoning today—but on the other hand the explanations of elite physicians were not centered on the will of gods or the power of sorcerers. The classical schemata were not self-consciously rigorous, as some of the medical philosophies of Greek antiquity strained with limited success to be.[58]

The classical medicine of China was as adequate as any system before the nineteenth century for thinking about particular instances of physical or mental suffering. The mind-body split is, of course, a Western dichotomy. Chinese doctors could perfectly well talk about physical symptoms that had no significant emotional consequences, or vice versa, but their holism (in the strict sense of the word) prevented their mistakenly assuming, as Europeans often did, that this is the norm.

Chinese doctrine remained intimately tied to concrete symptoms and therapies. This was not the case throughout the history of Western medicine. Galen of Pergamon (129/130 – 199/200) was equally concerned with theory and practice. After the fourth century, in the detritus of the Roman Empire, most classical learning stopped circulating. The handful of Galen's writings that survived in Western Christendom fell mainly into the hands of clergy and a very few secular scholars whose primary concern was to preserve them, not to apply and teach them. Over most of Europe, therapists did not have access to them, or to the education needed to put them into practice. The split continued when most universities from the twelfth to the nineteenth century based their curricula on mastery of

---

[56] For the formation in the Han of syntheses that made yin-yang and the five phases aspects of *qi*, see Lloyd & Sivin 2002, 253–271. On common misunderstandings, see Sivin 1987, 70–80.

[57] Various sixfold schemata that use yin-yang to discuss processes in the circulation tracts. See Sivin 1987, 80–87.

[58] On the Greek failure to establish conceptual rigor in medicine, see Lloyd & Sivin 2002, 168–169.

texts, while the majority of therapists learned their trades by apprenticeship. After a millennium and a half, medical thinkers have not yet overcome this split between theory and practice, nor the one between body and emotions—further complicated by the more recent one between the certainties of physical science and the unruliness of flesh and psyche.

In China there was no significant split between theory and practice. The great majority of medical authors were active as physicians. The classics gave them structures for making sense of and organizing their therapeutic experience. That experience gradually deepened their understanding of the abstract disquisitions they had memorized and the therapeutic techniques they had learned at the outset of their careers. The result, as the countless case records of late imperial times reflect, is an unending cycle of learning.

With this in mind, it is not surprising that even the elite writings most receptive to ritual and magical cures use the basic conceptual language of the classics when they explain health, medical disorder, and therapeutic action. Some doctors saw great conflict between popular beliefs and classical doctrines, and some none, but to the extent that they assimilated symbolic elements into their writings, they tended to interpret them in terms of classical concepts.

New drug remedies, no matter what their origin, had to be integrated into the conceptual structure of medicine if they were to be passed down in the materia medica. Scholars assigned medicinal substances to categories of physiological activity that corresponded to yin-yang and the five phases. The usual ones were "nature *(xing* 性)," expressed as heating or cooling function and allied to yang and yin, and "sapidity *(wei* 味)," functions abstracted from the classic five flavors, and corresponding to the five phases.

A simple notation that the sapidity of a given medicinal plant was Sour, far from being a simple description of its taste (which indeed need not be sour), succinctly indicated its characteristic action. "Sour" meant to the classical practitioner simply that a drug belonged to the phase Wood. Thus its action would directly affect the body's system of hepatic functions, also governed by Wood. Because the language of the five phases pervaded every aspect of Chinese writing, these associations, abstract though they were, spoke clearly to everyone who read a medical book. Of course, to half-educated practitioners, whose understanding lay closer to sensory experience, Sour might mean nothing more than sour. But everyone who ate Chinese food knew, at least, that sour flavors had to be balanced by others. Such abstract considerations frequently accounted for how drugs were combined in prescriptions, their dosage, and when they were administered.

The social milieu of classical medicine

I have noted that the ideas that evolved classical medicine belonged to China's tiny educated elite, distinguished by traditions of orthodox learning, access to official appointment, and landowning. What distinguished it most of all was a monopoly on the very high level of literacy that resulted from a classical education. Medical writing expressed the world views, traditions, convictions, preferences, and biases of that social stratum. What we understand about health care comes almost entirely from critically reading elite writings. Even for religious curing, all we have is documents by learned clerics and those by physicians and literati.

The social origins of physicians, and the standing of various sorts of doctors, changed continually as society transformed. Up to the Song period, as I noted at the beginning of this chapter, physic was a craft, and ideally hereditary, but it was from men of high birth who for one reason or another took up therapy that the medical literature came. The overwhelming majority of practitioners were still hereditary. Their gentry clients considered them a species of retainer (p. 57).

Through the eleventh century, the literati physicians remained too few for the competition to be intense, so there was little visible friction. It was changes at the end of the Northern Song period that sharpened the division between hereditary doctors and literati physicians. Emperor Huizong's efforts to raise the status of the latter, although short-lived, did make medicine attractive to more elite men. As their numbers increased the competition became sharper. We find more and more diatribes against doctors whose lack of foundation in the classics made them inadequate in the eyes of their betters.

In imperial China, there was no medical guild that included everyone, and no government regulation. People at every level of society above the lowest could practice some version or other of medicine, and call themselves doctor—and others could just as easily grumble at their effrontery. Everyone found his own level of income.

In the modern world, physicians are marked by a prescribed formal education and professional status. I understand the words "profession" and "professional" in the sociological sense of a group that can control admission of qualified beginners to its ranks, has the authority to eject the incompetent, and can set its own fees.[59] But that sense of "profession" holds only for a few countries in modern times. It has never been true of much of the world, and is quickly losing its currency. In China, from the earliest time to the present day, there has never been a group with such powers. What we find in the eleventh century is not a profession but an occupation with very loose borders. There was no group of doctors to prosecute malpractice; some dynasties enacted criminal laws against it as a subcategory of wrongful death.

Another source of frequent misunderstanding is the notion of a specialist. For modern readers, this word implies a physician more deeply educated than an ordinary M.D., more skilled, and paid higher fees. For medical sociologists, an equally important difference is that doctors in general practice depend primarily on referrals from patients, and therefore benefit by pleasing them. Specialists, on the other hand, are usually referred by other doctors, and thus are more likely to cater to colleagues rather than to patients. The kinds of ancient doctor that Sinologists often call a specialist—those who treated only external lesions, or diseases of children—ordinarily

---

[59] Sociologists differ. I find most useful the powerful argument of Eliot Freidson 1970; see also Freidson 2001.

did so because they were not broadly enough trained for general practice. Because our distinction between generalist and specialist did not exist, all practitioners depended primarily on referrals from laymen. All succeeded or failed depending on whether they satisfied patients.

The fact that physicians did not have a fixed place in society is reflected in a perennial theme, the lambasting of inferior doctors *(yongyi* 庸醫). *Yongyi,* like the English word "quack," is not the name of a defined social group, but an epithet that authors fire off in the general direction of people they despise but can't be bothered to identify accurately. For instance, in the *Imperial Grace Formulary* of 992, the term occurs three times in discussions of foot *qi* disorder *(jiaoqi* 腳氣). The symptoms of this group of disorders, common in the south, were highly variable. For instance, "In cases of young women, married women, or youthful scholars in the capital who contract these disorders, because they are not in the south, *inferior doctors* unfamiliar with [this group of diseases] diagnose them as other disorders and treat them erroneously; there are deaths [due to such errors]!"[60]

Although the economics of therapy and of competition between elite and rank-and-file physicians is an entirely unexplored topic, we can see it reflected in the frequent complaints of this kind.[61] Hilary Smith has made a case that the group of foot *qi* disorders entered classical nosology late, and was elaborated—related to general medical doctrines—only in the seventh century. To patients and minimally educated physicians, it was a disease of the south that caused swelling in the lower legs. The few medical authors fortunate enough to have read widely and deeply, and who knew other parts of the empire, disagreed. Their appeal to a clientele who insisted on, and could afford, the flower of the art depended on becoming known as superior doctors. In the absence of professional organization, a good way to do that was publicly to draw a sharp line between one's own learning and the inferior expertise of others. Doing so not only affected income, but persuaded balky patients and their relatives that they ought to accept the practitioner's judgment over their own non-technical common sense.[62]

Medicine and the Elite

We have seen (p. 64) that emperor Huizong took several new steps to tempt sons of elite families into medicine. At the same time, the character of medicine as an occupation remained extremely ill-defined, as befits a society in which the composition of the educated classes was changing quickly.[63] Social prestige aside, the civil ser-

---

[60] *Taiping sheng hui fang* 太平聖惠方, 45: 1355. For other examples also said to cause wrongful deaths see pp. 1356–1357. On *jiaoqi,* see chapter 3, p. 44.

[61] Grant 2003 contains some important observations about a later period.

[62] Smith 2008, 68–75.

[63] Goldschmidt 2009, 52–57; Chen Yuanpeng 1997. See, for instance, the sixfold classification of medical authors in Li Chan's 李梴 *Yixue rumen* 醫學入門, *"juanshou* 卷首," pp. 54a–80b.

vice grades (and salaries) of medical civil servants remained low. In other words, medical careers in the imperial palace became a route into the bureaucracy—which was attractive enough—but not a ladder to the top.

Despite the prestige of civil service, literati paid little attention to palace medical officials before, during, and after the Song. This was, I suspect, because of the social isolation of these functionaries. What gave doctors standing in the eyes of the gentry was their non-medical accomplishments, and palace physicians generally had none of note.

Beginning about the seventh century, the celebrities of medicine tended more often than before to be gentlemen of universal culture rather than career therapists or aristocratic enthusiasts. For instance, two of the best-read medical authors of the Song period were Shen Kuo 沈括 (also read Shen Gua, 1031–1095) and Su Shi 蘇軾 (1037–1101), both of them important officials and widely read authors.[64] The majority of physicians were, of course, neither palace officials nor celebrities. Most were still hereditary practitioners. The rest were increasingly people who had studied with an established physician. As printing became more common and books cheaper—roughly, from the mid fourteenth century on, well after the Northern Sung period—those used to learning from texts often did without teachers.[65]

When, from about A.D. 1000 on, the elite expanded greatly in size and the bureaucracy failed to grow proportionately, ambitious individuals' hopes of a high administrative post receded. The idea that medicine is a respectable career for someone of the ruling class began to take hold in the mid eleventh century. Emperor Huizong's initiatives were in part inspired by the reformist statesman Fan Zhongyan's 范仲淹 (989–1052) celebrated saying that "if you can't be a good prime minister, at least you can be a good physician." There were many other reasons for these changes, but Fan's declaration became proverbial. A famous anecdote about him makes his attitude clearer:

> Once, before Fan Zhongyan became prominent, he visited a temple known for the efficacy of its gods and prayed. He asked "Is it possible that at another time I will occupy the post of prime minister?" The answer was no. Praying again, he said "Well, if not, I am willing to be a good physician." Again the answer was no. At this he sighed and said "to be unable to aid the living can hardly fit the life's ambition of a magnanimous man!"
>
> At another time someone asked him "That a magnanimous man's ambition should aim at the post of prime minister makes obvious sense. But why should you be willing to practice the [mere] techniques of a good physician? Certainly that is aiming too low!"
>
> He replied "I'm sorry to say that it is not at all so simple as that. … A magnanimous man's attitude to study is that his heart is set on encountering a sage ruler[, becoming his advisor,] and thus being able to put his Way into practice. When he thinks of all the ordinary men and women whom he cannot benefit, he feels as though he himself has pushed

Although Sun Simiao is known for introducing popular and other ritual remedies into the classical tradition, and his biographies in the official histories appear among those of wonderworkers and recluses, in 1575 Li praised him as an exemplary "literatus physician." See Sivin 1968, 88–89.

[64] Not everyone agreed about Su's medical talent; see the scandalous anecdote by Ye Mengde 葉夢得 in *Bi shu lu hua* 避暑錄話, 1: 239.

[65] Wu Yiyi 1993–1994, a prosopographical study of the lineage of Liu Wansu 劉完素 (1120?–1200), traces what claims of membership over four centuries were based on.

> them into a ditch. Certainly, the ability to give life to [all] the people in a greater or smaller way can belong only to the prime minister. But when one cannot attain that position, the state of mind that makes it possible to save [individual] people and benefit [all living] things (? *li wu* 利物) is unsurpassable in a good physician. One who is able to become a good physician can treat his lord and his relatives above him, can rescue poor people from danger below him, and on his own level can protect and prolong his health. People in lowly positions who can affect both the great and the small, if it were not for good physicians, would never have existed."[66]

Fan, it is true, was not fated to become prime minister or physician, but he did become assistant prime minister. In that capacity he headed a group that began new government initiatives in many new directions, including the institution of the Imperial Medical Service to train doctors. Although his campaign of reforms was short and much of it was abortive (p. 64), it set the pattern for more lasting changes a generation later.

Doctor-Patient Relationships

A more or less representative literatus practitioner of the time was Xu Shuwei 徐叔微 (1079–1154). Xu was a southerner who passed the local civil-service examination but became a Presented Scholar only after the age of fifty. Up to that time, he supported himself as a physician, and wrote a great deal on medicine, becoming a leading authority on the classic *Treatise on Cold Damage Disorders*. He was an estimable member of the new class of literatus doctor who had to earn a living, did not come from a medical family, and could doctor the gentry as a peer rather than a retainer.

Neither the writings of physicians nor those of laymen looked systematically at doctor-patient relationships until a new literature of medical case records evolved long after the Song period. The first monographic collection of this kind was not published until 1531, but occasionally books of other kinds include accounts of medical cases.[67] One of Xu Shuwei's books is the richest source for the Northern Song period. *Ninety Discussions Based on the Treatise on Cold Damage Disorders (Shanghan jiushi lun* 傷寒九十論) brings together his case records involving this group of diseases, each followed by a discussion of the principles it embodies. He identifies more than half of his patients by name, which suggests they had some social standing, but others are "a city-dweller named Zhou," "a married woman of Yizhen," "a man," and "someone." What little we can learn about the relation between a patient and his doctor comes from entries like this one[68]:

---

[66] *Neng gai zhai man lu* 能改齋漫錄, 13: 5b–6a. For a memorial by Fan proposing an Imperial Medical Service for educating physicians see *Fan Wenzheng Gong ji* 范文正公集, *"Zouyi* 奏議," 2: 376–377. Goldschmidt 2009, 44–47, ably discusses the reforms. On Fan's career see Liu 1957.

[67] Cullen 2001.

[68] This and the next example are records nos. 6 and 7, p. 3.

A low-ranking military officer named Li, on garrison duty in Xuanhua 宣化 (modern Hebei province), had had a Cold Damage disorder for five or six days. There was no doctor in the town, so he sent someone to the prefectural capital to summon me. I examined him and said "His pulse is swollen, large, and long, he is constipated, and his body feels hot[69] but without sweating. This is a yang brightness syndrome. Bringing down[70] is essential." A member of the patient's family [who accompanied him] said "The patient is over seventy. I fear that bringing down will be impossible."

I said "When hot pathogens and toxic *qi* are both stored up in the yang brightness sector and, furthermore, in the yang brightness circulation tract there is more *xue* and less *qi* than normal, then no matter whether [the patient] is young or old, one ought to employ bringing down.[71] If you are unwilling, kindly ask some other doctor to treat him." The person in charge of the patient said "Now that I have given it some thought, you may proceed."

As soon as he assented, I gave the patient Greater *Qi*-calming Infusion. For half a day I had no idea what was happening. When I examined him and evaluated his symptoms, it seemed to me that [the disorder] was still present. I asked him "Did you finish the dose?" The patient replied "I was afraid that my *qi* was too weak to rule out [harm], so I only took half of it." I said "Take it again," and personally watched him drink it. In less than an hour, he was looking for a chamberpot. First he expelled between ten and twenty pieces of dried excrement, then he vented semi-liquid stool, so foul-smelling that I could not go near it, and in a short while he finally responded to the sudorific ingredient. The sweat poured out over his whole body. In a short while the perspiration stopped and his body cooled off. All of his suffering was soon gone.

The next day, as I was about to return from the town, the person in charge of the patient (?) asked for a tonic preparation. I replied "Now that he has recovered as a result of taking Greater *Qi*-calming Infusion, it is not a good idea to take any tonic preparation. If he stimulates [his system], the hot sensations will return. From now on all he need do is eat rice gruel for ten days."

During my whole career I have treated this disorder only with a dose of Greater *Qi-calming* Infusion, and [the outcome is always] recovery.[72] No other medication is as rapid.

As this account makes clear, physicians like Xu were not in a position to issue orders to their social peers and count on obedience. The ritual more usually took the form of a negotiation. At a time when members of the scholar-official class were increasingly knowledgeable about medicine, patients and their families were more apt than before to challenge the judgment of their doctor.

The patient in this case is socially near the lower end of officialdom. Still, a representative of the patient's family simply assumes that Xu had not taken the patient's age into account when prescribing, and the patient himself does not hesitate to take only half of Xu's purgative formula. Xu leads patients to recognize that his medical skill—in large part a matter of classical learning—exempts him from servility. In a highly competitive environment, he gets his way, but in the process has to demand that they either accept his judgments or go elsewhere.

Many of Xu's ninety patients belonged to official families, and he often found himself the last in a succession of therapists that they had tried (in fact this became a familiar refrain in later medical case records). The families called him in because

---

[69] I.e., the patient experiences hot sensations.

[70] *Xia* 下, purging with a laxative.

[71] Re the Six Warps sectors, see above, p. 116.

[72] The next excerpt does not fit this generalization.

his predecessors—presumably less expert or cheaper—had failed or had otherwise been unsatisfactory. Here is an example:

> In the second month of spring, 1170, [I saw] Ai Daoxian 艾道先,[73] who had caught a Cold Damage disorder. He had had it for nearly ten days. He felt hot sensations and sweated spontaneously. He could not defecate, but urination was normal. He was confused and slept a good deal. When I palpated his pulse, it was long and large but empty.
>
> I said "This is a yang brightness syndrome." At that point his older brother Jingxian 景先 asked "My brother seems to perfectly conform to the syndrome [diagnosed] by Dr. Li, which was also a form of yang brightness [syndrome]. Does this mean that Qi-calming Infusion can't be used?" I replied "Although this is yang brightness, one cannot use bringing down for this syndrome. In Zhang Ji's yang brightness syndrome with spontaneous sweating and diarrhea,[74] the dispersed body fluids *(jinye* 津液) have dried up inside. Even though they have solidified one cannot use attack therapy on them. One should guide them out with honey and white lead(?)[75] in three suppositories, used one at a time. First we bring down the dried excrement, next vent the semi-liquid stool, and finally [expel the pathogen with] a sudorific."

Here, as in many cases, a relative of the elderly patient is present, and challenges the physician by declaring greater confidence in a previous diagnosis by another doctor. Xu exhibits his fine clinical reasoning to convince those present that his prescription is superior. He implies (without taking the trouble to say so) that his solution worked.

Xu was not eminent in his time. He was a product of the Northern Song's new style of education—not of the imperial medical school, meant to train palace physicians, but of the new access to classics that made it possible for literati anywhere to educate themselves. The high level of competition and the need to exert authority by demonstrating individual learning are equally visible in the case records of later centuries.

Doctrine and Practice

In China, where theory and practice were not a dichotomy, most medical authors treated patients, using the classics they had memorized, along with later formularies, as guides. At the classical end of the spectrum of medicine, it makes sense to speak of doctrines that underlay healing rather than of theories that might or might not be applied. Let me offer a couple of examples, first of basic doctrine and then of approaches to treatment.

The notion that health depended on balanced body functions lay at the basis of all medicine. It depended on the equilibrium of *qi* and its vital processes in harmony

---

[73] Neither Ai Daoxian nor his brother Jingxian is otherwise known.

[74] Zhang was the author of the canonical *Shanghan za bing lun* 傷寒雜病論.

[75] *Dui* 兑 is an esoteric term that may have different denotations in different contexts. I do not know its meaning here.

with the seasons. Disease was an imbalance, to be cured by the correct conduct of life, regimen, or therapy.

We can find restatements of this principle in every formulary that pays attention to principles. An example is the *Compass formulary (Zhinan fang* 指南方, early twelfth century) of Shi Kan 史堪. Shi was a member of a medical family of Sichuan, practiced medicine himself, eventually attained the highest examination degree, and served as a local official. His "General Discussion of Medical Practice" begins with this meditation on cosmogony, which begins from undifferentiated primordial chaos[76]:

> As for the chaotic stage of the Way, no one can tell its origins. Once it had split [into yin and yang phases], change was endless, so that no one knows where [cosmic order] began. We can reason that in the midst of change, when [the basic stuff of the cosmos] congeals in tangible form (? *zhi* 值), the five phases provide it with names; when it metamorphoses into *qi*, the Five Circuit Phases furnish a system for it[77]; when it materializes as a human being (? *zhong er wei ren* 鍾而爲人), the Five Visceral Systems respond to it. From that point, [on the basis of] things that can be named, regularities that can be understood, principles that can be thoroughly explored, it becomes possible to discuss the traces of the Way. Whether [the object of thought is] as large as sky and earth, or as small as one person, the [underlying] principles remain true.

These few sentences link the clinical tasks of the doctor to the formation of an ordered universe from an undifferentiated chaos, and to the cosmology that analyzes patterns in the phenomenal world to find "traces of the Way." They assert that the classical physician's fivefold classification of vital processes comes directly from the inherent categories of cosmic process.

This cosmic view of the scope of medical practice also emerges in the writing of the polymath Shen Kuo,) for whom studying medicine was one aspect of unlimited curiosity about nature as well as a reason for activism in court politics. Here is an excerpt from his famous essay on the difficulties of medicine, which links principles to practice[78]:

> These days therapists, when carrying out an examination, read the [states of the] six circulation vessels in the *qi*-mouth pulse *(qikou* 氣口), and that is that.[79] When the ancients carried out an examination, they insisted on paying attention to every sound that the patient made, his complexion, his movements, the condition of his skin, his temperament, and his preferences. They asked about what he did, and investigated his behavior. That told them most of what they needed to know; but still they thoroughly read the man-welcome and inch-mouth pulses and all twelve pulsating vessels.[80] When disease breaks out in one of the five yin visceral systems, the five colors respond to it; the five sounds change accordingly; the five

[76] This statement begins j. 2, p. 74, of the critical edition I cite.

[77] "Five Circuit Phases" refers to Phase Energetics *(yunqi* 運氣), a system popular from the Song on that related disease to irregularities in climatic cycles. See Porkert 1974 and Despeux 2001.

[78] Shen's preface to his *Good Prescriptions (Liang fang* 良方 is reproduced in *Su Shen liang fang* 蘇沈良方.

[79] The radial pulse.

[80] "Man-welcome *(renying* 人迎)" originally referred to the carotid pulse, but in the system of the *Mai jing* it was the left radial pulse and *qikou* (or *cunkou* 寸口) was that on the right radius. In *Huangdi neijing ling shu* 黃帝內經靈樞 and other Han sources, doctors read the pulse on each of

tastes become correspondingly unbalanced; the twelve pulsating vessels move accordingly.[81] But detailed as the ancients' investigations were, still they feared that they might err. That is the first challenge, that of identifying the disease.

These days doctors when providing therapy select a couple of medicines, write down a regimen for taking them, hand it over, and that is that. Before the ancients treated patients, they became familiar with the cycles of yin and yang and of time, and with the exhalations [of *qi]* from mountain, forest, river and marsh. They discerned the patient's age, body weight, social status, style of life, disposition, likes, feelings, and state of debilitation. In accord with what was appropriate to these characteristics, and avoiding what was not, they chose among drugs, moxa (lit., "fire"), acupuncture, lancing with the stone needle, infusions, and extracts. They straightened out old habits, and manipulated patterns of thought and emotion.[82]

Trying every possibility as they inquired [? *dao er suo zhi* 擣而索之], missing no opportunity and constantly adapting, [they reasoned] without a hairsbreadth's gap. They would go on to regulate the patient's dress, rationalize his diet, change his living habits, and follow the transformation of his emotions [*or* circumstances], sometimes treating him according to heaven and sometimes according to the person [i.e., dealing with environmental vs. individual factors].

Note the unlimited breadth of what passes for therapy in this typically idealized picture of "the ancients."

Now let us look at three brief discussions of disorder and how to go about correcting it, so that we can understand the scope with which doctors applied basic doctrines. All three come from the *General Record of Sagely Benefaction (Sheng ji zong lu* 聖濟總錄, 1117), an enormous formulary compiled by order of the emperor Huizong.

First, consider *huangbing* 黃病, an internal disorder that, unlike many, is more or less identical to a biomedical symptom, namely jaundice (although *huangbing* can also be a syndrome or a disease):

Discussion: According to the *Inner Canon,* "when the eyes are yellow, that is *huangbing*." It also says "if the pulse is at an abnormally high level *(sheng* 盛) when the patient lies at ease, that is called *huangbing*."[83] External symptoms include yellow coloration of the body, face, eyes, fingernails and urine. Internal symptoms include feeling famished immediately

---

the twelve circulation tracts (which they also called the "six vessels," since there are six on each side of the body).

[81] Here Shen concisely outlines correspondence theory along the lines of *Ling shu,* 4.3, to explain why observations of many kinds are pertinent. The doctor cannot see the functional changes in the visceral systems, but they stimulate visible pathological alterations (according to Five-Phases correspondences) in the patient's complexion, voice, breathing and other sounds, and appetite (seen in preferences for foods and flavors associated with one of the phases). These external changes are open to the physician's view, but he can also read disturbed inner states directly through abnormalities in the pulse.

[82] *Ye* 液, which I tentatively translate "extracts," ordinarily occurs in combination with *tang* 湯, and otherwise refers mainly to exudates. I do not find this usage documented elsewhere. As for *baimo* 捭摩, the two characters mean literally "pull open with the hands" and "rub." Since they refer to the patient's mind, and the context is the physician's active stance rather than his cognitive activity, I provisionally take them to mean something like "manipulate." This phrase is thus parallel to the preceding one.

[83] The first quotation is from *Su wen*, 18.3.5, and the second from 18.3.3, but that source actually identifies this symptom as that of yin *qi* prostration (*tuo xue* 脫血), serious debilitation of yin vitality, not *huangbing*. This is thus almost certainly a misquotation from a corrupt passage; see the

> after eating. This disorder is due to overindulgence in alcohol or food, so that there is heat in the spleen and stomach. It may also be due to attack by wind or damp *qi*. When a stasis forms and will not disperse, the hot *qi* may cause stagnant steaming, which [also] gives rise to this disorder.
>
> If the face is faintly yellow, and gray, red, and black discolorations are visible on the body, this is not the same as the syndrome due to pure hot *qi*. One should look for it in a patient with a persistent damp disorder.
>
> If the various types of *huangbing* become manifest in the yin aspect, the patient is certain to vomit; if in the yang aspect, the patient will shiver and feel slight hot sensations at the same time. *Huangbing* without thirst is curable; thirst accompanied by *huangbing* is difficult or impossible to treat.[84]

It is clear that the underlying pathology has to do with a buildup of hot *qi*, particularly in the spleen and stomach systems. The twenty formulas that follow take various approaches to overcoming it. The choice between them is mainly a matter of identifying particular symptoms. The first is for "*huangbing*: eyes yellow, urine the color of blood, worry, agitation, mental upset, and feelings of tension, a bitter taste in the mouth, and headache," the second for "*huangbing*: heat built up in the splenetic and stomach systems, skin and flesh yellow, agitation and mental upset, bitter taste in the mouth, urine red and produced with difficulty,"[85] and so on. In other words, although in this compendium therapeutic strategies are holistic, derived from doctrine, tactics depend on running down lists of symptoms.

For a second example, here is Nasal Obstruction Disorder—not mere stuffiness, but an abnormal reflection of the overall state of the body:

> Discussion: When the nose functions harmoniously, it senses odors, pleasant and unpleasant. The nose is the orifice that corresponds to the pulmonary functions; it is unable to harmonize itself. It is essential that the pulmonary *qi* be flowing freely; only then is the nose usable for detecting pleasant and unpleasant odors. If the cardiac circulation tracts pass hot [pathogens] to the pulmonary tracts, causing the lungs' visceral functions to lose their harmony, their orifice too will be unable to allow free passage [of *qi*], and the result is nasal obstruction. This is what the Inner Canon means by "when there is a disorder of the cardiac and pulmonary functions, the result is that the nose cannot maintain a free flow."[86]

The point of this passage is that merely cleaning out or forcing open clogged nasal passages will not necessarily restore free breathing or the sense of smell. An underlying lung dysfunction, even one involving cardiac functions as well, may need to be treated. As one of the six formulas recommended for this ailment points out, their purpose is "to make the pulmonary *qi* concordant."

This treatment of a nasal disorder through its ties with the pulmonary functions is typical. Analogously, the normal approach to dealing with tooth decay is based on the passage of the large intestine system's circulation tract through the lower

---

discussion in Shandong Zhongyi Xueyuan 山东中医学院 & Hebei Yixueyuan 河北医学院 1982, p. 250, n. 3.

[84] *Sheng ji zong lu*, 60: 1100–1103.

[85] Literally, "rough, harsh *(se* 澀)."

[86] *Su wen*, 11.2. This discussion also draws on *Ling shu*, 17.2. The passage is from *Sheng ji zong lu*, 116: 1981–1982.

teeth, and that of the stomach through the upper teeth. One simply treats the underlying dysfunction in the corresponding visceral system.[87] The most common explanation of caries was that worms of some kind were eating the substance of the teeth. The literatus physician's immediate question was why the normal invulnerability of the teeth failed.

Finally, let us look at injury from falls and other traumata that brings on vomiting with loss of blood *(shang duo zhi sun tutuo chu xue* 傷墮致損吐唾出血)[88]:

> Discussion: Falls and other traumatic injuries produce internal change in the cardiac *qi*, so that the constructive and defensive *qi*, and *qi* and *xue,*[89] do not go [where they are needed], with many undesirable consequences. If there is violent damage to the chest or ribs, the *qi* will remain in the diaphragmatic membranes *(mang mo* 盲膜), and the *xue* damaged [by it] will enter the stomach, where it accumulates and cannot exit. When this situation is serious, there will be coughing, spitting, and vomiting of blood. The method of therapy should be adjusting the constructive and defensive *qi* and moderating the medial aspect[90] to expel the damaged *xue*.

Although there is no doubt that the cause of the disorder is external, reasoning on therapy begins as usual within the skin; that is, with the effects of injury on the body's internal systems, in this instance the inevitable interference with the cardiac functions that direct the *qi* circulation. The choice between the eleven formulas given for this disorder depends, among other things, on symptoms that indicate difficulties in the other internal systems. The first, for example, is for "falls with damage to the pulmonary *qi*, coughing, spitting, and loss of blood," and the second for "all injuries in which there is coughing, spitting, and loss of blood, so that day by day the body becomes weaker and more debilitated."

To sum up, the need for experience is obvious, particularly in recognizing symptoms, choosing the most appropriate formula, and modifying it to generate a prescription for the individual patient. Overarching doctrines tied what the doctor sensed into a coherent understanding of the body, health, illness, and therapy. The early classics crystallized these doctrines, on which elite physicians' educations were based, and later writings elaborated or modified them. But this was not simply a theory of the body, and doctors were experts on more than therapeutic knowledge.

The Physician as Cosmologist

The identification of the body and the state as microcosms made the doctor a cosmologist in the same sense as a statesman was one. Both, by education and activity, could think of themselves as attuned to the rhythms of the universe, able to find and

---

[87] *Ling shu,* 10.2.2–3. The circulation passes through the teeth, not the gums.

[88] *Sheng ji zong lu,* 145: 2386–2388.

[89] See the preface, p. 41.

[90] I.e., the visceral systems of function that control the *qi* and *xue* circulation.

restore equilibrium in disordered health or flawed state policy. Whether or not they had skills and tools equal to the task at hand, that is how they claimed authority. Just as today's M.D. uses the symbology of science and the rituals of his profession to do legally what is forbidden to others—prescribe toxic substances, cut into the living body—the eleventh-century doctor called upon his knowledge of the universe to validate what only he was allowed to do. Today, whether one calls this cosmology or science is a matter of taste.

Let me give a single example of reasoning on cosmic principles to explain an unusual therapeutic decision. It comes from the memorial inscription of the physician Hao Yun 郝允, who was practicing between 1049 and 1053.

> When a prefectural Army Supervisor became ill from grief and worry, Hao told the man's son "According to the correct method, we must greatly alarm him, and then he will recover." The Vice Governor at the time, the Censor Li Songqing李宋卿, was a martinet. The Army Supervisor inwardly feared him. Hao and his son asked Li to visit [the Army Supervisor], inquire into his faults, and castigate him. The Army Supervisor, terror-struck, broke out in sweat. He recovered from his illness.

A twelfth-century collection of jottings records this case. The inscription's author explains the cure: "It would seem that as a result of grief and worry the *qi* congeals, but that as a result of fright or terror the *qi* floats up. When that happens it can no longer congeal. This too is an instance of one emotion overcoming another."[91] No physician would have found this enigmatic; it is a simple deduction from well-known five-phases relationships. Worry and grief are seated in the splenetic functions, which correspond to the phase of Earth. The Wood phase (in the hepatic functions) overcomes Earth, so its corresponding fright or anger overcomes worry or grief.[92] The therapist is simply applying the cosmological principles that Shi Kan summarized in his "General Discussion of Medical Practice." They are the same principles that a philosopher used to explain the alternation of the seasons, or a policy advisor to reason about military strategy.

Thus the classical physician's power to cure, he and his patients agreed, came from the fact that the human body is a microcosm, and that he had mastered cosmology. In the eleventh century his authority was more potent than in earlier or later periods. The rebirth of cosmological medicine gave him new stature. Later, this ebbed as the encounters of most doctors with patients became more overtly commercial, and the seclusion of women barred physicians' physical access to half the population.

There is nothing exotic about classical medicine. It differs fundamentally from biomedicine, but its underlying doctrines are not utterly dissimilar to early elite medicine in Europe and other parts of the world. At the same time, the parallels between the bodily and political microcosms, the understanding of body dynamics in terms of *qi* that was at the same time the material and energetic basis of all

---

[91] *Henan Shao shi wenjian hou lu* 河南邵氏聞見後錄, 29: 226. The inscription on which this anecdote is based gives several other stories that illustrate Hao's skill in avoiding the unnecessary use of drugs. Cf. Lincoln 2001.

[92] For details see Sivin 1995b. Zhang 2007 discusses aspects of interaction between a TCM physician and his patient that may be pertinent to earlier times.

things, formed reasoning about what could go wrong with the body and how to repair it. This made it possible to apply a very large materia medica, as well as a broad array of other therapies, to restore the balance characteristic of a healthy body. The classical basis of its doctrines and the literature it generated limited its practice to an extremely small part of the population. This made its role small in the health care of China's population. But it did enrich popular medicine, and adapted fresh ideas from it.

References

Abbreviations

DZ = Volume number in *Daozang*
ES = *Ersishi shi* 二十四史 of Zhonghua Shuju, 1959–1977.
HY = text in Harvard-Yenching Concordance series
j. = *juan* 卷 (chapter)
RW = published by Renmin Weisheng Chubanshe 人民衛生出版社, Beijing
S = Title number in Schipper 1975
SQ = Siku quanshu 四庫全書
SV = Schipper & Verellen 2004
T = *Taishō shinshū Daizōkyō* 大正新修大藏經
UP = University Press
YZ = Yi tong zheng mai quan shu 醫統正脈全書
ZD = Volume, item, *juan,* and page numbers in *Zhonghua daozang* 中华道藏
ZS = published by Zhonghua shuju 中華書局, Beijing
ZZ = Zhongyi zhenben congshu 中醫珍本叢書 ed.

Classical Chinese Sources

Bei ji qian jin yao fang 備急千金要方 (Revised formulas worth a thousand, for every urgent need). Sun Simiao 孫思邈. 650/659. Taipei: Guoli Zhongyao Yanjiusuo reproduction of Edo Igaku ed. of 1849.

Bi shu lu hua 避暑錄話 (Anecdotes set down while avoiding the summer heat). By Ye Mengde 葉夢得. Completed 1135. In *Quan Song biji* 全宋筆記 (Complete jottings of the Song period; Zhengzhou: Da Xiang Chubanshe), series 2, vol. 10, 1: 239.

Boji fang 博濟方 (Broadly helpful formulas). Wang Gun 王袞. Author's preface 1047. Preface in Yan Shiyun 严世芸 1990–1994, 2180–2181, s.v. *Wang shi boji fang* 王氏博濟方. Lost, quoted in *Yongle da dian* 永樂大典.

Fan Wenzheng Gong ji 范文正公集 (Collected writings of Fan Zhongyan). Fan Zhongyan 范仲淹. Compiled 1053? In Sibu congkan 四部叢刊 (Taibei : Taiwan Shangwu Yinshuguan, 1979).

Henan Shao shi wen jian hou lu 河南邵氏聞見後錄 (Sequel to Things Heard and Seen by Mr. Shao of Honan). Shao Bo 邵博, posthumously compiled 1157. Beijing: Chung Hwa Book Co., 1983. Sequel to Shao's father's *Wen chien lu.*

Huangdi bashiyi nan jing 黄帝八十一難經 (Canon of Eighty-one Problems in the Inner Canon of the Yellow Emperor). Anonymous. Probably 2nd C. A.D. In YZ under title *Nan jing.*

Huangdi jiayi jing 黃帝甲乙經 (A–B Canon of the Yellow Emperor). Huangfu Mi 皇甫謐. Compiled 256/282. In YZ under title *Zhenjiu jiayi jing* 鍼灸甲乙經.

Huangdi neijing. See *Huangdi neijing su wen* and *Huangdi neijing ling shu*.

Huangdi neijing ling shu 黃帝內經靈樞 (Inner canon of the Yellow Emperor: Divine pivot). Anonymous. First century B.C. or first century A.D. In *Ling shu jiao shi* 靈樞校釋 (2 vols.; RW, 1982).

Huangdi neijing su wen 黃帝內經素問 (Inner canon of the Yellow Emperor: Basic questions). Anonymous. First century B.C. or first century A.D. Taipei: Xuanfeng Chubanshe, 1973.

Huangdi neijing tai su 黃帝內徑太素 (Inner canon of the Yellow Emperor: Grand basis). Yang Shangshan 楊上善. 666/683. In *Tōyō igaku zempon sōsho* 東洋醫學善本叢書 (Collected rare books on Oriental medicine). Osaka: Tōyō igaku kenkyūkai.

Hsu, Elisabeth, ed. 2001. *Innovation in Chinese Medicine*. Needham Research Institute Studies, 3. Cambridge UP. Papers, varying in quality, from a memorial conference in honor of Lu Gwei-djen.

Jin gui yao lue 金櫃要略 (Essentials in the Golden Casket). Attributed to Zhang Ji. In present form by 1057. YZ.

Jing shi zheng lei Daguan bencao 經史正類大觀本草 (Materia medica of the Great Prospect era, classified and verified from the classics and histories). Tang Shenwei 唐慎微. 1108. Tokyo: Hirokawa Shoten, 1970.

Li ji 禮記 (Record of rites). Anonymous. Early second century A.D. HY.

Neng gai zhai man lu 能改齋漫錄 (Desultory records from the Studio of Corrigibility). Wu Zeng 吳曾. 1157. SQ.

Qian jin yi fang 千金翼方 (Revised formulas worth a thousand). Sun Simiao. Late 7th century. RW, 1955, reproduction of 1307 ed.

Shanghan lun 傷寒論. See *Shanghan zabing lun*. In YZ.

Shanghan zabing lun 傷寒雜病論 (Treatise on Cold Damage and miscellaneous disorders). Attributed to Zhang Ji 張機. 198–220. Divided into *Shanghan lun* and *Jin gui yao lue* by 1057.

Shen yi pu jiu fang 神醫普救方 (The divine physician's formulary for universal relief). Jia Huangzhong 賈黃中 et al. Compiled and promulgated by imperial order, 986. A mammoth compilation, in 1010 *juan*. Lost.

Sheng ji jing 聖濟經 (*Canon of Sagely Benefaction*). Compiled by order of Emperor Huizong. Promulgated 1118. In Zhenben yishu jicheng 珍本醫書集成, vol. 9.

Sheng ji zong lu 聖濟總錄 *(General Record of Sagely Benefaction)*. Shen Fu 申甫 et al., compiled by order of Emperor Huizong. 1117. RW ed. of 1952, reprint of 1982.

Shennong bencao 神農本草 (The Divine Farmer's materia medica). Anonymous. Late first or second century A.D. Lost; of the many reconstructions, that in Ma Jixing 1995 is superior.

Su Shen liang fang 蘇沈良方 (Superior formulas by Su & Shen). Su Shi 蘇軾 & Shen Kuo 沈括; anonymously compiled, 1141/1151; combines Shen's *Liang fang* with some unpublished medical writings by Su. In *Zhi buzu zhai congshu* 知不足齋叢書.

Sun Zhenren bei ji qianjin fang 孫真人備急千金方 (Formulas worth a thousand for urgent need, by Sun the Realized Immortal). Compiled anonymously. Date unknown. S1162–1163, DZ 799–820. A conflated version of Sun Simiao's *Beiji qianjin yao fang* and *Qianjin yi fang*.

Taiping sheng hui fang 太平聖惠方 (Imperial grace formulary of the Great Peace and Prosperous State era). Compiled by Wang Huaiyin 王懷隱, printed, and promulgated by imperial order. 992. RW, 1958.

Xin Tang shu 新唐書 (New history of the Tang period). Ouyang Xiu 歐陽修 et al. 1060. ES.

Yixue ru men 醫學入門 (Introduction to medical studies). Li Chan 李梴. Preface 1575. Tailian Guofeng Chubanshe reprint of 1973.

Yixue yuanliu lun 醫學源流論 (Topical discussions of the history of medicine). Xu Dachun 徐大椿. 1757. In *Xu Dachun yishu quanji* 徐大椿醫書全集 (Complete collected medical writings of Xu Dachun), RW, 1988).

Zhenghe xin xiu jing shi zheng lei bei yong bencao 政和新修經史證類備用本草 (Revised materia medica of the Regnant Harmony Era, classified and verified from the classics and histories, for every use). Cao Xiaozhong 曹孝忠. 1116. Extant only in the slightly revised *Chong xiu Zhenghe jing shi zheng lei bei yong bencao* 重修政和新修經史證類備用本草 of 1249, Beijing reproduction of 1957. For differences see Unschuld 1986, 77–82.

Zhinan fang 指南方 (Compass formulary). Shi Kan 史堪. Early twelfth century. Also called *Shi Zaizhi fang* 史載之方; under that title in Liang Song ming jia fangshu jing xuan 两宋名家方书精选 collection (2003).

Zhouhou jiu zu fang 肘後救卒方 (Emergency remedies ready to hand). Ge Hong. Ca. A.D. 340. Survives only in form revised by Tao Hongjing 陶弘景 as *Zhouhou beiji fang* 肘後備急方. RW reprint of 1574 ed., 1956.

Zhu bing yuan hou lun 諸病源候論 (Origins and symptoms of medical disorders). Chao Yuanfang 巢元方. Completed 610. RW, 1955.

Other Sources

Chao, Yuan-ling. 2000. The Ideal Physician in Late Imperial China: The Question of *San-shih* 三世. *East Asian Science, Technology, and Medicine* 17: 66–93.

Chen Yuanpeng 陳元朋. 1997. *Liang Sung de "shang yi shi ren" yu "ruyi." Jian lun qi zai Jin Yuan de liubian* 兩宋的「尚醫士人」與「儒醫」. 兼論其在金元的流變 ("Elite enthusiasts of medicine" and "literati physicians" in the Northern and Southern Song, with a discussion of changes in the Jin and Yuan periods). *Guoli Taiwan Daxue wen shi congkan* 國立臺灣大學文史叢刊, 104.

Cho, Philip S. 2006. Ritual and the Occult in Chinese Medicine and Religious Healing: The Development of Zhuyou Exorcism. Ph.D. dissertation, History and Sociology of Science, University of Pennsylvania.

Cullen, Christopher. 2001. From Case Records to Case Histories: The Modernisation of a Chinese Medical Genre, 1912–49. In Hsu 2001: 324–336.

Despeux, Catherine. 2001. The System of the Five Circulatory Phases and the Six Seasonal Influences *(wuyun liuqi)*, a Source of Innovation in Medicine under the Song (960–1279). In Hsu 2001, 121–165.

Farquhar, Judith. 1994. *Knowing Practice. The Clinical Encounter of Chinese Medicine.* Studies in the Ethnographic Imagination, 4. Boulder: Westview Press.

Fang Xiaoyang 方晓阳 & Chen Tianjia 陈天嘉, eds. 2009. *Zhongguo chuantong keji wenhua yanjiu* 中国传统科技文化研究 (Cultural Studies of traditional Chinese science and technology). Beijing: Kexue Chubanshe.

Freidson, Eliot. 1970. *Profession of Medicine. A Study of the Sociology of Applied Knowledge.* New York: Dodd, Mead and Company.

Freidson, Eliot. 2001. *Professionalism: The Third Logic.* University of Chicago Press.

Furth, Charlotte. 1999. *A Flourishing Yin: Gender in China's Medical History, 960–1665.* Berkeley: University of California Press.

Goldschmidt, Asaf. 2009. *The Evolution of Chinese Medicine. Northern Song Dynasty (960–1127).* Needham Research Institute Series, 8. London: Routledge.

Grant, Alicia, & Bo-Ying Ma. 2013. The Safe Use of Difficult and Dangerous Acupuncture Points. *Journal of Chinese Medicine in the UK* 2 (Supplementary issue): 47–51.

Grant, Joanna. 2003. *A Chinese Physician. Wang Ji and the 'Stone Mountain Medical Case Histories.'* Needham Research Institute Series, 2. London: RoutledgeCurzon.

Hinrichs, TJ. 2003. The Medical Transforming of Governance and Southern Customs in Song Dynasty China (960–1279 C.E.). Ph.D. dissertation, East Asian Languages, Harvard University.

Hymes, Robert P. 1987. Not Quite Gentlemen? Doctors in Sung and Yuan. *Chinese Science* 8: 9–76.

Lee T'ao. 1940. Ten Celebrated Physicians and their Temple. *Chinese Medical Journal* 58: 267–274. On state cult and popular cults.
Legge, James. 1885. *The Texts of Confucianism,* parts 3–4. *The Lî Kî.* Sacred Books of the East, 28. 2 vols. Oxford UP. Reprint, Delhi: Motilal Banarsidass, 1968.
Leung, Angela Ki Che. 2003. Medical Learning from the Song to the Ming. In Smith & von Glahn 2003, 374–398, 510–512.
Levine, Ari Daniel. 2009. The Reigns of Hui-tsung (1100–1126) and Ch'in-tsung (1126–1127) and the Fall of the Northern Sung. In *The Cambridge History of China.* Vol. 5, part 1. *The Sung Dynasty and its Precursors,* 556–643. Cambridge UP.
Liang Jun 梁峻. 1995. *Zhongguo gudai yizheng shi lue* 中国古代医政史略 (Outline history of ancient Chinese medical administration). Hohhot: Neimenggu Renmin Chubanshe.
Lincoln, Bruce. 2001. Revisiting 'Magical Fright.' *American Ethnologist* 28. 4: 778–802.
Liu Shufen 刘淑芬. 2008b. *Zhonggu de fojiao yu shehui* 中古的佛教与社会 (Medieval Buddhism and Society). Shehui, jingji, guannian congshu 社会. 经济. 观念丛书. Shanghai Guji Chubanshe.
Liu, James T. C. 1957. An Early Sung Reformer: Fan Chung-yen. In *Chinese Thought and Institutions,* ed. John K. Fairbank, 105–131. Comparative Studies of Cultures and Civilizations, 8. University of Chicago Press.
Lloyd, G. E. R., & Nathan Sivin. 2002. *The Way and the Word. Science and Medicine in Early China and Greece.* New Haven: Yale UP.
Meng Yongliang 孟永亮 & Liang Yongxuan 梁永宣. 2014. Bei Song Jiaozheng Yishuju bian jiao yi ji gai shu 北宋校正医书局编校医籍概述 (An overview of the collation and editing of medical books by the Bureau for Revising Medical Books of the Northern Song dynasty). *Zhonghua yishi zazhi* 中华医史杂志 44. 4: 206–210.
Miyasita [Miyashita] Saburō. 1976. A Historical Study of Chinese Drugs for the Treatment of Jaundice. *American Journal of Chinese Medicine* 4. 3: 239–243.
Miyasita Saburō. 1977. A Historical Analysis of Chinese Formularies and Prescriptions: Three Examples. *Nihon ishigaku zasshi* 23. 2: 283–300.
Miyasita Saburō. 1979. Malaria *(yao)* [i.e. *nue* 瘧] in Chinese Medicine during the Chin and Yuan Periods. *Acta Asiatica* 36: 90–112.
Miyasita Saburō. 1980. An Historical Analysis of Chinese Drugs in the Treatment of Hormonal Diseases, Goitre, and Diabetes Mellitus. *American Journal of Chinese Medicine* 8. 1: 17–25.
Needham, Joseph, et al. 1954– . *Science and Civilisation in China.* 24 vols. to date. Cambridge UP.
Porkert, Manfred. 1974. *The Theoretical Foundations of Chinese Medicine: Systems of Correspondence.* MIT East Asian Science Series, 3. Cambridge: The MIT Press.
Scheid, Volker. 2002. *Chinese Medicine in Contemporary China: Plurality and Synthesis.* Durham: Duke UP.
Shandong Zhongyi Xueyuan 山东中医学院 (Shandong Provincial College of Chinese Medicine) & Hebei Yixueyuan 河北医学院 (Hebei Provincial Hospital). 1982. *Huangdi neijing Su wen jiaoshi* 黄帝内经素问校释 (*Inner Canon of the Yellow Emperor, Basic Questions,* with critical and explanatory notes). RW.
Shinno, Reiko. 2007. Medical Schools and the Temples of the Three Progenitors in Yuan China: A Case of Cross-Cultural Interactions. *Harvard Journal of Asiatic Studies* 67. 1: 89–133.
Sivin, Nathan. 1968. *Chinese Alchemy: Preliminary Studies.* Harvard Monographs in the History of Science, 1. Harvard UP.
Sivin, Nathan. 1987. *Traditional Medicine in Contemporary China.* Science, Medicine, and Technology in East Asia, 2. Ann Arbor: Center for Chinese Studies, University of Michigan.
Sivin, Nathan. 1995a. *Medicine, Philosophy and Religion in Ancient China. Researches and Reflections.* Variorum Collected Studies Series. Aldershot, Hants: Variorum.
Sivin, Nathan. 1995b. Emotional Counter-therapy. In Sivin 1995a, chapter 2.
Smith, Hilary. 2008. Foot Qi: History of a Chinese Medical Disorder. Ph.D. dissertation, History and Sociology of Science, University of Pennsylvania.

Taylor, Kim. 2004. Divergent Interests and Cultivated Misunderstandings: The Influence of the West on Modern Chinese Medicine. *Social History of Medicine* 17. 1: 93–111. On the origin of the term "Traditional Chinese Medicine."

Unschuld, Paul Ulrich. 1986. *Medicine in China. A History of Pharmaceutics.* Comparative Studies of Health Systems an Medical Care, 14. Berkeley: University of California Press.

Unschuld, Paul Ulrich. 1989. *Forgotten Traditions in Ancient Chinese Medicine. The I-hsueh Yüan Liu Lun of 1757 by Hsü Ta-Ch'un.* Brookline, MA: Paradigm Publications.

Unschuld, Paul Ulrich. 2003. *Huang Di nei jing su wen. Nature, Knowledge, Imagery in an Ancient Chinese Medical Text.* Berkeley: University of California Press.

Wang Zhenguo 王振国. 2006. *Zhongguo gudai yixue jiaoyu yu kaoshi zhidu yanjiu* 中国古代医学教育与考试制度研究 (A study of medical education and the examination system in ancient China). Jinan: Qi-Lu Shu She.

Weerdt, Hilde de. 2006. Byways in the Imperial Chinese Information Order: The Dissemination and Commercial Publication of State Documents. *Harvard Journal of Asiatic Studies* 66. 1: 145–188.

Wu Yiyi. 1993. A Medical Line of Many Masters: A Prosopographical Study of Liu Wansu and his Disciples from the Jin to the Early Ming. *Chinese Science* 11: 36–65.

Xue Qinglu 薛清录 et al. 1991. *Quanguo Zhongyi tushu lianhe mulu* 全国中医图书聯合目录 (National union catalogue of primary sources for Chinese medicine). Beijing: Zhongyi Guji Chubanshe.

Yan Ruixue 閻瑞雪. 2009. Songdai yixue zhishi de kuosan 宋代医学知识的扩散 (Spread of Medical Knowledge in the Song Period). In Fang Xiaoyang 方晓阳 & Chen Tianjia 陈天嘉 2009, 63–85.

Yu Gengzhe 于赓哲. 2011. *Tangdai jibing yiliao shi chu tan* 唐代疾病医疗史初探 (Preliminary historical studies of illness and therapy in the Tang period). Beijing: Zhongguo Shehui Kexue Chubanshe.

Zhang Haipeng 張海鵬. 2014. Cong Songren dui yizhe de jishu kan zhishi chuancheng moshi de zhuanbian 从宋人对医者的记述看医学知识传承模式的转变 (On changes in the model of medical knowledge in Song period depictions of physicians). *Zhonghua yishi zazhi* 中华医史杂志, 44. 6: 329–334.

Zhang, Yanhua. 2007. *Transforming Emotions with Chinese Medicine: An Ethnographic Account from Contemporary China.* Albany: State University of New York Press.

Zhang Zuoji 张作记 & Zhang Ruixian 张瑞贤, eds. 1995. *Yaowang quan shu* 药王全书 (Collected books of the King of Medicine). Beijing: Huaxia Chubanshe. Collected works of Sun Simiao.

Chapter 5
Therapy in Popular Religion

Abstract The great majority of the Chinese population depended on religious ritual, which often incorporated materia medica, for its health care. Of the therapeutic rituals available, those of popular religion—popular in the sense of participation by all social strata—were most accessible. Its priests were usually neighbors, farmers or craftsmen who performed their liturgical duties as they were needed, often qualified by their ability to be possessed by spirits. Here too the government shaped popular religion, partly by registering temples whose deities its functionaries judged morally orthodox and effective, and in part by periodically persecuting those it did not register. People at every level of society believed that the gods were a bureaucracy, which supervised the operations of sky and earth. Laymen measured the efficacy of individual deities by their ability to meet people's needs, the curing of ailments prominent among them. The gods enforced conventional morality, rewarding what the community valued and preventing or punishing what it feared. This chapter studies popular ritual therapies, examines their role in curing medical disorders, and explains why and how many medical authors adapted them.

By "popular religion" I mean forms of religious activity in which people of every social stratum took part, distinct in that sense from rites of worship by Buddhist and Daoist clergy, and the state's religious activities. It often took place in local temples—the main public buildings in villages and towns.[1] Its priests or "ritual masters *(fashi* 法師)" conducted some ceremonies in private houses or elsewhere. They were usually farmers or craftsmen, performing their liturgical duties part time, often qualified by their ability to be possessed by spirits.

It would be difficult to find a more confused topic in studies of China than popular religion. What specialists describe as an "enormously heterogeneous jumble of rites, cults, texts, feasts, habits, processions, pilgrimages, economies, organizations, ways of speaking, modes of sociality, and styles of thought" boils down to acts of religious worship as individuals experienced them.[2] Literate practitioners (and scholars) after the eleventh century used the distinction between the

[1] As Susan Naquin points out, temples were the main places where ordinary people could experience the wider culture (2012, 194). Government offices were not open to the public.

[2] Mueggler 2003. Nickerson evidently restricts popular religion to commoners, equating it with folk religion (Pregadio 2008, 146–147).

© Springer International Publishing Switzerland 2015
N. Sivin, *Health Care in Eleventh-Century China*, Archimedes 43,
DOI 10.1007/978-3-319-20427-7_5

Three Religions—Confucianism (a flagrantly vague term), Daoism, and Buddhism—to mark their own learning. That distinction meant nothing to most laymen, for whom the issue was worship, not learning. Mu-chou Poo has posed a question with an obvious answer: "what is more important for a commoner: the distinction between one religious persuasion and another, or the distinction between effective and ineffective ways of warding off evil ghosts?"[3]

Scholars of religious studies have constructed an incomprehensible rat's nest of terminology. They have not even agreed on what to call popular religion. Specialists refer to it, according to individual taste, as folk religion, popular religion, the common religion, local religion, folk Daoism, popular sects, local cults, shamanism, shamanic possession of mediums, and various other equally offhand names. Since such authors do not explain how the term they prefer is related to any that others use, all this leaves curious readers with the impression of roiling, miscellaneous activity that does not add up to anything.[4]

But inquiry by students of religion beginning in the 1960s has gradually begun to cohere. Once we brush aside the irrelevancies, it is adding up to a new perspective on Chinese religion.[5] It looks as though the many varieties of worship were invented, evolved, reinvented, and kept vital by communities of the uneducated, not by imperial officials, erudite monks, or philosophers. Popular religion, whatever we choose to call it, formed the historical backbone of religious life. The Three Religions of the textbooks are elite growths out of it. I will look at elite religious therapy in the next two chapters. In this one I will discuss the symbolic therapy available to the whole population, high and low. By "symbolic therapy" I mean treatments that invoke the meaning response. It is of course possible for a given remedy to be both ritually and pharmacologically effective.

I refer to the therapy of popular religion, because that is an accurate term. Unlike "folk religion," which implies that it had nothing to do with the literate minority who ruled the empire, "popular religion" rightly implies that everyone knew about it, and that all the Han people, high and low, made use of it. Even the officials who denounced it in essays and memorials as "vulgar customs *(su* 俗*)*" learned about it, sometimes from their fathers, and more often from their mothers (who were likely to be illiterate) and the servants who raised them. When in their native place, they supported and worshiped in the local temple. As we will see, in the eleventh century they were required to perform services of worship on behalf of the government in state-registered temples of popular gods. Many of them also carried out rites of exorcism as useful administrative tools.[6]

Rank-and-file ritual masters became possessed to receive revelations from the gods, carried out exorcisms, purified houses to keep out demons, determined propitious locations for tombs, and led community rituals. They were not full-time clerics

---

[3] Poo 2010, 1076.

[4] Sivin 2010 and 1995c, 31. I cite all of these terms from recent reference works on Chinese religion.

[5] Sivin 1979.

[6] Chapter 7, p. 251, below, and Boltz 1993.

or priests. Nor were most of them independent operatives. They generally acted on behalf of a community, whether that of a village, a town, or part of a city. Sinologists often refer to them as shamans, a name in the Tungusic Evenk language for Siberian political leaders who gained their authority by taking spirit journeys to the realms of the gods. Shamans are, in that sense, the opposite of mediums, whose bodies gods took over.[7] Because of this confusion, I prefer to use the term ancient Chinese used, *fashi,* or its literal translation "ritual master." I sometimes refer to part-time clerics who served their own communities as "popular priests."[8] The writings of literati often refer to them as "wizards *(wu* 巫)," a grab-bag epithet for all sorts of religious operatives that many elite authors usually looked down upon.

Transitions

Two important transitions in religion took place in the Northern Song period, one due to state involvement and one due to the growth of commerce. In earlier dynasties, the state had formally recognized only nature deities and ancient heroes and sages. At the whims of rulers, it had occasionally granted patronage to popular temples. This was on a much smaller scale than imperial largesse to Buddhist and Daoist institutions. In the eleventh century official recognition for popular gods and their temples considerably increased, especially in the reigns of Shenzong 神宗 (1067–1085, 152 temples registered) and Huizong 徽宗 (1101–1126, 764 temples), continuing at a high level for another century.[9]

The procedure for registration required an application from a local official. He in turn normally responded to encouragement—or pressure—from gentry or wealthy merchants, who were avid for this imperial recognition of their home place. Claims that the god was efficacious *(ling* 靈) had to be fully documented, and were often double-checked. Efficacy meant a god's proven ability to answer prayers, with those for healing prominent. A great deal of the time, the prayers had come from commoners, and the gods had in life been commoners or civil servants who had served locally. Particularly in the newly settled south, whose ancient heroes and meritorious officials the government did not know about, the only well-documented gods were the recent dead. What mattered was not pedigree but miracles.

---

[7] Heavenly Masters priests, who ritually undertake spirit journeys to the celestial court to present written memorials, are in this crude sense shamanic. For certain rites they used mediums, since they themselves were not allowed to be possessed.

[8] Sometimes *fashi* was also used for Buddhist or Daoist clerics.

I have not taken up the sects to particular gods that began to establish themselves in wide areas about this time or a little later, and became an important component of popular religious life. See, for instance, the discussion of "local cults" by Paul Katz in Pregadio 2008, 152–156. The article on "popular sects" by Philip Clart in the same source, pp. 150–152, deals with the same phenomena in late imperial China.

[9] For incomplete figures given in *Song hui yao ji gao* 宋會要輯稿, tabulated by province, see Sue 1994, 119. See also Hansen 1990, 80–84 and 94, Liao 2007, and Iiyama 2010.

If this application succeeded,[10] officials enrolled the temple as an orthodox shrine *(zhengsi* 正祀) in the Register of Sacrifices *(sidian* 祀典). The government undertook to pay for maintenance and to have officials perform rites there in the spring and fall. It also granted a plaque to be placed over a doorway, and awarded a title to the temple's main god—to whom it often later gave higher titles. In other words, the government claimed the authority to decide what was divine and what was demonic in popular religion, to establish bureaucratic criteria for assigning existing temples to one side or the other, to subordinate widely worshiped gods to the state's authority, and to promote (and occasionally demote) them.[11] What it wanted in return was for divinities "to conform to official norms, serve needs of the state, bring popular welfare, becoming subordinates of the mundane authority."[12] It was also assembling a pantheon that would protect the state from the northern peoples who threatened it, and attract more enthusiastic support from the upper classes.

Government recognition was a matter of considerable local prestige. Inscriptions on large stone monuments, paid for by the gentry, commemorated exceptional feats of the god or receipt of official titles. They not only "conveyed a deity's power and the extent of support for him" to posterity, but informed the god of honors granted in the hope that this would elicit more miracles. Most inscription texts were based on oral accounts of the time.[13]

Persecution of ritual masters and other local religious curers not protected by registration was a natural result of the Northern Song government's religious ambitions.[14] As the government chose which temples it would make officially respectable, those it rejected became "illicit cults *(yinsi* 淫祀)." Pressure from local officials encouraged centrally ordered campaigns to close them or tear them down—which seldom succeeded for long if the local people strongly supported them. Most of these persecutions (but not all) responded to reports about the demonic activities of wizards in the southern coastal provinces and Sichuan in the far southwest.[15]

It turns out that most of the officials who instigated such persecutions on a large scale came from the south themselves. Bureaucrats from old official families of North China often resented southerners as arrivistes. Some of the latter felt the need to demonstrate their rectitude, destroying unregistered temples and smashing their images, issuing medical handbooks to local masters and brutalizing them despite their illiteracy if they did not promptly learn and begin practicing classical medicine.[16]

---

[10] Sue 1994, 103–106, gives examples of the intricate paths taken by applications.

[11] Cai Xianghui 蔡相煇 1994, 437–454, has traced 22 successive titles awarded to one goddess in the Southern Song period.

[12] Liao 2007, 134.

[13] Hansen 1990, 14–16.

[14] Persecution of popular priests was not new. For a prominent instance in the second century A.D., see Lagerwey 2010, 27.

[15] See the detailed compilations of reports and campaigns of suppression based on them in Nakamura 1978 and Han Yi 韓毅 2007.

[16] Hinrichs 2003 is a detailed study of this topic's medical dimension. Among the southerners whose careers benefited by their reports of persecuting ritual masters were Li Weiqing 李惟清 (944–999) and Xia Song 夏竦 (985–1051) of present Jiangxi, Cai Xiang 蔡襄 (1012–1067) of Fujian (p. 80), Zhou Bangshi 周邦式 (Presented Scholar 1079) of Hangzhou, and in the Southern

This does not mean that such persecutions were a simple matter of self-promotion. The south, rising quickly to preeminence in the civil service, was as culturally varied as the rest of China. Officials were usually assigned to a series of local posts outside their own native places. What they had learned about popular religion when growing up often failed to prepare them for the varied kinds of worship they encountered. Zhu Yu 朱彧, himself a native of today's Zhejiang province, made this uncomprehending but not untypical generalization about the whole lower Yangzi region in 1119:

> In Jiangnan, the common people worship the gods. When confronted with illness or official matters they only seek the help of the gods. Their wizards vary. Some, called "incense spirits," worship the heavenly bodies and do not use aromatic vegetables [in their rites]; others, called "ministerial spirits" or "immortal spirits," use animal sacrifices. They all use wine, and go by many names. I have seen in temples to their gods *(shentang* 神堂) the name tablets of "immortal emperor spirits." They have such appellations as Emperor Chai 柴, Emperor Guo 郭, Emperor Shi 石, and Emperor Liu 劉. These, it seems, are [the family names of the emperors of] the [Later] Zhou 周, [Later] Jin 晉, and [Southern and Northern] Han 漢 [periods] of the Five Dynasties era. I have no idea why they are worshiped! The words of their rituals make no sense at all. ...[17]

Ordinary people made up their own minds about the efficacy of their gods. For most worshipers, registration of their temple meant not only local prestige but safety from harassment by the state. They often did not accept rejection passively, for the local temple was the focus of their community. Persecution, and even demolition, seldom meant that the temple disappeared permanently. The regular repetition of large-scale campaigns against wizards indicates that, despite the condemnatory tone of the edicts that ordered them, the outcomes were short-lived. The first was announced three years after the beginning of the dynasty, in 963, and the last of more than a dozen campaigns in 1117, a decade before its end.[18]

The second significant change was due to what Stephen Teiser has called "a new morality, commercial in tone and optimistic in outlook." Donations that earlier had gone to temples were spent instead on token paper money burnt to remit it to the account of the dead in the otherworld. This and other changes lessened the income and the economic power of the temples.[19]

A third change began too late in the Northern Song period to affect this analysis. Up to that time, ordinary people in villages and small towns were used to worshiping the gods of the place they lived. As merchants and others began increasingly to

---

Song, Zhang Guimo 張貴謨 (Presented Scholar 1169) of Zhejiang. On Zhou, see Zhong Jingwen 钟敬文 2008, 254.

[17] *Pingzhou ke tan* 平洲可談 (1119), 3: 161. Avoiding meat, alcohol, and onions, garlic, etc., is a standard part of purification rituals; not using them in offerings also implies purity. This taboo is standard among Buddhist and Daoist clerics, whom some pedants considered wizards. The imperial connection is an uncomprehending guess on Zhu's part. All the surnames he mentions are extremely common. It may be that this southerner's problem is not ignorance but a desire to distance himself from commoners.

[18] Han Yi 2011, 114–117.

[19] Teiser 1993, 132–134.

travel beyond their native places, they took their gods with them. The result was the beginning of regional cults, some of which eventually became empire-wide. From then on, widespread cults competed with those of local gods.[20]

Why was the eleventh century a watershed for popular religion? What facilitated the changes that took place beginning then was, as Terry Kleeman puts it,

> the rapid economic development and societal transformations during the Song. They are also the product of a rising concern with moral conduct, an expanding program of government ennoblements that encouraged redefinition of local cults in moralistic terms, the profusion of new sacred technologies such as spirit writing [by mediums] that expanded communication between commoners and the gods, the rise of the examination culture and its focus on supernatural aid as key to success, and the religious reforms of Emperor Huizong, which had a lasting effect on the Chinese religious world.[21]

How We Know about Popular Religious Curing

The vitality of popular religion came from the illiterate majority, who left no written records. Nevertheless, there is ample written evidence from which we can learn about the therapy of local ritual masters. In the Song everyone knew about their curative skills. With the exception of a few elite skeptics, and officials who favored persecuting the unregistered as "wizards," everyone acknowledged their power.[22]

Three kinds of sources describe in detail popular religious methods of curing: Daoist scriptures, medical manuals, and informal writings by gentlemen. The first adapted and transmogrified popular practices. Daoist clerics often claimed that their own rites were superior to everyone else's, which, for the sake of such comparisons, they duly described in their scriptures. The third reflected the manifold interests of their authors, who often described remarkable religious phenomena. The collection most used in recent research is *Records of the Listener,* whose author compiled hundreds of anecdotes about exceptions to the conventional separation between the spiritual and human worlds. Informal collections of jottings rich in information about religious health care multiplied quickly in the Song period.[23]

The presence of popular symbolic therapies in handbooks of classical medicine calls for a little more explanation.

Despite the abstraction and rationalism of traditional medical doctrine, we find in the clinical literature a remarkably rich variety of therapies. We can learn a great deal about popular medicine from classical formularies *(fangshu* 方書) and

---

[20] A number of Japanese scholars have documented this change; their work is summed up in Matsumoto 2006, chapter 1. The topic has been studied in English in Hansen 1990, chapter 6. On the situation in the Jin, Yuan, and southern Song, see Iiyama 2010.

[21] Kleeman 2005, 108.

[22] Liao 2007 has documented the ubiquity of "ghosts and demonic forces in the lives of the Song elite."

[23] *Yijian zhi* 夷堅志; Inglis 2007. Tao Yufeng et al. 1988 compiles medical jottings.

writings on materia medica *(bencao* 本草) if we pay as much attention to the apparently superstitious parts as to the parts that seem naturalistic. Both genres accommodated popular therapy because their authors were convinced it had value in curing disease.

A number of formulas include some information about the rites with which they were used. A good example is Vermilion and Honey Pellets, which the government's drug handbook of 1108 recommended for preventing Warm Factor Epidemic disorders[24]:

> Take 13 gm of first-quality vermilion, grind finely, and mix with white honey to form pellets the size of sesame seeds. At dawn of every day that corresponds to Great Year,[25] the whole family, large and small, without having had anything to eat, is to face east. Each swallows 21 pellets. None will ever catch an epidemic disease.

This tells us nothing about who the ritualist was, or what rites he performed, but it indicates that the remedy originated in popular or Daoist therapy. (I will discuss an analogous procedure, with fuller details, below, p. 121.) Despite the ritual content of this formula, the functional classification of vermilion[26] fits such therapy seamlessly into the materia medica: vermilion's sapidity is sweet (although mercuric sulfide is tasteless), it is slightly chilling, and it contains no toxicity.

Ritual therapies and what a modern doctor would consider empirical remedies were both easily adapted to the abstract formal categories of classical medicine. For example, cow bezoar *(niuhuang* 牛黃, bovine calculi) is solid secretions, often biliary, which come from animals but resemble minerals. They are prominent among the Chinese materia magica that I discuss below (p. 115). The government-sponsored drug handbooks of the Song period follow earlier sources in recommending cow bezoar for, among other things, driving ghosts out of the body. They add that "if taken for a long time, it lightens the body, adds to the lifespan, and keeps people from being forgetful." The handbooks say nothing about its preparation or the ritual circumstances in which practitioners used it for these purposes. Classical pharmacognosy recognizes the activity of drugs by three abstract variables: sapidity[27] (bitter), which aligns them with the five phases; nature, or heating or cooling virtue (neutral), related to yin-yang activity; and toxicity (slightly toxic), which indicates that they were potent when used against invasive pathogens.[28]

There is reason to believe, in view of its usefulness for expelling ghosts, that the use of cow bezoar also began in popular therapy, where it would naturally be accompanied by rites that revealed its symbolic meaning. When a physician appropriated it, he would use his own therapeutic rituals, which might or might not treat it like

[24] *Daguan bencao,* 3: 3b and *Zhenghe bencao,* 3: 4b, paraphrasing with credit *Waitai mi yao* 外臺秘要, 4: 130b–131a.

[25] An astrological determination, based on the computed motion of *tai sui* 太歲, the invisible counter-rotating correlate of Jupiter (Ho 2003, 32–33).

[26] The term that I translate "vermilion *(zhusha* 朱砂)" is often used for man-made mercuric sulfide, and *dansha* 丹砂 (cinnabar) for the natural substance, but this is far from universal.

[27] See chapter 3, p. 118.

[28] *Daguan bencao,* 16a.

any other drug. That would doubtless affect its efficacy, in ways that only detailed knowledge of the circumstances could reveal.

The efficacy of symbolic therapies, I will argue below, depends on specific social circumstances and beliefs. But in the absence of critical experimental tests—of which there were none anywhere in the eleventh century—symbolic therapies would appear to function in much the same way as herbal remedies. The distinction was even less clear when some doctors used elements of popular rites when administering drugs, as we have seen in the case of Vermilion and Honey Pellets. Sometimes, from the biomedical point of view, this would be validated by the success of the drug. In other cases a pharmacologically useless herb gained credence from the healing virtue of the ritual—or, of course, from the body's own curative power, which even today is responsible for the prosperity of companies that manufacture remedies for the common cold.

Gods, Ghosts, and Ancestors

What were the gods to the people who experienced them?

In the eleventh century, humans and spirits lived side by side. China was governed not only by an imperial administration but by the cosmic divinities and officers who ruled the otherworld. The gods, from the viewpoint of the government and that of clerics, were a bureaucracy.[29] The Jade Emperor governed the cosmic civil service. Its personnel were commissioned to superintend the operations of earth and sky, to staff the supernal palaces, and to judge, reward, and punish the living and the dead. This celestial government was organized with a symmetry and efficiency that terrestrial administrations could never attain. It appointed, banished, promoted, and reassigned spirits as the needs of the service demanded and the quality of their performance—their efficacy—merited. The terrestrial government attempted to take over this authority, but in the long run was overruled by folklore.

The gods worshipped in a given temple were not the state's choice, nor even that of the local gentry. It was a matter of whom ordinary people prayed to. Although they did not change their minds lightly, from time to time new gods joined the old ones in the temple, often as the result of changes in the human population. We have already seen that, when outsiders brought regional cults with them, the result could be new temples spreading a network. In some localities their gods found a place in an established temple.

It casts no doubt on the spiritual character of the gods to think of them collectively as an ideal model of human relations, a great symbolic creation. They were

[29] There is no comprehensive source on the divine hierarchy in any Western language. See Zong Li & Liu Qun 1987 for data from primary sources on a couple of hundred popular gods. For a comparative study of early accounts of a pantheon's organization see Ishii 1968, 135–182. The most pertinent of recent Western accounts are Hansen 1990 and the essays by Katz and Nickerson in Pregadio 2008, 145–150, 152–159.

not simple, objective, or mechanical symbols, but rather an articulated and abstracted vital embodiment of experience and aspiration, rich enough to respond to every predicament and need brought to it. The Divine Order gave meaning to anything that people did together, to how they perceived not only their community but themselves.

The gods were, like officials, enforcers of conventional morality, offended by infringement, and tireless—more tireless than most government officials—in rewarding what the community valued and punishing what it feared.[30] In the popular imagination, the gods could be mischievous and evasive, even drunken and lascivious, just as imperial officials sometimes were.[31] Life was like that. That the gods were multi-dimensional increased their power to heal and grant blessings.

Why did Chinese gods take this form? That question is best asked in another way: Why do some humans become gods?

Everyone is born with a certain endowment of vital energy *(qi*氣, or, in more technical contexts, *yuanqi* 元氣), some with more than others. The wear and tear of life gradually uses it up. Profligate living wastes it; self-control preserves it; and personal cultivation adds to it. When one's spiritual vitality is gone, one dies a natural death.

By the eleventh century, most new gods were people who died before their time. What was left of their vitality, after death, caused manifestations among the living. The most prominent of these was cures resulting from prayer. If they happened often outside the dead person's family, they could lead to worship by what became a cult. Sustained demonstrations of charisma (or, looked at on another plane, growth of the cult until it could sustain itself economically) led to recognizing the shade as a god, and incorporating it in the local hierarchy. A few new gods, as their worship and patronage spread, joined the orthodox pantheon.[32] The latter was much larger than the list of gods the government recognized and registered.

Not many who died became a god, only those who found a stable cult of worshippers beyond the individual family that sustained its own ancestors. A niche in the celestial table of organization required exceptional virtue, and often exceptional attainment through a variety of arcane means (alchemy was one). Did medium cults

[30] One need not assume that every individual believed in all of the collective representations of his culture. Robin Horton (1973, 272) suggested the crux is not whether people believe in the same symbolic structures—their accounts of them are never identical—but whether they are convinced that their community does. "One may further define 'traditional' societies as those whose members believe that they are living in the light of such representations, and 'modern' societies as those whose members no longer have any such illusion." Of course it is rejection that makes it an illusion.

[31] Shahar & Weller 1996 documents the unruliness of gods in popular lore (particularly noticeable from the fifteenth century on); Bokenkamp 2010, 1169–1174, explains it.

[32] I use "shade" to denote spiritual presences that may manifest themselves as either gods or ghosts.

Elliott's classic field study of 1955 documented the establishment and expansion of organizations around a possessed Chinese curer in Singapore. Schipper 1985 has explored the incorporation of individual cults into the village hierarchy, and of local gods into pan-Chinese hierarchies organized by Daoists. On the multiplicity and diversity of pantheons, see Bokenkamp 2010.

form only around figures so qualified, or did the qualifications appear as the cult established its claims to legitimacy? That is the sort of crude either/or question that makes it impossible to understand how complex traditional mores were.

The lingering presence that became a god could as well become a ghost. The difference, like so many differences in Chinese thought, was a matter of function. Those dead who were not laid to rest—because they had no survivors, or because their survivors did not provide ritually for their sustenance in the spirit realm—became free-floating malignancy *(xie* 邪 or *xieqi* 邪氣, literally "deviant *qi").* This malignancy became a ghost or demon when it made itself felt among the living, when it insinuated itself among them as a source of ill will or disharmony. It could also become a pathogen, possessing people and causing sickness.

One might put it a little too simply that the memory of a dead person can unite a family as an ancestor, serve a community as a god, or cause disharmony and distress as a ghost. Rites for the dead integrate and provide continuity between generations in the consciousness of the living, and teach them to live with their own inevitable deaths. A proper funeral is indeed a harbinger of social concord, for it demonstrates publicly that a family is willing and able to play a part that its neighbors expect of it, and that it expects of its neighbors.

It is impossible for an individual to be sure exactly what his recently deceased relations have become. If one can afford the elaborate funerary rites, if they are performed punctiliously, if there is no defect in the sincerity of mourning, if the shade is reasonable and does not expect more than the family can give, one can at least do one's best and cope with the consequences. But one can have no confidence at all about what demons *other families* may be generating by their carelessness, lack of discipline, defective filial piety, or poverty. One man's deified ancestors may well be another man's hobgoblins. As Stephan Harrell puts it, "the fact that efficacy means more to most people than logical consistency means . . . there is nothing wrong with treating a spirit who was originally or properly [a ghost] as if he were [a god]; if he acts like a god and people fare best by treating him as they would a god, then he must be a god."[33]

What defines "ghost" is troublesome manifestations among the living, not a distinct order of being. As anthropologists have found in one culture after another, shades are potentially both benevolent and dangerous. Gods and ghosts, like people and everything else in the Chinese world, were kinds of *qi* function rather than separate species of being. Ghosts could become gods. A group of worshipers builds a shrine or otherwise affirms that it has experienced, and expects to experience, only good. The state formally registers an existing temple, based on documented efficacy. The issue is whether people encounter shades as representatives of the Divine Order acting in their proper capacities and thus benign, or as malevolent forces of disorder. What matters to the living is not what category of being shades belong to, but how they behave toward humans.

Ursula-Angelika Cedzich has studied an ancient cult of mountain demons *(shanxiao* 山魈) widely worshiped in south central China. These goblins originally

[33] Harrell 1974, 204. Cf. the arguments in Wolf 1974b.

inspired dread; people worshiped them to placate them. But as monks and priests carried Buddhism into the areas where this cult was prominent, the clergy domesticated the demons. People came to think of them as docile and benevolent supporters of the Buddhist faith. Buddhists named them "Spirits of the Five Penetrations (*wutong* 五通)" after the remarkable powers of the Buddha and certain other spirits. Beginning perhaps in the tenth century and definitely by 1035, we find the Five Penetrations cult attached to popular as well as Buddhist temples.[34]

Government acceptance came in 1109, as the registration of popular gods was greatly accelerating. The spirits of the Five Penetrations of a temple in Wuyuan 婺源, in one of China's richest prefectures (in present-day Jiangxi), were officially recognized as the Five Manifestations *(wuxian* 五顯) . Merchants worshiped them in the first temple networks to spread widely along China's waterways.[35] Cults of the *wutong* not directly connected with that of Wuyuan, and thus not registered, became "illicit cults," occasionally persecuted, or their temples torn down, by zealous officials. Many of the cults that the government rejected remained strong, not only in the countryside but in the capital, other cities, and towns. Popular religion, after all, has never followed the fault lines of legislation.

Daoists, on the whole, disapproved of the whole complex—mountain demons, spirits of the Five Penetrations, and the Five Manifestations—but could not turn a blind eye to the state's recognition. After all, they considered themselves, and wanted others to recognize them as, organizers and custodians of the divine hierarchy. Long after the eleventh century, they incorporated the various forms of the Five Penetrations spirits into their own pantheon as the Five Manifestations. These—like many other reformed demons—became Heavenly Marshals, military enforcers of divinely decreed order.

For commoners, the bureaucracy of the gods was more familiar than that of the political order. Contact with the representatives of either order was rare and expensive for the ordinary family. Someone of low station and little property seldom saw even the underlings of the imperial government's local office, and then only when they showed up in connection with demands concerning taxes, contracts, labor service, or judicial matters. Chances are that he never saw any centrally appointed official, unless—as he could anticipate only with dread—he was brought before the bench for judicial interrogation.

The world of spirits did not extract military or labor service regularly, as the government did. People merely had to support the shared religious activity of the community. The impost usually depended on wealth and standing but, for people who rarely had money to spend, a very small contribution usually satisfied the expectations of their neighbors.

People saw the local gods every time they went to the temple. They often installed images of gods above the spirit tablets of their ancestors in the main room of their

---

[34] Cedzich 1995, especially pp. 152–182; Szonyi 1997; von Glahn 2004. For another example, see Kleeman 1994.

[35] Hansen 1990, 140. Ter Haar 2007, 256–257, has argued that the relationship between Wuyuan and Wuxian was more complicated than this.

house. Every important family occasion took place in the presence of those deities. Other gods, for instance the Stove God, lived in every house; the Earth God governed the locality; even in cities the City Wall God *(Chenghuang* 城隍) was the divine counterpart of the local magistrate, keeping order among the denizens of the spirit world. People heard the voices of certain gods speaking through mediums, and saw their handwriting traced out by the planchette *(fuji* 扶乩 or *fuluan* 扶鸞).[36]

The gods gave as good as they took, which was not always the case with the yamen. Supernal bureaucrats responded to gifts as readily as local functionaries, but after the gods had imbibed the subtle essence of the food offerings, the worshipers could take the material residue home and feast on it. That was memorable in a peasant society where people rarely had meat to eat. For the poor and unconnected, consulting a ritual master—a local part-time priest—who knew his way about in the Divine Order and could intercede on one's behalf was easier than finding someone who could put in a good word with the magistrate's clerk in the nearby city.

Health Care in Popular Religion

The prevention and cure of illness played a central role in people's relations with the spiritual world. I will describe this role in a very general way.

Medical and religious sources reveal essentially the same notions of illness, although their orientations toward therapy differ. Authors and readers considered it appropriate for religious and medical therapies to sit within the covers of the same book. Many liturgical and historical documents in the Daoist scriptures cited below have, for instance, been quoted in medical books. A number of important medical books were included in the Daoist Canon.[37]

We have seen that marginal figures of the Divine Order could invade the human body and feed upon its sources of vitality, causing illness. Even classical physicians recognized the sort of possession disorder in which shades took over the body under such titles as "infusion *(zhu* 注, 疰)," "attack by noxious agents *(zhonge* 中惡)," "assault by demons *(guiji* 鬼擊)," "occupation by a perverse agency *(kewu* 客忤 or *ganwu* 感忤,)," and "Cadaver Vector Disorder *(chuanshi* 傳尸)."[38] In a second type of illness the soul *qi (hun* 魂, *hunpo* 魂魄) of the individual left his body.[39] The sick person lost his vitality and intelligence, entering a state that a modern doctor might

[36] On the planchette, known in the West in conjunction with the oujia board, see Chao 1942.

[37] From the late fourteenth century on, the skepticism that state-sponsored neo-Confucianism encouraged (re non-political matters) lessened this tolerance. That often led to doctors' reliance on drugs useless by themselves, where their use in ritual might have been able to provoke the meaning response. On medical books in the Daoist Canon, see Kohn 2000, 89–94.

[38] These terms all occur in *Zhu bing yuan hou lun* 諸病源候論, 610. "Infusion" is a literal translation, but the word denotes spirit possession.

[39] *Hun* or *hunpo* was not conceptually close to the European theological term "soul," although Sinologists often translate it that way. I translate it "soul *qi*" as a reminder of the difference. For a penetrating discussion of the conception see Baldrian-Hussein 2008.

describe as withdrawn or call chronically depressed. This condition might easily be mortal, especially in children, who were most susceptible to it. In classical medicine, loss of the soul *qi* is known by the technical term "fright" (*jing* 驚 or *jingji* 驚悸).

Psychiatrists who work with Chinese patients recognize certain forms of this disorder, which does not occur among other peoples. They have coined the English term "Fright Syndrome" for it.[40] In many cases this type of disease may have been the result of possession, the invading spirit driving out the soul *qi*.

There was also a third version, in which a shade, because of some animus against a living person, harasses him until disease results. This often happened in cases treated by thunder rites, in which the priest, after identifying the shade that was oppressing the patient, often forced it to enter *the patient's* body so that he could interrogate it and drive it away. If the patient was too weak to cope with possession, the priest might use a surrogate. In other words, possession in this instance was not the cause of the illness but a stage in the cure.[41]

In classical medicine, possession disorders were only a small part of the spectrum of disease (what part I will discuss anon). Information about them generally shows clear traces of popular origin. But the impression conveyed by the sources that tell us most about popular curing—liturgical texts, classical therapeutic manuals that preserved ritual cures, scholars' reports of "vulgar customs," later repertories of curers who did not fit the usual elite pattern—is that on the whole sickness is spirit possession or harassment by spirits. This notion of spiritual causation shaped popular convictions about how people fall ill and how they recover.[42]

What made people in eleventh-century China ill? There are two problems to consider, what brings the disease about and what makes the patient susceptible to it. The popular conception of pathological agents is far from simple. It will be best to begin by studying the ambiguities.

When someone fell seriously ill, the first assumption was usually that a resentful ghost or demon had invaded his body. The immediate question was what shade in his family or a related or nearby family had felt offended, and for what reason.[43] Some popular priests, especially mediums, made it their business to help the patient identify the resentful shade. As we know from many accounts, this investigation often brought to light disturbed relations between the patient and living relatives

---

[40] P. M. Yap 1960, 1969. See also the important anthropological study in Topley 1970. For a detailed ethnographic record of a ceremony used by a popular sect in modern Taiwan to cure Fright Syndrome, see Liu Zhiwan 劉枝萬 1974b.

[41] Davis 2001, 196–201.

[42] There were other conceptions of etiology; the possession model was only the predominant one among those we find at various times in various parts of China,, especially in various ethnic, marginal, transitional, and acculturating groups. Another particularly interesting cause of disease, often cited in the Six Dynasties but less frequently in the Song period, was that the guilt of an ancestor had made his descendants susceptible to illness. See the discussion of "ancestral etiology" in chapter 6, p. 156.

[43] The frequency with which this question arises in cases of disease or other troubles may be seen from Elliot 1955 and Jordan 1972, passim, as well as from more generally oriented studies of Chinese villages.

and neighbors. Such revelations happened often, for the setting was not a private interview between curer and patient, like that of psychiatrist and patient today. The séance was more of less open to the public; it involved not only the immediate family but relatives, neighbors, and others familiar with the family's affairs.[44]

Sometimes the illness turned out not to be an affair of one or two families, but a matter of offense to some tutelary deity of the community (always through antisocial conduct of some kind). It was therefore important for the therapist to elicit from those present what the patient (or another member of the household) had done that was wrong. Diagnosis in this sense was usually a collective act. The patient, and others present, were involved in negotiating it. This could happen even without intervention by the medium in trance. His ability to embody the voice of a god, at least, gave him the final word on the diagnosis.

Once the ritual master knew what the disorder was, the cure usually meant learning the location of the possessing shade in the spiritual hierarchy and interceding with its superiors to make it behave. Getting rid of a possessing shade was thus like dealing with a yamen official who pressed a commoner family for bribes beyond the bounds of reason. That was very much the way ordinary people experienced possession. But the parallel goes deeper than that.

In the mundane world, families generally needed a mediator to right wrongs. I have noted that ordinary people had little or no contact with the government, and reason to regret it when they did. Because they were dealing with a bureaucracy, the only recourse for most people was someone who knew his way around the structures of authority—a relative, a friend of a friend, or someone who was content with a small gift—who could find his way to someone in the yamen who could straighten the matter out if persuaded to be helpful.

Because in China the divine world was a bureaucracy, the work of the ritual curer—popular priest, Daoist, Buddhist, even official—was the same sort of mediation. His qualifications were precisely his knowledge of structures of authority, access to them, and mastery of rites that urged the possessing spirit to accommodate, or that brought to bear power over it. Popular priests could only mediate with higher powers; Buddhists could request help from their own powerful deities; Daoists, as initiates into the Divine Order, could issue orders in writing. That made the latter substantially more expensive.

The problem became more complicated when a widespread outbreak of disease suggested divine resentment against a whole community. When a mass of spirits descended at once, as in epidemics, it was proper for the curer to approach the Epidemic God. And who is the Epidemic God? He is the leader of the epidemic demons! He was responsible either directly or indirectly for the group invasion by his subordinates, so his sympathetic concern had to be aroused. When a priest installed him in the main temple of a village or ward at one step in the ritual,

[44] Potter 1974 gives a perceptive account of this social process. I. M. Lewis considers it cross-culturally, in certain situations, to be a regular feature of mediumistic seances (1971, 158–170).

he—that is, his function—was transformed. In the eyes of the local people he became the Epidemic God.[45]

Spiritual beings are thus ambiguous, potentially both benevolent and dangerous. What matters to the living is not what classification shades fall into, but what they do. Their functional character—potentially either protective or punitive—emerges clearly from some of the earliest ample records of widespread popular beliefs, the documents of Daoist millenarian cults from the third century on. Here is the picture sketched in the *Divine Incantations Scripture,* a writing of the Heavenly Masters from the early fifth century[46]:

> The Dao says: Sexagenary year 21 is about to arrive. The flood will not be long in coming. Now, there are epidemic ghosts *(yigui* 疫鬼) who are killing people. The world abounds in vice and lacks goodness. The people do not recognize the truth. The Three Caverns (san dong 三洞) revelations[47] have been spreading for a long time, but the people don't know enough to seek out and accept them. [Such people] bring suffering on themselves. What can be done? The people are to be pitied. I will now send eight units of palace guards to annihilate the epidemic spirits, and dispatch an order to banish them. Let Daoist masters convert people and make them accept the Three Caverns revelations.
>
> The Dao says: From now on, for those who accept this Scripture of Divine Incantations, thirty thousand celestial crack troops will protect you. Convert all the unenlightened day by day on behalf of all the living. If the unenlightened persist in their confusion and ridicule people who do good, Heaven will send epidemic spirits to kill these people. The souls of such people will enter the three evil paths of rebirth, with no prospect of egress.
>
> The Dao says: In sexagenary years 18 and 19, eighty million great spirits will come to annihilate bad people. As for those with forked tongues, those who slander the law of the Dao, those who refer to their masters by their taboo names,[48] those who dispute the scriptures, those who have no faith in the Three Caverns revelations, and those who are unwilling to accept the Dao, the great spirit kings will come and annihilate all of them.
>
> The Dao says: From now on, if there is a place where Daoist masters obediently follow the Three Caverns revelations, practice the Dao, and teach the people, I will send a multitude of 90 billion great soldiers of the ninefold heaven to come all at once and protect you. If there is [even] a single spirit who won't leave, the divine protectors of the ten regions will come down immediately to arrest it. …

The demon kings and their ghostly subordinates sow disease to slaughter all those who disdain the worship that this scripture prescribes. They are also responsible for saving those who reform, and are harshly punished if they fail them. As their activity becomes merciful and contributes to social welfare, they become heavenly beings, to be recognized by promotion in the celestial order.

---

[45] Li Fengmao 李豐楙 1993, 1994.

[46] *Taishang dongyuan shen zhou jing* 太上洞淵神咒經, 2: 2b–6a. See the study in Mollier 1990. Although this and other sources cited in this chapter are Daoist, many of the conceptions of the spiritual world they contain were much more widely current. Those in this passage are consistent with those in similar texts discussed at length in Kaltenmark 1968 and Seidel 1969–1970. In the eleventh century the boundaries between Daoist and popular practice were particularly porous.

[47] *Sandong* means "three caverns"; here it refers to the Divine Incantation scripture.

[48] I.e., their formal names; see chapter 2, p. 26. Among literate people, calling someone with whom one was not intimate by the given name was insulting.

Later chapters of the same scripture make the implications clearer: once sick society is cured, personal illness will be no more. Religious worship is therapy, and those who are incurable because they do not accept the Way of this sect will be annihilated. In the new order spiritual and physical health will be identical.[49]

Now that I have argued for the centrality of possession and the ambiguity of spiritual beings in popular healing, I will look at how people became susceptible to medical disorders, and how ritual masters cured them. Those topics lead to three subsidiary but important issues: the relationship of drugs and rituals, the use of drugs and drug formulas as talismans, and the ritual matrix of drug therapy.

Immunity and susceptibility

If disease is possession, its predisposing condition is contamination, which people thought of as impurity or wrongdoing. The distinction between impurity and wrongdoing is only apparent. The state in which man has nothing to fear from wild beasts, natural catastrophes, or demonic forces depends upon a spectrum of factors including uprightness, conformity to community norms, purity of heart, cleanliness of body, and possession of esoteric knowledge. These were also conditions for the effectiveness of medicines.[50] In other words, one did much the same thing to keep possessing spirits away and to drive them out—to exorcise them—if they had entered the body. Interdiction *(jin* 禁) is a kind of rite directed toward both goals. Individuals carried it out for their own sakes, and practitioners did so for individual clients, or it might be part of communal liturgy. This special understanding of *jin* was fully developed in the first millennium A.D. and did not change markedly thereafter.

Upright conduct is the point of writings that see moral fault as leading to illness or shortened life. *Formulas Worth a Thousand* (650/659) of the eminent physician Sun Simiao 孫思邈 notes in a chapter on cultivating one's nature that conduct and purity are more essential for longevity than drugs: "One who has cultivated his nature not only ingests medicines and imbibes the roseate clouds, but depends also on good conduct.[51] If he is thorough about good conduct, that alone will be enough to prolong his life, even though he has stopped taking medicines. If he is deficient in virtuous conduct, even if he ingests jade potions and the golden elixir, they will not extend his life."[52]

Purity of heart is the object of the *zhai* 齋, the normal purification rites for any important ceremony. The dictionary definition "fast" or "vegetarian meal" ignores

[49] See especially 5: 2a, 6a, and 9: 2b, 5b.

[50] See "The ritual matrix of drug therapy," pp. 118 ff.

[51] The context (particularly the last sentence of this translation) suggests that by "medicines" Sun means alchemical preparations, either alone or in combination with conventional drugs.

[52] *Bei ji qianjin yao fang* 備急千金要方, 27: 1b–2a, p. 476. In *Xuandu lü wen* 玄都律文, 4b–11a, right conduct is medicine.

the diversity that makes up the *zhai:* observance of taboos, especially those against dirt, and seeing or being seen by ritually unclean animals, menstruating women, and so on; abstinence from sex; limitations on diet and dress; concentration, self-examination, and meditation. In popular belief, purity of heart implies sincere faith in the gods.

An alchemical commentary probably of the seventh century, arguing that seclusion is necessary when making an elixir, draws attention to some contemporary pharmaceutical and artisans' taboos that it calls mandatory for ritual purity: "Today, when mixing the physicians' fine drugs, one also does not want chickens, dogs, women and small children to see them. Drugs which have been so seen are not effective when they are used. Also, in the practice of dyers, when evil eyes see the fabric it loses its color. How much truer this is of great medicines of immortality and eternal life!"[53] Such taboos typically protected the work not only of the pharmacist but of the builder, the dyer, the miner, the smith, the vintner, and other craftsmen. This alchemist was also typical in thinking of his elixir as a medicine.

Symbolic aids to invulnerability include talismans (*fu* 符), exorcistic spells and incantations *(zhou* 咒, *zhu* 呪),[54] visualization of divinities, and even drugs. The use of all these is described in the *Inner Chapters of the Master who Keeps to Simplicity* (ca. 320), which promises the aspirant that by visualizing the *qi* of his five visceral systems in their proper colors as a mist emanating from his eyes and surrounding his body "he will be able to share the bed of an epidemic victim. Some do the Steps of Yu, *(Yubu* 禹步 which ritually pace out cosmic configurations), calling out the name of the Jade Girl [i.e. the celestial attendant] on duty that day. Some shut in their breath and visualize a hundred twenty mighty guardian spirits *(lishi* 力士) wielding one-ton hammers who surround them. Some use Ghost-shooting Pills, Crimson-carriage Emissary Pills, Commander Pills, Xu Changqing's 徐長卿 Powder, Jade Casket Seminal Sublimate, the Gray-ox Daoist's (Qingniu daoshi 青牛道士) Body-smoking Pills, Cui Wenhuang's 崔文黄 Powder, Herbal Jade Wine, Yellow Court Pills, Imperial Talismans, Laozi's Collar Talisman, or Crimson-beard's Peach-blossom Talisman. All of these give good results."[55]

The idea of *fu* talismans—fantastic characters written on a strip of paper—evolved from contractual pledges (Fig. 5.1).[56] They were, in other words, a means of establishing or affirming a secure relationship with the Divine Order. The other party to the agreement was the community, with its ritual master as mediator.

The idea that medicinal formulas in pill and powder form can serve as talismans pops up in popular religious practice. It is a key to comprehending symbolic health care, and calls for separate examination below.

---

[53] *Huangdi jiu ding shen dan jing jue* 黄帝九鼎神丹經訣, 4: 2b.

[54] See Sawada 1984.

[55] *Baopuzi nei pian* 抱樸子内篇, 15: 11b; cf. Ware 1966, 260.

[56] Bokenkamp 2008 and the less satisfactory Gai Jianmin 2012. On the structure of talismans, see Ch'en 1942.

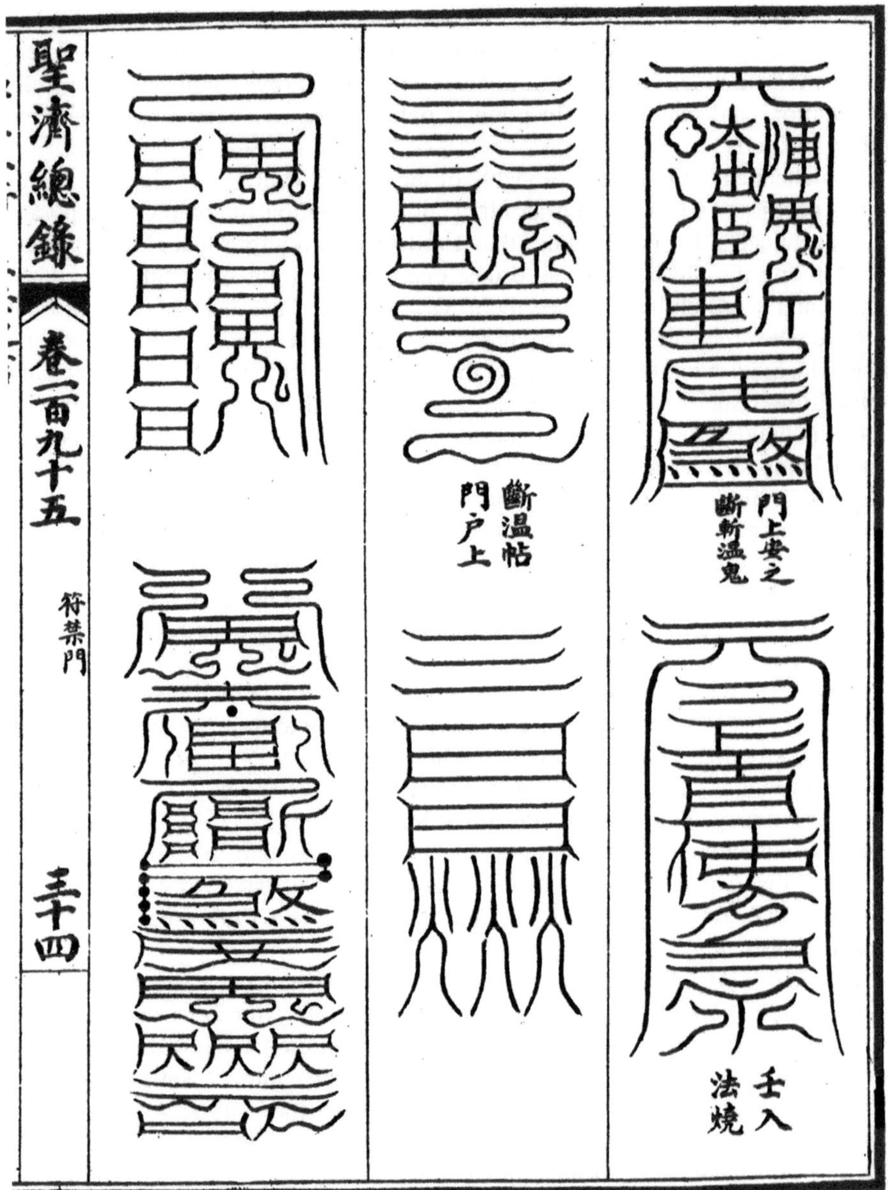

Fig. 5.1 Six talismans, to be affixed to the door to interdict demons that cause Warm Factor disorders (from *Sheng ji zong lu,* 295: 34a)

The ritual attainment of invulnerability boils down to the symbolic restoration of order.[57] What underlies it is the conception of a universal, hierarchic and harmonious

[57] My hypothesis owes a great deal to the pioneers of social anthropology, and in some respects extends the analysis of pollution ideas in Douglas 1966 and her later writings.

realm that unites the celestial government, nature, the world of human affairs, and the human body (which itself contains a replica of the world and the divine hierarchy).[58] That meaning gives ritual interdiction its power.

These four aspects of the realm are exactly mirrored in the objects against which the individual seeks protection using the means I have just outlined: ghosts and spirits in the Divine Order; wild beasts, snakes and poisonous insects in nature; grasping officials, thieves, bandits and bullies in society; and diseases in the microcosm of the body. These are all parts of what exists, but people experience them as disorderly parts, as out of line.

Unlike the elite physician, the popular curer, lay or religious, was not confronting an impersonal and self-regulating cosmos. He dealt, rather, with a spiritual authority that at one moment precipitates the disturbance and at another relieves it. The rites in which the ritual master, the patient, and others participated drew on the remarkable ability of symbols to convey deep meanings, to call forth belief, to change behavior, and to heal. Curing, in other words, was one among many applications of symbolic behavior intended to maintain and restore order in society. But there is more evidence to consider before I can draw the full implications of this hypothesis.

Cure of illness

Medical disorders were not only prevented by order, they were treated by order. Ritual masters applied all of the techniques of interdiction to the restoration of health. Themes of ritual purification and taboo, as we have seen, are common in records of popular remedies.

Rituals were necessary conditions of therapy as well as techniques of curing. This can be seen first of all in an early Daoist scripture, the *Five Talismans*. It appropriated southern spiritual traditions of personal cultivation that originally had nothing to do with any Daoist movement.[59] It typifies religious writings that taught the believer the secret names of his internal gods so that he could summon them. These writings told the adept how, when ill or in pain, to call upon the god or gods of the part affected to cure it.

Similar name magic was used on days of transition (new and full moons, solstices and equinoxes) to prevent loss of one's soul *qi (ju hun zhi po* 拘魂制魄). The Divine Incantations sect of the late fourth century whose beliefs I have already examined (p. 107) controlled disease-bearing shades by invoking their secret names in spells. This symbolic exposure was effective, the scripture informs us, because the

[58] On the Interior Gods in Daoist belief see Schipper 1982.

[59] Documented by Isabelle Robinet 1984, 1:11–34. *Taishang lingbao wufu xu* 太上靈寶五符序 (compiled 317/420), 1: 21b.

ghosts whose names were called were ashamed at the thought that their bureaucratic superiors would learn about their misdeeds.[60]

A possessing spirit is able to cause illness and other functional anomalies because it is itself anomalous. To know its name (and the schedule that constrains its activity) is to know what it is and where it is, to exert over it the authority of knowledge—to share that of its supervisors in the Divine Order. The knowledge of names, in other words, gave power that trumped the power of shades.

Countless popular cures that appear in the medical literature reflect, directly or indirectly, the view of the world and of disease that I have sketched. The conception of medicine that all reflect seems to be the same: Violation of taboos or ethical norms—disorderly behavior—is contaminating, and leaves one susceptible to disease.

Priests in the eleventh century dealt with disease as possession or harassment by shades, which may or may not involve loss of the client's own soul *qi*. Illness was both prevented and cured by interdiction, which makes possession impossible. Purification ritual accompanying the interdiction cancels out the original violation.

Drugs and rituals

Before further probing the experience of popular curing it is worth while to ponder the connections of symbolic therapy—which elicits the meaning response—and drug therapy. Were there two distinct kinds of classical remedies, namely symbolic practices that elicited the meaning response, and drug therapy that, though not specific in the biomedical sense, controlled symptoms and sometimes did more? The classical therapeutic compendia combine many religious and other ritual remedies with medicinal formulas. Such combinations imply that often the uneducated discovered and tried *both* before literati adapted them to the high tradition.

Let us consider two perennial motifs among many in discourse on the connection between materia medica and popular thought. One, plentifully recorded in the classic therapeutic treatises, is that drugs themselves can be talismans. Certain drug formulas were meant not to be ingested but instead hung up in one's house, worn in packets on one's person, or burnt as incenses or fumigants. These uses are parallel (rites included) to applications of more conventional talismans written on paper. The second theme resonant in accounts of popular curing is the use of rites when drugs and prescriptions are being prepared and administered in familiar medical applications. I will now examine, in other words, drugs used for rituals and rituals used for drugs.

[60] *Taishang dongyuan shen zhou jing*, 7: 6b, 11: 5b–9b.

Medicines as talismans

In the third century B.C., in a work which blends geography with cosmography, we see the beginning of a curious but persistent idea, namely that certain medicinal substances protect one from disease when not ingested but rather worn on the person *(pei 佩)*.[61]

Ge Hong 葛洪, in the early fourth century A.D., began to elaborate the idea of drugs carried on the person to confer a general sort of invulnerability. He stipulated preparing them under the same ritual conditions as other talismans, and they had much the same range of powers. Ge richly depicted the matrix in which these drug talismans evolved. He recommended that travelers use them to protect themselves from the physical and spiritual hazards of wild places. "Take Chinese anise and aconite and pound them into a rough powder. Make a triangular crimson gauze bag, put the powder in it, and wear it on your head. Snakes will not dare approach you."[62]

The range of interdictory use of medicines continued to widen. *Effective Formulas* (ca. 620) describes a complicated preparation of inorganic and herbal ingredients meant to be worn in a black bag tied under the left arm when traveling, to be painted on the door at home, and to be affixed over snake or insect bites.[63]

Sun Simiao, whose writings transmit many popular beliefs, provides in his *Essential Formulas for Oral Transmission from the Alchemical Canons* elaborate instructions for pellets with some of the same ingredients as his predecessors used, to keep demons away from his alchemical laboratory. Sun does not indicate how the pellets are to be used, but the *Handy Oral Instructions for Medicines by the Red Pine Master,* a century or so later, directs the alchemist to hang swords and anti-demon talismans at the sides of the laboratory, and to burn pills which largely agree in composition with Sun's demon-killing pellets.[64]

Among the many prophylactic and curative drug talismans in medical writings, the variety of ingredients is enormous but there is considerable duplication. The substances that often turn up fall into several groups that we might call (although Chinese did not) the departments of Chinese materia magica.[65]

---

[61] In *Shan hai jing* 山海經, 1: 3a ff. Ogawa Takuji 小川琢治 1935 notes that a couple of dozen of the minerals enumerated in that book overlap listings in the *Divine Farmer's Materia Medica,* the oldest pharmacognostic manual, but that medicinal applications coincide in only one or two cases (1935, 305–306).

[62] *Baopuzi nei pian,* 抱樸子内篇, cited in *Ishin hō* 醫心方, 26: 610b, but missing from the received text of the former book.

[63] *Gu jin lu yan fang* 古今錄驗方, lost but cited in *Ishin hō,* 26: 608b. In the recent reconstituted version of the former, see 41–45: 386. The binding of drugs on the body to serve as talismans is documented as late as the eighteenth century. See, for instance, *Wu li xiao zhi* 物理小識 (1643), 5: 18a; and *Chuan ya, wai pian* 串雅外篇 (1759), 3: 189.

[64] *Taiqing dan jing yao jue* 太清丹經要訣, 27a, tr. Sivin 1968, 208–209; see also Needham 1954– , 5:2, 149–150; and *Chisongzi zhouhou yao jue* 赤松子肘後藥訣, pp. 13b–14a.

[65] This is not a distinct category in the sources.

There are, in the first place, a number of toxic drugs, even corrosives and vesicants such as the root of bitter crowfoot *(maojian cao* 毛建草, *maogen* 毛茛, *Ranunculus japonicus)*. This subclass includes poisonous inorganic substances, especially mercury and arsenic compounds basic in alchemical elixirs of immortality, as well as toxic botanicals with such suggestive names as Demon's Mortar *(gui jiu* 鬼臼, a *Hosta* rhizome) and Demon's Arrow-feathers *(gui jianyu* 鬼箭羽, *Euonymus alatus, Regel,* spindle-tree wings). Parts of dangerous animals probably were used for analogous reasons. In pharmacognostic thought, the idea of toxicity *(du* 毒; see p. 99) was ambiguous. Physicians believed that certain ingredients could cure acute disorders precisely because their toxicity was effective against pathogens.[66]

Pure mercuric sulfide, whether as natural crystals of cinnabar or artificial vermilion, is so barely soluble that normally it is excreted before it can have any perceptible effect on the body. Its association with mercury and poisonous substances made from it, however, put it in the same class of powerful drugs as realgar and orpiment, both arsenic sulfides. The *Divine Farmer's Materia Medica (Shennong bencao* 神農本草), of the late first or early second century A.D., listed cinnabar as a non-toxic immortality drug. But from at least the eighth century on, the writings of alchemists (who could not chemically distinguish mercuric sulfide, *dan* 丹, from poisonous red substances made from it) influenced physicians.[67] This literature considered cinnabar potentially harmful to the body unless "cyclically transformed *(huan* 還)" by heat. According to an alchemical source of 758 or 759, when correctly prepared, elixirs of immortality (also called *dan*) produced such reactions as "an itching over the body and face as though insects are crawling on them; edema of the arms and legs; revulsion at the sight of food, nausea and vomiting after eating; weakness of the limbs; diarrhea or vomiting; headache or abdominal pain. But please do not think that something has gone wrong. This proves the elixir is effectively driving out the disorder."[68]

A second class of drugs found in almost every pharmaceutical talisman was aromatics, from musk to benzoin. These were familiar as ingredients of incense, the most usual means of contact with the Divine Order.[69]

A third class I cannot resist, despite the anachronism, calling psychotropic drugs. These were botanicals generally believed to improve perception, intelligence, and will, "cure forgetfulness, settle the soul *qi*, and prevent confusion." They were often used in medicine, particularly for the failure of memory that accompanies old age. In exorcistic formulas the common ones, such as various products of cannabis and

---

[66] The same ambiguity persists in the beliefs of twentieth-century Hong Kong women (Topley 1974). Ho and Needham (1959, 232–233) have noted that in imperial times the toxicity concept was ambiguous; Obringer 1997 has studied it in depth.

[67] The eleventh-century imperial formulary *Sheng ji zong lu* 聖濟總錄 contained three chapters on "food for immortals 神仙服餌" (j. 198–200). They offered many alchemical formulas recommended by the compilers for medicinal use.

[68] *Taiqing shi bi ji* 太清石壁記, 2: 7a.

[69] See the study of incense ingredients in Needham 1954– , 5. 2: 134–147.

the rhizome of sweet flag (Acorus calamus), appear together. The pharmacognostic manuals did not consider them toxic, but instead classed them as benign substances that can lead to immortality.[70]

Finally there are a number of what we might call liminal ingredients, which cross the borders between classes. Rhinoceros horn and cow bezoar (p. 149) resemble minerals, but originate in animals, and ginseng was a botanical root whose shape resembled that of the human body.

We can see these four classes—toxic, aromatic, psychotropic, liminal—combined in a formula that, among other things, cures several kinds of possession. "The Great One's Divine Broken Ice Pellets *(Taiyi shenming xianbing yuan* 太一神明陷冰圓)," includes among its twenty-two ingredients centipede *(wugong* 蜈蚣) and the Chinese cantharides beetle (*banmao* 斑貓, *mylabris cichorii),* poisonous insects; vermilion and realgar, inorganics classed as toxic; the botanical devil's mortar; musk, an aromatic; and the three liminal substances just listed.[71] The accumulation of such ingredients in medical writings over the centuries demonstrates the interpenetration of classical and popular therapies.

The ritual matrix of drug therapy

Not only in popular and Daoist records, but here and there in the medical literature, one finds with unexpected frequency that people used rites when gathering or buying, processing, compounding, and administering drugs. The ritual elements, especially the use of secret names and times—keys to authority in the Divine Order—are again consistent with what we know of popular curing.[72]

To take a simple example, Ge Hong's *Handy Formulas,* of the early fourth century A.D., requires secrecy in both the preparation and administration of senega root *(yuanzhi* 遠志, literally, "mind set on what is distant"), a common remedy in Japan, China, India and other parts of the world for forgetfulness due to old age: "For a tendency to forget and make errors: On the thirty-fourth day of the sixty-day cycle, go secretly in person to the market and buy senega there. Carry it home in a corner of your kerchief. When you get home, powder it and take it without letting anyone know." Perhaps someone would need a tolerably good memory in order to maintain such secrecy. It is obvious that what the patient does is as important as the drug.[73]

---

[70] *Daguan bencao,* 6: 69a, s.v. senega root *(yuan zhi* 遠志), citing *Yao xing lun* 藥性論.

[71] In the imperial formulary *Taiping sheng hui fang* 太平聖惠方, 56: 1723.

[72] Like the names of inner gods, the schedules of their rotation through different parts of the body could be used to control them.

[73] Cited in *Zhenghe bencao,* 6: 46a, from Ge's *Zhou hou jiu zu fang* 肘後[救卒]方 (early fourth century). This formula is not found in the extant expanded version, called *Zhou hou beiji fang* 肘後備急方, but has been passed down in later compilations. *Ishin hō,* 17: 601a, cites an analogous remedy: "On the seventh of the seventh month, if one take some cobweb and put it in the collar of one's robe without letting anyone know, one will no longer be forgetful."

When curing others, one sometimes also had to dose them unbeknownst. A frequently quoted remedy incorporating "the 'river halfway in the sky *(bantian he* 半天河)'—water that collects in bamboo or hollow trees—kills demons. For patients who are confused and talk wildly, give them some to drink without letting them know, and they will recover."[74] Here the point seems to be that the afflicted person is not to be warned, so that the possessing shades will be taken by surprise.

Gathering drugs in the wild and buying them were not always distinct. Rituals acknowledged that, like other products of the earth, they were the property of local gods. Symbolic acts to propitiate the spirits of the place are sometimes recorded, and herb-gatherers went to considerable trouble to make sure that they were entitled to what they took. Here is one report, from the writer on classical materia medica, Chen Cangqi 陳藏器 (fl. ca. 725): "In Guiji [near modern Nanking] there is a place called Liao 蓼 which produces limonite *(yuliang* 餘糧). The people of the place, when they are about to dig it up, offer articles with which they ask permission to buy it. There is a set compensation *(shu* 數) for the quantity they request, and if they provide this compensation they are sure to find [the quantity of mineral requested]. They cannot find it on their own whim."[75]

Rites for gaining possession of drugs, special days for collecting them and for mixing the formula, special times of day for its administration, the need to conceal it, the requirement that it be taken in silence: these rules hardly suit the temper of traditional medicine, and are not the norm in the classical treatises. Still, the passages I have quoted from medical writings of the high tradition are far from unique. Authors chose them and others like them from popular sources. The formulas in which such requirements occur—and the labored rationales that literati construct for them—make their popular origin plain.

There was always a tension in Chinese communities between the desire to maintain concord with nature in order to survive and prosper, and the desire to exploit nature—to violate its spontaneous order and rhythms—to meet human needs. Every farmer had to respect the soil and seasons. His community's rituals shaped the modes by which he imposed his will on his land. Among craftsmen the need to go against the grain was especially poignant for those who manipulated the time dimension of natural processes. The miner collaborated with the smith in wresting ores from the womb of the earth and maturing them by art into metals at a pace immensely quicker than they matured when left alone. The vintner controlled the time-bound cycle of fermentation. The therapist interfered with the course of sickness by accelerating recovery.

As Mircea Eliade observed with respect to metal-workers, technicians were the vanguard of their society's encounter with natural forces. In doing their work they took upon themselves spiritual danger. That is why in one culture after another technicians protected their activities by taboos and by rites that maintained their purity of mind and heart, and thus symbolically made their work part of the natural order while they were violating it.[76]

---

[74] *Daguan bencao,* 5: 20b, citing *Yao xing lun.*

[75] *Daguan bencao,* 3: 28a.

[76] Eliade has shown the importance of this theme the world over (1962, 1968).

The rites and abstinences that ensured purity if performed sincerely were essentially those used to prepare for active participation in any sacrament (see p. 108). Any contact with the holy, after all, requires that one be not only pure in mind but in a correct relationship with the Divine Order. This was as true for the emperor, who ritually maintained a cosmic alignment that corresponded to that of the Pole Star, as for a popular priest.[77] How people used rites in different circumstances reflected their social viewpoints and world-views.

I have outlined patterns of overlap between symbolic and pharmacologic aspects of classical therapy. From the fourth century on, a number of physicians, eminent enough for their writings to survive, reconciled the idea of curing as restoring cosmic order with the idea of curing as restoring harmony with the hierarchy of the gods. The beliefs about drugs that they record belong in part to popular religion. Daoist writings also include remedies of the same sorts as those, also taken from popular usage, as we will see in chapter 6.

Popular beliefs about health, illness, and curing incorporate beliefs about drugs. For the Chinese villager before modern times, what moderns see as pharmacodynamically effective substances were as tied to the divine order as talismans and incantations.

Why Medical Authors Accepted Popular Therapies

I will now argue that many ritual remedies are in classical handbooks because sensible people were convinced that they cured illnesses.

Chinese physicians were aware in a general way that people recover from sickness or injury mostly because their bodies heal themselves. In the eleventh century, that did not lead most physicians to minimize drug or other therapy. Nor, when health returned, did they decline the credit. Doctors from earliest times were aware of the danger of malpractice, and even of iatrogenesis, causing disease by erroneous treatment. A good deal of both has been documented over the centuries.[78] We have no reason to expect ancient doctors' judgments of success in ordinary clinical practice to be more accurate than our own. Still, the desire to succeed is one of many reasons that we can expect them to recognize what worked regularly, and what consistently did not work.

The meaning response played a perceptible part in recovery often enough that some classical physicians took religious healing seriously. They did so even when other literati contemptuously dismissed it (usually on social rather than empirical grounds) as mere "customs of the vulgar." This openness is no small matter, since large parts of the belief pattern underlying popular remedies could never be entirely assimilated to that of classical theory. But the framework of Chinese medical learning has always maintained space for contradictory ideas. That is a corollary of valuing

---

[77] The classical authority for such practices is the *Analects (Lunyu* 論語), 2/2/1, 31/15/5.

[78] Xu Fulin 徐复霖 et al. 1985 is an anthology of medical error. See also Sivin 1987, 197–199, and Scheid 2002, 10–13.

doctrine for its fertility rather than its logical rigor. Even today the looseness remains, and shows no signs of disappearing. The fact is that classical therapy drew freely on popular visions of health and sickness.

Doctors frequently reinterpreted popular ideas as they applied them. This they did in several ways, which their writings reflect. They translated religious and vitalistic notions into their own abstract conceptual language (discussed in chapter 4). While in popular therapy a medicine, as we have seen, may have played only a small part in a complex interdiction, classical therapy often magnified the importance of the drug while abridging the rite or discarding it. Medical authors usually ignored the rites that accompanied the mundane gathering and use of drugs in the villages. They made possession and harrassment by demons and loss of soul *qi* (p. 157) only three causes of illness among many. In explaining how a disorder comes about, they shifted their focus from the invading spirit to changes in the body's functional systems that leave it open to invasion, as well as those that the pathogenic agent brings about.

Here is a typical example, from the classical handbook *Origins and Symptoms of Medical Disorders*. The subject is the very large class of infusion (that is, possession) disorders *(zhu)*. The book is typical in its vagueness about the character of the causative agent, for which it uses the conventional term "pathogenic *qi*" (*xieqi*), that is, vitalities different in kind from those of the body and therefore antagonistic to them.[79]

> *Zhu* is a way of saying *zhu* 住, "to reside," because the pathogenic *qi* takes up residence within someone's body. This happens when yin and yang fail in their responsibility [to maintain a dynamic balance], so that the circulation tracts develop vacancy and depletion. [Possession] may be brought on by wind, cold, heat, damp, or exhaustion pathogens. In cases of Cold Damage Disorders *(shanghan* 傷寒), when sudorifics are not given in a timely way to drive them out with perspiration, or when, although this has been done, the result is not true perspiration [capable of flushing out recently entered pathogens], the disease will be transmitted from the yang circulation tracts to the yin [inner] tracts, and thence to the visceral systems of function. If a lingering pathogen is not expelled in a timely way, or in cases of Overnight Food Accumulation Disorder[80] when hot and cold foods have not been regulated, the pathogenic *qi* may circulate and reside [in the body]. Being suddenly affected by the *qi* of the newborn or the newly dead, or offending the ghosts or shades, may bring about this disease. Its transformations are so manifold that one finds as many as thirty-six or ninety-nine types, although not all the therapeutic formulas specifically name them.

Because popular curing depended so greatly upon meaning, therapies effective in their own cultural milieu may have been less successful when tried on conventional officeholders than on their uneducated wives or their open-minded children. But classic and popular medicine overlapped and blended insensibly into each other along an extended spectrum. Considering the many social levels at which people calling themselves physicians *(yi* 醫) subsisted, and the differing beliefs of their patients, it is not surprising that verifications of symbolic cures should have continued to pour in.

---

[79] *Zhu bing yuan hou lun,* 24: 130a.

[80] *Su shi* 宿食 is stasis of alimentary matter in the stomach or intestinal system due to overeating or unbalanced diet.

Finally, Daoist, Buddhist, and popular practitioners continually plundered each other's rites and methods. Those of the two elite religions were in large part adaptations and transformations of what ordinary people did. Despite the efforts of Buddhists and Daoists to separate themselves from what went on in the popular temples and shrines, the ritual masters in the latter delightedly made use of anything that they believed would help people avoid misery.

Illness as Learned Behavior

A culture (or subculture) defines disorders in ways that depend on how people in it understand order. This is a familiar theme in the anthropology and sociology of medicine.[81] It is another way of saying that, as people grow up, they learn not only how to tell they are sick but how to be sick. The tension headache is one response to stress in modern societies; the fainting spells of the Victorian lady are out of style.

P. M. Yap catalogued a few of what he called "culture-specific syndromes": syndromes that are coherent, well-defined, and recognized in certain societies but not found elsewhere. A modern example is South Chinese *so-lò,* a painful disorder of males in which the testicles retract into the abdomen, sometimes eventually causing death. When observed in Hong Kong, it is usually caused by violation of some sexual taboo. A certain number of people who know about *so-lò* (from those around them, not from medical books) behave in accordance with it; they get sick. Their physical symptoms are in no sense imaginary. If belief can make them sick, belief can cure them. Recorded formulas specify the conditions of cure, and symbolically enact the expulsion of the pathological agent.[82]

Here is an example well-known in the eleventh century in which the theme of sickness as learned social behavior appears clearly. Among the dangerous disorders women may contract after childbirth is one called "post-partum dizziness and nausea with abnormal blood loss" *(chanru xue yunmen* 產乳血運悶), and by various shorter names. Chao Yuanfang's *Origins and Symptoms of Medical Disorders* (610) described and explained this illness in classical terms. Its author, an imperial physician, focused on the balance of yin *(xue* 血) and yang *(qi* 氣) vitalities in the circulatory system:

> The manifestations of [this] dizziness and nausea are upset and inner tension, to the extent that one's *qi* feels about to expire. There are also instances in which excessive bleeding or extremely scanty bleeding may bring on dizziness. If in childbirth bleeding is excessive, so that the *xue* is deficient and *qi* exhausted [that is, yin and yang vitalities are greatly below normal], there will be only feelings of upset and tension. When bleeding is too scanty, so that the *qi* reverses its normal flow, the *xue* will follow it, pressing upward against the heart. The result is not only dizziness and nausea but tension, sensations of fullness, and anxiety.

[81] Sivin 1977.

[82] Yap 1969; Lebra 1976; Topley 1970, 424 and 429. Later authors have pointed out that some syndromes Yap considered unique actually turn up in more than one culture. Retraction of the testicles appears often in the classical medical literature *(nang suo* 囊縮 or *luan suo* 卵縮), but as a symptom of serious illness rather than as a disease.

> Thus one distinguishes the two types. One should note how much the woman has bled, in order to anticipate whether post-partum dizziness is likely. If feelings of upset and tension persist unabated, they may kill the patient.

As Chao goes on, we can recognize from his description that he sees the ultimate cause as wrong behavior, namely breaking a taboo:

> If a woman violates the prohibitions concerning the direction she should face when sitting or lying down during labor, dizziness will usually result. The downflow of blood will be either excessive or deficient. When her direction violates a prohibition, this will usually bring on dizziness and nausea, and bleeding may be overly copious or scanty. On account of this, where childbirth takes place, and whether she lies down or sits up, must be appropriate to the season and the direction, to avoid infringing prohibitions according to the five phases. Violations will generally call down disaster.[83]

Here is an instance of translation from one medical world view into another. What obviously began as a taboo in popular curing becomes meaningful in classical thought when educated physicians relate it to the cyclical sequence of compass directions that govern activity according to the five phases doctrine—east in spring, south in summer, and so on. Dizziness, nausea, and changes in blood flow, as biomedical physicians would put it, are common symptoms of stress and anxiety. If a woman in labor were unexpectedly warned by her midwife or her mother-in-law that she was facing in the wrong direction and thus might have contracted a dangerous disease, the results are likely to be heightened anxiety and, ultimately, the symptoms that constitute the disorder.[84]

Among the 34 formulas for post-partum dizziness with abnormal blood loss in the *Imperial Grace Formulary* is Black Gold Powder (Wu jin san 烏金散). Its nine ingredients include scales from a red carp *(chi liyu lin* 赤鯉魚鱗), oily human hair *(you toufa* 油頭髮), leeches *(shuizhi* 水蛭), horseflies *(mengchong* {蝱蟲), amber *(hubo* 琥珀), and musk *(shexiang* 麝香). These seven are redolent of the materia magica already discussed (p. 113).

It is not a good idea to dismiss this medicine as an ignorant and deluded substitute for modern drugs. Medicines were not only, as we experience them, something swallowed with a glass of water during a moment's respite from more productive activities. Therapists used them to embody powerful symbolic themes in elaborate patterned action. Bearing in mind the range of ritual situations in which popular practitioners originally would have administered this remedy, it is possible that the total constellation of treatment would have lessened the patient's stress and thus cured her vertigo. But in this instance we can go no further, for the formulary has not recorded the context.[85]

---

[83] *Zhu bing yuan hou lun,* 43: 230b, paraphrased in the tenth-century *Taiping sheng hui fang*, 80: 2526. On the complementarity of *qi* and *xue* in classical medicine, see chapter 2, p. 19.

Kleinman (1980, 135) has discussed Chinese terms in twentieth-century Taiwanese usage like those for upset and tension, which refer to something midway between symptoms of depressive emotional states and physical feelings. It is impossible to be sure, for instance, whether *ji* 急 refers to a physical sensation of urgent pressure in the chest cavity, to vague and ambiguous discomfort, or to a feeling of anxiety. I have tried to maintain some of this ambiguity with "tension."

[84] On directional and other taboos see Furth 1999, 110–111.

[85] *Taiping sheng hui fang*, 80: 2524. The disorder is cited as *chan yun* 產運.

A procedure for interdicting post-partum dizziness in advance can teach us something about the content and significance of such rituals. It comes from the *Canon of Interdiction (Jin jing* 禁經), a handbook of exorcism for Heavenly Masters Daoists, that found its way into one of Sun Simiao's seventh-century medical formularies:

> Take seven cloves of garlic. On the first day of the first month, facing due east, have the wife recite [the following interdiction] once; then the husband is also to chant it once. One at a time, the husband is to swallow a clove of garlic and seven sesame seeds. Then he is to walk due east and repeat the formula a full seven times. They may not see anything polluting or loathsome. In learning and practicing [this interdiction] avoid seeing corpses or mourners, or it will not be effective:
>
> I tread the mainstays of the sky, roam the Nine Realms.
> Hearing of your difficulty in childbirth, I come in search,
> To tear apart and slaughter the inauspicious,
> Replace them by every felicity.
> To mother and child, long life in mutual regard.
> Impermissible [for shades] to tarry long.
> Quickly, quickly, by lawful order.[86]

The prospective parents, directed by a Daoist exorcist, speak themselves what we recognize to be the words of a member of the Divine Order. The last two lines send the unwanted demons on their way, invoking the authority of the celestial bureaucracy. Here is the crux of symbolic cure: the performance, directed by the ritualist, transforms the client from an isolated and passive victim of malevolent possession into a person protected by hierarchic authority and thus able to drive out menacing demons.

A mundane consequence of this ritual is equally important. It focuses the husband's concern upon the dangers which his wife will face in childbirth, and lets him express his concern in the interdiction. If he does this sincerely, a lasting reduction of the wife's stress would be a natural by-product.

Custom did not encourage husbands to be aware of their pregnant wives' anxiety. Many no doubt showed that they cared, and others did not, to avoid offending elders with whom they lived, for instance, or because they lacked feeling. There was little or nothing in Chinese social practice—that is, in what we know of its many variations—to focus a husband's concern for his wife, except rites like this one.

After all, what a change in one's relations to the Divine Order is supposed to cure is often, by the lights of modern psychology, a result of defective relations with the people around one. I. M. Lewis has demonstrated that in many African societies possession is an effective means of dealing individually or institutionally with social predicaments. His conclusions were foreshadowed by half a century in the neurologist Andrew H. Woods' early clinical studies of spirit possession in China. As Woods puts it,

> Usually, the motives were obvious. The victims were girls who had been seduced and disgraced, wives who had been badly treated, or persons who had substantial reasons for desiring revenge; and the demon always acted in a way to cause the greatest possible uneasiness and discomfort to the alleged aggressors. In brief, the [therapists'] performances gave

[86] *Qian jin yi fang*, 29: 22b–23a. On the celestial mainstays, the cosmic meridians that bind the stars together, see Schafer 1977, ch. 12. The Nine Realms are archaic divisions of China. The point is that the god summoned by the exorcism ranges freely through sky and earth.

respite and satisfaction to the patients. Nearly all the victims were women. The exorcisms were always accompanied by the impressive and dramatic presentation to the victims' minds that a deity superior to the demon which was then present had issued orders that the demon must depart.[87]

The "respite and satisfaction" of which Woods writes is not necessarily a momentary matter. The outcome may be familial solicitude that was not forthcoming earlier despite less desperate efforts. It may be relatives and neighbors who are present insisting that some settlement be found for an untenable situation, overruling the inclination of many Chinese families to put up with internal problems that seem out of its control.[88]

My larger point is that religious exorcism, whatever else it may be, and regardless of who performs it, is an institution, sometimes the only one, for dealing with abrasive human relations within a family that cannot be resolved without outside help. Possession thus signals social disorder which the symbolic procedures of the exorcist—oriented as they are about images invoking a universal order—are designed to put right.

Investigators influenced by psychiatric thought have proposed that mediumistic curing is a kind of folk psychotherapy, effective within the structure of Chinese social norms because it calms anxiety.[89] We can consider this one function of the medium's rites, as my examples indicate, but only by defining "psychotherapy" vaguely enough to include diverse emotional manipulation. As a general explanation of symbolic therapy, however, anxiety reduction is inadequate. A great deal more is involved than the patient's anxiety.

I have already noted (p. 106) that popular curing rites, unlike those of modern psychiatry, were performed in public places. The practitioners who depended on this therapy applied it to the whole range of ailments. They sought out and dealt with kinked personal relations in the presence of a family, and often members of the community unrelated to it.

The rites made the illness comprehensible by relating it to views of life which the patient shared with the other people he knew. They have that much in common with psychiatry. They actively focused the support of the patient's family and neighbors toward his health, or toward his reintegration into his social nexus after disease has changed his pattern of participation—as most varieties of conventional psychiatry do not.

To say that Chinese culture defines emotional illnesses as demon possession can be misleading unless we are aware that the concept of emotional illness is also culture-bound. It is based solidly on the values of twentieth-century secular society,

[87] Lewis 1971; Woods 1929, 68.

[88] Kleinman has discussed social interactions at mediumistic sessions he observed in modern Taiwan (1980, 219 and elsewhere). He notes on p. 205 that "the entire family may be labeled sick or inharmonious and treatment directed to it or to key family members."

[89] This generalization is often found in accounts meant to encourage sympathetic study, such as Torrey 1974. Torrey speaks of his subjects as "true psychotherapists playing the same role as psychiatrists play" (p. 330). Anxiety reduction or catharsis is a central explanation in Erwin Ackerknecht's work and in the studies of Chinese folkways by the psychiatrist Tseng Wen-shing.

with its special notion of individuality. In Western medicine the idea of emotional disorder largely replaced those of insanity and mental illness, which had in turn replaced the spiritual disorders of a previous era.

In eleventh-century China, if a young woman began having visions that a god had entered her body, her family would be responsible for her care. If necessary they could call on the aid of a priest or some other curer. If these visions continued, she might gradually learn to control their onset and termination and become a curer herself, more or less independent of her family. A small cult might grow up around her. In modern Japan, major new religions have evolved from such beginnings.[90]

In some parts of Western Europe or North America today, diagnosticians would consider visions nothing more than symptoms of illness. Therapy would ordinarily be centered about the therapist's professional, one-on-one relationship with the patient. Some therapeutic movements involve members of the family in formal treatment, but others rigorously exclude them.

No undergraduate who has studied the historical sociology of medicine would claim institutions that isolate the patient with the therapist were generated by the unfolding essence of scientific psychiatry, or were the only conceivable basis for its development. Early psychiatrists adapted a pattern already formed for biomedical practice, in which they were trained.

Biomedicine's evolution has accompanied changes in the values of practitioners, patients and their families over the past century and a half. The success of aggressive professionalizing movements concentrated health care in the hands of scientifically and clinically trained doctors of medicine. They moved their work into surroundings designed to symbolize scientific objectivity and efficiency, and to give priority to efficient use of the therapist's time and rapid access to advanced technology. The physician's authority, and thus his freedom of action, were enhanced in surroundings that encouraged the patient to become a passive object of examination and manipulation. Assimilation of the M.D.'s role to that of the physical or biological research scientist—a role given great prestige from the late nineteenth century on—persuaded the public to endorse the institutional transformation of medicine.

Conclusion

To recapitulate, social norms shape abnormal behavior into symptoms, and symptoms into disorders, in categories that reflect every culture's perceptions of the moral as well as physical conditions underlying each disease, and the resources of each society for helping patients. This is as true of modern psychiatry (with its reliance on psychopharmacology) as of ritual curing in China (with its dependence on the

[90] Lewis has examined in detail the process by which mastery of possession makes it possible to become a healer (1971, ch. 3, 7). The varieties of mediumism in Japan and their connections to the founding of religions have been investigated in McFarland 1967, Blacker 1975, Kotaki 1997, and Clarke 2000. Elliott 1955 has remarked on the games of South Chinese children in Singapore that identified and encouraged a predisposition toward possession—analogous to the children's games that favor marksmanship in the United States.

celestial bureaucracy) a millennium ago. There is every reason to believe that the conceptual structure underlying popular therapy was as much in tune with the reality experienced by its own patients as are modern medical theories. We cannot assume, in our ignorance, that popular healing is less effective. Psychotherapists may remind us that their understanding of emotional dysfunction is bound to be more penetrating than that of a medium in trance; but that difference does not translate in any simple way into better functioning for their patients. And popular therapies treated the whole range of ailments. Their effectiveness has to be evaluated one case at a time.

Setting aside for the moment the perspectives of the modern physician and psychiatrist for that of the ancient Chinese physician is not retrogression, but rather making use of a viewpoint more meaningful in its time and place. That effort of the imagination *before* we ask our own questions is a great help in making sense of the kinds of health care I have explored in this chapter.

References

Abbreviations

DZ = Volume number in *Daozang*
ES = *Ersishi shi* 二十四史 of Zhonghua Shuju, 1959–1977.
HY = text in Harvard-Yenching Concordance series
j. = *juan* 卷 (chapter)
RW = published by Renmin Weisheng Chubanshe 人民衛生出版社, Beijing
S = Title number in Schipper 1975
SQ = Siku quanshu 四庫全書
SV = Schipper & Verellen 2004
T = *Taishō shinshū Daizōkyō* 大正新修大藏經
UP = University Press
YZ = Yi tong zheng mai quan shu 醫統正脈全書
ZD = Volume, item, *juan,* and page numbers in *Zhonghua daozang* 中华道藏
ZS = published by Zhonghua shuju 中華書局, Beijing
ZZ = Zhongyi zhenben congshu 中醫珍本叢書 ed.

Classical Chinese Sources

Daguan bencao 大觀本草. See *Jing shi zheng lei Daguan bencao.*

Gu jin lu yan fang 古今錄驗方 (Register of Effective Medical Formulas Old and New). Chen Quan 陳權 & Chen Liyan 陳立言 (?). Ca. 620. Lost. Reconstituted version, ed. Xie Pangen 谢盘根. Beijing: Zhongguo Yiyao Keji Chubanshe 中国医药科技出版社, 1996.

Huangdi jiu ding shen dan jing jue 黃帝九鼎神丹經訣 (Canon and oral instructions for the divine elixir of the Yellow Emperor's nine ritual cauldrons). Anonymous, j. 1 probably of Han period, remainder probably of seventh century. S885, DZ584–585.

Jing shi zheng lei Daguan bencao 經史正類大觀本草 (Materia medica of the Great Prospect era, classified and verified from the classics and histories). Tang Shenwei 唐慎微. 1108. Tokyo: Hirokawa Shoten, 1970

Pingzhou ke tan 平洲可談 (Acceptable chats from Pingzhou). Zhu Yu 朱彧. Author's preface 1119. Critical ed. in Tang Song shiliao biji 唐宋史料筆記, ZS, 2007.
Qian jin yi fang 千金翼方 (Revised formulas worth a thousand). Sun Simiao. Late 7th century. RW, 1955, reproduction of 1307 ed.
Shan hai jing 山海經 (Classic of mountains and seas). Anonymous. 290/240 B.C.? SQ. The layers in this work and their dates are contentious. See Riccardo Fracasso in Loewe 1993, 357–367.
Sheng ji zong lu 聖濟總錄 *(General Record of Sagely Benefaction).* Shen Fu 申甫 et al., compiled by order of Emperor Huizong. 1117. RW ed. of 1952, reprint of 1982.
Taiqing dan jing yao jue 太清丹經要訣 (Essential formulas for oral transmission from the alchemical canons). Sun Simiao, late 7C? Critical ed. and translation in Sivin 1968.
Taiping sheng hui fang 太平聖惠方 (Imperial grace formulary of the Great Peace and Prosperous State era). Compiled by Wang Huaiyin 王懷隱, printed, and promulgated by imperial order. 992. RW, 1958.
Taiqing shi bi ji 太清石壁記 (Records from the stone wall, a Great Purity canon). Anonymous. 758/759. S882, DZ582–583. Alchemical formulary. See SV 381.
Taishang dongyuan shen zhou jing 太上洞淵神咒經 (or *shen zhu jing* 神祝經; Scripture of Divine Incantations of the Cavern Abyss of the Most High). Anonymous. Accreted between the early fifth century and 900. S335, DZ 170–173.
Yijian zhi 夷堅志 (Records of the listener). By Hong Mai 洪邁. Written over the period 1157–1202. 4 vols. ZS, 1981. Only 207 of the original 420 j. survive.
Zhu bing yuan hou lun 諸病源候論 (Origins and symptoms of medical disorders). Chao Yuanfang 巢元方. Completed 610. RW, 1955.

Other Sources

Anonymous, ed. 1994. *Minjian xinyang yu Zhongguo wenhua guoji yantaohui lunwen ji* 民間信仰與中國文化研討會論文集 (Proceedings of an international conference on popular beliefs and Chinese culture). Center for Chinese Studies Research Series, 4. 2 vols. Taipei: Hanxue Yanjiu Zhongxin 漢學研究中心.
Baldrian-Hussein, Farzeen. 2008. *Hun* and *Po.* In Pregadio 2008, 521–523.
Blacker, Carmen. 1975. *The Catalpa Bow.* London: Allen & Unwin.
Bokenkamp, Stephen R. 2008. *Fu* 符. In Pregadio 2008, 35–38.
Bokenkamp, Stephen R. 2010. Daoist Pantheons. In Lagerwey & Lü 2010, 1169–1203.
Boltz, Judith Magee. 1993. Not by the Seal of Office Alone. New Weapons in Battles with the Supernatural. In Ebrey & Gregory 1993, 241–305.
Cai Xianghui 蔡相煇. 1994. Yi Mazu xinyang wei li, lun zhengfu yu minjian xinyang de guanxi 以媽祖信仰為例論政府與民間信仰的關係 (The relation between government and popular beliefs, using belief in Mazu as an example). In Anonymous 1994, 437–454.
Cedzich, Ursula-Angelika. 1995. The Cult of the Wu-t'ung/Wu-hsien in History and Fiction. The Roots of the *Journey to the South.* In David Johnson 1995, 137–218.
Chao Wei-pang. 1942. The Origin and Growth of the Fu Chi 扶乩. *Folklore Studies,* 1: 9-27. On the planchette.
Ch'en Hsiang-ch'un. 1942. Examples of Charm against Epidemics with Short Explanations. *Folklore Studies,* 1: 37–54.
Clarke, Peter B., ed. 2000. *Japanese New Religions: In Global Perspective.* Curzon Studies in New Religious Movements. Richmond: Curzon.
Davis, Edward L. 2001. *Society and the Supernatural in Song China.* Honolulu. University of Hawai'i Press.
Douglas, Mary. 1966. *Purity and Danger.* London: Routledge & Kegan Paul.
Eliade, Mircea. 1962. *The Forge and the Crucible,* tr. Stephen Corrin. New York.
Eliade, Mircea. 1968. The Forge and the Crucible: A Postscript. *History of Religions* 8: 74–88. New York: Harper & Row.

Elliott, Alan J. A. 1955. *Chinese Spirit Medium Cults in Singapore.* London: Royal Anthropological Institute.
Furth, Charlotte. 1999. *A Flourishing Yin: Gender in China's Medical History, 960–1665.* Berkeley: University of California Press.
Gai Jianmin. 2012. Study of the Medical Elements in Taoist Healing: The Use of Talismans and Incantations. In Mou Zhongjian 2012, 293–308. Condescending, poorly informed.
von Glahn, Richard. 2004. *The Sinister Way. The Divine and the Demonic in Chinese Religious Culture*: University of California Press.
Haar, Barend J. ter. 2007. Review of von Glahn 2004. *Journal of Sung–Yuan Studies* 37: 250–258.
Han Yi 韓毅. 2007. *Songdai yixue zhaoling nianbiao yu ziliao huibian* 宋代医学诏令年表与资料汇编 (Chronology and compilation of Song imperial edicts on medicine). Beijing: Zhongguo Kexueyuan, Ziran kexueshi yanjiusuo.
Han Yi 韩毅. 2011. Bei Song zhengfu dui wuyi de kongzhi yu gaizao 北宋政府对巫医的控制与改造 (The Northern Song government's control and reform of wizard curers). *Zhongguo kejishi zazhi* 中国科技史杂志 (Studies in the history of natural sciences) 32 (supplement): 106–130.
Hansen, Valerie. 1990. *Changing Gods in Medieval China, 1127–1276.* Princeton UP.
Harrell, C. Stevan. 1974. When a Ghost Becomes a God. In Wolf 1974a, 193–206.
Hinrichs, TJ. 2003. The Medical Transforming of Governance and Southern Customs in Song Dynasty China (960–1279 C.E.). Ph.D. dissertation, East Asian Languages, Harvard University.
Ho Peng Yoke (= Ping-yü, He Bingyu 何丙郁). 2003. *Chinese Mathematical Astrology. Reaching out to the Stars.* Needham Research Institute series, 3. London: RoutledgeCurzon.
Ho Ping-yü & Joseph Needham. 1959. Elixir Poisoning in Mediaeval China. *Janus* 48. 4: 221–251, reprinted in Needham 1970, 316–339.
Horton, Robin. 1973. Lévy-Bruhl, Durkheim and the Scientific Revolution. In Horton & Finnegan 1973, 249–305.
Horton, Robin, & Ruth Finnegan, eds. 1973. *Modes of Thought. Essays on Thinking in Western and Non-Western Societies*. London: Faber and Faber.
Iiyama, Tomoyasu. 2010. Maintaining Gods in Medieval China: Temple Worship and Local Governance in North China under the Jin and Yuan. *Journal of Song–Yuan Studies* 40: 71–102.
Inglis, Alister D. 2007. *Hong Mai's Record of the Listener and its Song Dynasty Context.* Albany: SUNY Press.
Ishii Masako 石井昌子. 1968. *Shinkō* no seiritsu o meguru shiryōteki kentō 真誥の成立をめぐる史料的檢討. (Documentary investigation of the formation of the *Declarations of the Realized Immortals*). *Dōkyō kenkyū* 道教研究 (Études taoistes) 3: 79–195.
Johnson, David, ed. 1995. *Ritual and Scripture in Chinese Popular Religion. Five Studies*. China Popular Culture Project, 3. Berkeley: The Project.
Jordan, David K. 1972. *Gods, Ghosts, and Ancestors*. Berkeley: University of California Press .
Kaltenmark, Max. 1968. Notions sur quelques grands sutras Taoïstes (sommaire). Unpublished paper read at 1st International Conference on Taoism, Bellagio, Italy.
Kleeman, Terry F. 1994. *A God's Own Tale. The* Book of Transformations *of Wenchang, the Divine Lord of Zitong*. SUNY Series in Chinese Philosophy and Culture. Albany: State University of New York Press.
Kleinman, Arthur. 1980. *Patients and Healers in the Context of Culture: An Exploration of the Borderland between Anthropology, Medicine, and Psychiatry.* Comparative Studies of Health Systems and Medical Care, 3. Berkeley: University of California Press.
Kleeman, Terry. 2005. The Evolution of Daoist Cosmology and the Construction of the Common Sacred Realm. *Taiwan Journal of East Asian Studies* 2. 1: 89–110.
Kohn, Livia. 2000. *Daoism Handbook.* Handbook of Oriental Studies, section 4, vol. 14. Leiden: Brill.
Kotaki Tōru 小滝透. 1997. *Kamigami no mezame: kindai Nihon no shūkyō kakumei* 神々の目覚め: 近代日本の宗教革命 (Awakening of the gods: religious revolution in modern Japan). Tokyo: Shunjūsha, 1997.
Lagerwey, John. 2010. *China. A Religious State.* Hong Kong UP. Four lectures.
Lebra, William P., ed. 1976. *Culture-Bound Syndromes, Ethnopsychiatry, and Alternative Therapies.* Mental Health Research in Asia and the Pacific, 4. Honolulu: University Press of Hawaii.

Lewis, I. M. 1971. *Ecstatic Religion. An Anthropological Study of Spirit Possession and Shamanism*. Harmondsworth: Penguin.

Li Fengmao 李豐楙. 1993. Daozang suo shou zao qi dao shu de wenyiguan 道藏所收早期道書的瘟疫觀 (Views of epidemics in early Daoist books in the Daoist Canon). *Bulletin of the Institute of Literature and Philosophy, Academia Sinica* 3: 1–38.

Li Feng-mao 李豐楙. 1994. Xing wen yu song wen. Daojiao yu minzhong wenyiguan de jiaoliu yu fenqi 行瘟與送瘟. 道教與民衆瘟疫觀的交流與分歧 (Parading the epidemic gods and sending them off. The interaction and divergence of Daoist and popular views of epidemics). In Anonymous 1994, 372–422.

Liao Hsien-huei. 2007. Encountering Evil: Ghosts and Demonic Forces in the Lives of the Song Elite. *Journal of Song–Yuan Studies* 37: 89–134.

Liu Zhiwan 劉枝萬. 1974a. *Zhongguo minjian xinyang lun ji* 中國民間信仰論集 (Essays on Chinese Folk Belief and Folk Cults). Institute of Ethnology, Academia Sinica, Monographs, 22. Nankang: Academia Sinica.

Liu Zhiwan. 1974b. Lüshan jiao zhi shou hun fa 閭山教之收魂法 (The method of retrieving the soul in the Lüshan sect). In Liu 1974a, 207–378.

McFarland, H. Neill. 1967. *The Rush Hour of the Gods: A Study of New Religious Movements in Japan.* New York: Macmillan.

Matsumoto Kōichi 松本浩一. 2006. *Sōdai no dōkyō to minkan shingyō* 宋代の道教と民間信仰 (Daoism and folk belief in the Song period). Tokyo: Kyuko Shoin.

Mollier, Christine. 1990. *Une apocalypse taoïste du Ve siècle. Le livre des incantations divines des grottes abyssales.* Mémoires de l'Institut des Hautes Études Chinoises, 31. Paris: L'Institut.

Mueggler, Erik. 2003. Review of Stephan Feuchtwang, *Popular Religion in China: The Imperial Metaphor* (Richmond, Surrey: Curzon Press, 2001). *American Anthropologist,* n.s., 105. 2: 410–411.

Nakamura Jihei 中村治兵衛. 1978. KitaSōchō to fu 北宋朝と巫 (The Northern Song dynasty and wizards). *Chūo Daigaku Bungakubu kiyo. Shigaku ka* 中央大學文學部紀要. 史學科 23: 63–78.

Naquin, Susan. 2012. Temples, Technology, and Material Culture in Shouzhou 壽州, Anhui. In Schäfer 2012, 184–207.

Needham, Joseph, et al. 1954– . *Science and Civilisation in China.* 24 vols. to date. Cambridge UP.

Needham, Joseph, et al. 1970. *Clerks and Craftsmen in China and the West. Lectures and Addresses on the History of Science and Technology.* Cambridge UP.

Obringer, Frédéric. 1997. *L'aconit et l'orpiment. Drogues et poisons en Chine ancienne et médiévale*. Penser la médecine, 4. Paris: Fayard.

Poo, Mu-chou. 2010. Images and Ritual Treatment of Dangerous Spirits. In Lagerwey & Lü 2010, 2:1075–1094.

Potter, Jack M. 1974. Cantonese Shamanism. In Wolf 1974a, 207–231.

Pregadio, Fabrizio, ed. 2008. *The Encyclopedia Of Taoism.* 2 vols. New York: Routledge.

Robinet, Isabelle. 1984. *La revelation du Shangqing dans l'histoire du Taoisme.* 2 vols. Paris: Ècole Française d'Extrême-Orient.

Sawada Mizuho 澤田瑞穗. 1984. *Chūgoku no juhō* 中国の咒法 (Chinese incantations). Tokyo: Hirakawa Shuppansha.

Schäfer, Dagmar, ed. 2012. *Cultures of Knowledge. Technology in Chinese History.* Sinica Leidensia, 103. Leiden: Brill.

Schafer, Edward H. 1977. *Pacing the Void. T'ang Approaches to the Stars.* Berkeley: University of California Press.

Scheid, Volker. 2002. *Chinese Medicine in Contemporary China: Plurality and Synthesis.* Durham: Duke UP.

Schipper, Kristofer M. 1982. *Le corps taoïste. Corps physique–corps social.* L'espace intérieur, 25. Paris.

Schipper, Kristofer M. 1985. Taoist Ritual and Local Cults of the Tang Dynasty. In Strickmann 1981–1985, 3:812–834.

Schipper, Kristofer, & Franciscus Verellen, eds. 2004. *The Taoist Canon. A Historical Companion to the* Daozang. 3 vols. University of Chicago Press.

Seidel, Anna K. 1969–1970. The Image of the Perfect Ruler in Early Taoist Messianism. Lao tzu and Li Hung. *History of Religions* 9: 216–247.
Shahar, Meir, & Robert P. Weller, eds. 1996. *Unruly Gods. Divinity and Society in China.* Honolulu: University of Hawaii Press.
Sivin, Nathan. 1968. *Chinese Alchemy: Preliminary Studies.* Harvard Monographs in the History of Science, 1. Harvard UP.
Sivin, Nathan. 1977. Social Relations of Curing in Traditional China: Preliminary Considerations. *Nihon ishigaku zasshi* 23: 505–532.
Sivin, Nathan. 1979. Report on the Third International Conference on Taoist Studies. *Bulletin,* Society for the Study of Chinese Religions 7: 1–23.
Sivin, Nathan. 1987. *Traditional Medicine in Contemporary China.* Science, Medicine, and Technology in East Asia, 2. Ann Arbor: Center for Chinese Studies, University of Michigan.
Sivin, Nathan. 1995c. Taoism and Science. In Sivin 1995a, chapter 7.
Sivin, Nathan. 2010. Old and New Daoisms. *Religious Studies Review* 36. 1: 31–50.
Sue Takashi 須江隆. 1994. TōSōki ni okeru shibyo no byogaku hogo no kashi ni tsuite 唐宋期における祠廟の廟額封号の下賜について (On the conferral of temple plaques and ranks for spirits on temples in the Tang and Song periods). *Chūgoku shakai to bunka* 中国社会と文化 (Chinese society and culture) 9: 96–119.
Szonyi, Michael. 1997. The Illusion of Standardizing the Gods. The Cult of Five Emperors in Late Imperial China. *Journal of Asian Studies* 56. 1: 113–135.
Tao Yufeng 陶御风, Zhu Bangxian 朱邦贤, & Hung Pimo 洪丕漠. 1988. *Lidai biji yi shi bielu* 历代笔记医事别录 (Classified anthology of medical matters in the collected jottings of various periods). Tianjin: Tianjin Kexue Jishu Chubanshe. About 2000 jottings from the *biji* literature, arranged by topic; some censorship.
Teiser, Stephen F. 1993. The Growth of Purgatory. In Ebrey & Gregory 1993, 115–145.
Topley, Marjorie. 1970. Chinese Traditional Ideas and the Treatment of Disease: Two Examples from Hong Kong. *Man,* n.s., 5: 421–437.
Topley, Marjorie. 1974. Cosmic Antagonisms: A Mother-Child Syndrome. In Wolf 1974a, 233–249.
Torrey, E. Fuller. 1974. Spiritualists and Shamans as Psychotherapists: An Account of Original Anthropological Sin. In *Religious Movements in Contemporary America,* ed. Irving I. Zaretsky & Mark P. Leone, 30–37. Princeton UP.
Ware, James R. 1966. *Alchemy, Medicine, and Religion in the China of A.D. 320. The Nei P'ien of Ko Hung.* Cambridge, Mass. Translation of *Baopuzi nei pian.*
Wolf, Arthur P., ed. 1974a. *Religion and Ritual in Chinese Society.* Stanford UP. Essays on contemporary Hong Kong and Taiwan.
Wolf, Arthur P. 1974b. Gods, Ghosts, and Ancestors. In Wolf 1974a, 131–182.
Woods, Andrew H., M. D. 1929. The Nervous Diseases of the Chinese. *Archives of Neurology and Psychiatry* 2: 542–570.
Xu Fulin 徐复霖, Tian Weijun 田维君, & Wu Shijiu 吴仕九. 1985. *Gu jin jiu wu* 古今救誤 (The correction of medical errors in ancient and modern times). Changsha: Hunan Kexue Jishu Chubanshe. Anthology of therapeutic errors.
Yap, P. M. 1960. The Possession Syndrome: a Comparison of Hong Kong and French Findings. *Journal of Mental Science* 106: 114–137.
Yap, P. M. 1969. Classification of the Culture-bound Reactive Syndromes. *Far East Medical Journal* 7: 219–225.
Zhong Jingwen 钟敬文, ed. in chief. 2008. *Zhongguo minsu shi (Song Liao Jin Yuan juan)* 中国民俗史 (宋辽金元卷) (The history of Chinese folklore: Song, Liao, Jin, and Yuan periods). Guojia sheke jijin chengguo wenku 国家社科基金成果文库. Beijing: Renmin Chubanshe.
Zong Li 宗力 & Liu Qun 刘群. 1987. *Zhongguo minjian zhu shen* 中国民間诸神 (Popular gods of China). Shijiazhuang: Hebei Renmin Chubanshe.

Chapter 6
Therapy in Elite Religions

Abstract This chapter examines ritual curing by Buddhists and Daoists. These two religions were based on the use of written texts. The curing of medical disorders was important to both as a means of spreading the faith. They freely adapted techniques from each other as well as from medicine and popular therapy. Certain techniques were peculiar to each. Buddhists in the eleventh century used mantras, rituals of repentance, and drugs energized by incantations or by invocations of divine beings. Buddhists established early hospitals, and often staffed those set up by the government. They originated the notion of karmic disease, the result of immoralities committed in earlier incarnations. Laymen often resorted to Buddhist meditation or prayer for the relief of disease. All the emperors of the Northern Song dynasty patronized Daoist movements and included their liturgy in that of the state; Huizong attempted to make China a theocracy based on the Divine Empyrean movement. The state's policy of registering popular temples lessened the opposition of the Daoist movements to the worship of popular gods. Daoists' initiations made them members of the bureaucracy of the gods. They were distinct from other clergy in their use of bureaucratic documents in curing and other rites. They also employed talismans (exorcistic graphs signed with the priest's official seal). They used their powers to diagnose sickness due to the sins of a dead father or other relative and to take action against it in the courts of the otherworld. Their great rituals sometimes also had curative aims.

By elite religions I mean those that differed fundamentally from popular religion in that they depended on canons written in classical Chinese, the touchstone of the governing class, and reflected that class's ways of conduct.[1] Three of them were most important: the state cult that was the ceremonial pillar of each dynasty, the varied Daoist movements from the second century A.D. on, and the adaptations of the Indian Buddhist religion that began to appear in the first century B.C., but that

[1] Not every Buddhist or Daoist priest or monk was a literatus. Some came from peasant families, and got what education they had in monasteries; but even those with no opportunity or aptitude for language had to memorize rites that came from books.

© Springer International Publishing Switzerland 2015

N. Sivin, *Health Care in Eleventh-Century China*, Archimedes 43,
DOI 10.1007/978-3-319-20427-7_6

broadly affected Chinese society only from the fifth century A.D. on.[2] The healing practices that each offered were distinct from those of classical medicine, but overlapped with those of local religion.

Three Religions?

The old clichés about the Three Religions—Confucianism, Daoism, and Buddhism—have long muddied our understanding of Chinese worship, all the more so since Occidentals tend to assume that everyone in China belonged to one or the other. Actually, Chinese people did not believe one had to choose and join one religious organization. They believed that gods were by nature benevolent, and that some were more powerful than others. Gods who were able would help those who sincerely asked them to do so, and their potency grew as humans' faith in them increased. Most eleventh-century Chinese, when they became ill, were inclined to pray to more than one god. They were looking for efficacy (*ling* 靈), which did not depend on which pantheon their object of worship belonged to. Ordinarily, the differences between religions mattered only to clerics, scholars, and gentry enthusiasts.

Sinologists apply the tag "Confucianism" to the teachings of the master and various of his successors, to the state ideology (which claimed to embody, but which conflicted in important ways with, the Confucian teachings), to conventional standards of conduct and sentiments of the gentry, or to a couple of dozen other vague entities that they seldom bother to specify.[3] But the state religion is none of these. It is rather the sum of diverse rites of worship performed by the ruler, by appointed ritualists, or by local officials, as part of their duties.

State religious activities need to be analyzed separately. I will take up that task in chapter 7. As we saw in the last chapter, the government also regulated other religions, their personnel and their practices. The state was in principle totalitarian, in the sense that its bureaucrats believed it was their duty to control not only what its populace did but what they thought, all in the service of social harmony and stability.[4] Imperial China never had the tools to wield that control effectively. Even today, when the aim remains much the same, the Party can silence those who (in the often questionable judgment of its officials) threaten it but, despite modern psychology and mass communication, does not seem able to convert them. Like its imperial predecessors, it ignores those who pose no perceptible threat.

In imperial times, that endlessly frustrated dream of control led to edicts, laws, and statutes on every aspect of human activity and thought about it. Bureaucrats

[2] I will not discuss other religions that affected Chinese health care only in minority communities, such as Manicheanism and Nestorian Christianity.

[3] Sivin 1978.

[4] See, among other sources, Yu 2006.

tried again and again to regulate every sort of private association. Birth, marriage and death, relationships with parents, children, spouses, siblings and other relatives, friends, and associates: they prescribed the details of all these meticulously and repeatedly. They strove not only to perpetuate and improve upon ancient elite ritual forms, but to regulate the priestly performance of Buddhist and Daoist rites.

Enforcing this all-encompassing thrust was another matter. As Patricia Ebrey has put it, "Even when the state discouraged a practice, it did not do so consistently. Through its laws, its administrative apparatus, its publication programs, and the example of the throne, the Sung state unintentionally conveyed several conflicting messages, outlawing particular practices but not enforcing the laws, [and] performing both Buddhist and Confucian ceremonies for the dead .... In other words, imperial example showed how to cope with inconsistency."[5] Given the enormous population and its diversity, the bureaucracy's cross-purposes, and the social isolation of most local officials, enforcing edicts and statutes was at best fitful.

Buddhism and Daoism were two collections of disparate movements, defined by their objects of devotion. Neither was a discrete, centrally controlled religious organization like Europe's Roman Catholic church. Robert Campany's apt description of Daoism as a "loose assemblage of repertoires, lineages, ideas, values, figures, and texts" fits Buddhism equally well.[6]

In the period this book is about, Buddhists and Daoists differed in their understandings of religious transcendence, about what it is and how one reaches it. They also differed in their primary objects of worship and in the ends of religious cultivation. But that did not affect the similarity of many of their curing practices to each other, or to those of popular priests. Stephen Bokenkamp describes "the interplay of Buddhism and Daoism ... as a complex dance of appropriation and accommodation, interspersed with periods of suspicion and antipathy."[7]

Two of the Song state's initiatives substantially affected the status of Buddhist and Daoist clerics. One, from the second half of the eleventh century on, was to raise revenue by selling blank ordination certificates at high prices. The other, from 1108, was to restrict ordination of Buddhist and Daoist clergy to those who passed a written examination. In fact, one could no longer even enter a monastery as a novice without governmental approval. This was not the first time the government imposed registration of monks, but by the Southern Song period, either buying a certificate or taking an examination became the preponderant means of becoming a priest. This ruled out official status except for those who had a substantial scriptural education, wealth, or a generous patron. The new moves (discussed in chapter 5) to register large numbers of popular temples and their gods paralleled the earlier registration of Daoist and Buddhist temples and monasteries.[8]

[5] Ebrey 1993, 229–230.

[6] Campany 2005, 177.

[7] Bokenkamp 2004, 198. On appropriation, see also Orzech 2002.

[8] Tang Daijian 唐代劍 2003, 111–123.

Among the results of this crushing embrace, even before 1127, unordained priests (called "ritual masters, *fashi* 法師," like popular priests) became an increasing presence.[9] They lacked the concern for orthodoxy of their initiated rivals. An anecdote dated just after the end of the Northern Song period suggests that an enterprising curer who lacked registration could eventually find his way to high status[10]:

> In the 1130s, to the west of Mt. Bian in Hu prefecture 湖州卞山 (in present Zhejiang), there lived a devotee of the Way (*daoren* 道人), one Shen Chongzhen 沈崇真. He got hold of a miracle-working image of Zhenwu 真武, and built a hermitage there to serve it. He also knew how to use use talisman water to control demons and treat illness. His success with these was exceptional, so that the common people there called him a Realized Man (*zhenren* 真人). Later he added a temple [to the hermitage], and by buying a state certificate of ordination became a Daoist (*daoshi* 道士). [Ultimately] he had dozens of disciples who followed him.
>
> Suddenly one day there were four rays of red light shining from the back of his temple. If you looked closely [at where the light came out], there was nothing to be seen. After a week or so, Shen tried digging at [the source of] the light. He obtained a greenish stone, ten yards long and a foot thick, on which was engraved a gate of heaven and, intersecting it, an earthly pole. There were two suns, the light of which flickered. He built a niche [in which to display the stone]. From then on the faith of gentlemen and ladies was double what it had been. They worked with him to transfer the signboard [i.e., the official marker of status] from the distant, derelict Yuanfeng Abbey (Yuanfeng guan 元峯觀) to mark his temple.
>
> When Shen Gai 沈該, as prime minister,[11] was in charge of the empire (1152–1155), a memorial [from him] arranged for a new signboard that said "Palace of the Protective Sage." Since Shen Chongzhen's death, his grandsons are in charge of [the temple].

Whether Shen Chongzhen initially thought of himself as a cleric is not certain—"*daoren*" is not specific—but he was clearly not ordained. His main source of income at the outset was curing and exorcism, at which his skill led people to regard him as an immortal. They paid to build a temple and then to certify him as a cleric. Realizing the virtues of expansion, he dug up next to his temple a charismatic artifact of a kind that would make his franchise an object of pilgrimage. He was able eventually to register his temple, which required not only money but the help of pious gentry and the sponsorship of an official. This evidently happened in one of the periods of the Southern Song when the only way to register a new temple was to transfer the name of a defunct, orthodox one. As the charisma of his abbey spread, he attracted high enough sponsorship to have it promoted. The tale ends by informing us that his industry outlasted him; he had created a family enterprise.

It is often impossible to say whether a given *fashi* was popular, Daoist, or Buddhist, or whether that was a distinction that he or his admirers cared about. In another tale from the collection just quoted, the key ritual was the Great Rites of the

[9] Hansen 1990, 40–43; Kleeman 2005, 101–102, calls them a "new class of religious professionals."

[10] *Yijian zhi, zhi ding* 夷堅志, 支丁, 3: 989. For an overview of information about Daoist curing in *Yijian zhi*, see Zhuang Hongyi 莊宏誼 1999. The basic elements of this anecdote hold equally for the late Northern Song.

[11] His official title was Senior Grand Councilor (*Shangshu zuo puye* 尚書左僕射). For the dates, see *Song shi* 宋史, 31: 585, 592.

Divine Treasure (*Lingbao da fa* 靈寶大法). By the early fifth century, the Lingbao movement had incorporated elements of the Buddhist rites of universal salvation, the merit of which depended on "the cooperative efforts of a host of divine forces representing the spirit realms of diverse Taoist, Buddhist, and local traditions."[12] This story is dated in the late twelfth century, but, like the last one, it could as easily have taken place a hundred years earlier[13]:

> When Zhao Shandao 趙善蹈, [a distant relative] of the imperial family, was young, he encountered a Master Zhou of the Jiuhua mountains (Jiuhua Zhou xiansheng 九華周先生), who transmitted to him the Great Rites of the Divine Treasure.[14] When [Zhao] performed them, in most cases they were conspicuously successful.
>
> The wife, née Wang 王, of Dong Song 董松, a gentleman of Fenghua (present Zhejiang province), was beautiful and self-indulgent. She had been possessed (*ping* 憑) by a demon.
>
> When this first happened, at dusk [members of her family] saw a lavishly dressed young woman, following a maidservant who carried a dark parasol, enter from outside the house. When she got closer [to Wang] she transformed into a fine young [man] wearing a black outer robe. His speech was sarcastically joking. Wang was powerfully attracted to him. She felt "he is just what I want," so she went to bed with him. Suddenly Dong Song entered the room, got into bed as he would any other night, went to sleep—and fell out of bed. This continued for several months. …
>
> All this happened at the end of winter in 1181. Her family was quite miserable because of it. Someone told them that they should politely persuade Master Zhao to visit them. When Zhao arrived, [the wife] Wang did not appear in the least apprehensive. Zhao took a dharma-seal and impressed it on her chest; it was as though she suddenly gone from drunk to sober.[15] She said that she had just been drinking with the young man when suddenly an emissary dressed in red, holding a sword, appeared right in front of them. The young man avoided her, and then followed the emissary back from where he came. That night the demon did not appear. After three days he appeared again.
>
> This time Zhao set up an altar and carried out the ritual. He burnt incense and did the Steps of Yu.[16] He told the boys of the Dong household to watch with care what appeared in the rising smoke of the incense. It would seem that he had a technique to make the smoke reflect an image like a mirror. It gradually broadened until it was the size of a winnowing basket, and then until it was as broad as a table. Gods and ghosts and their attributes[17] appeared, and it was possible to converse with them.
>
> The eleven-year-old son of Mr. Guo 郭, a nephew of the family, saw a godlike figure with flames enveloping his body, sitting on a throne,[18] with officials and soldiers arrayed at

[12] Boltz 2008.

[13] *Yijian zhi, bu* 補, 23: 1759–1761. Cf. the paraphrase in Davis 2001, 159–160.

[14] *Lingbao da fa* 靈寶大法 is an eclectic ritual collection assembled ca. 1200. The reference here is probably to an earlier partial compilation. Daoists of different movements widely used it for curing, exorcism, and salvation of the dead (Skar 2008). The Jiuhua mountains in Anhui are celebrated as a Buddhist center, but as usual Daoist monasteries were found there as well.

[15] This is a talismanic seal, an emblem of authority, and could be applied to the body as to a document on paper. On the use of seals in interdiction, see Katz 2008 and Strickmann 1993.

[16] The Steps of Yu (*Yubu* 禹步) is an ancient ritual dance by which the ritualist aligns himself with the cosmos.

[17] *Qiwu* 器物, the material objects that made it possible to identify them.

[18] *Huchuang* 胡牀, literally "barbarian bed," was what people called chairs shortly after they were introduced into China. In the twelfth century they were still uncommon (Fitzgerald 1965).

his sides—an awesome sight. Guo[19] bowed and asked the god's name and position. It replied "I am General Deng of the Celestial Origin (Tianyuan Deng jiangjun 天元鄧將軍), in charge of investigating and summoning [miscreant spirits]." Guo said politely "This demon has not come for three nights, but all of a sudden it's here again. I request that the general quickly discipline it." …

Guo saw a soldier drag in the black-robed young man. The general shouted an order to him to quickly regain his original form. The young man hesitatingly changed into a big black dog. The general again spoke to Guo: "I hope that the master (*fashi* 法師) will send a memorial about this to the Highest Lord."[20]

The next day Zhao performed the ritual of presenting a document. After midnight, a yellow-robed Daoist master riding a white crane slowly descended from the sky, his hand grasping a written message that looked like the memorial. At the end of it were written four characters. Guo, on seeing it, asked what the writing [of this endorsement] said. The general read it: "According to regulations, he is sentenced to truncation." A sword-wielding [spirit] soldier at his side immediately cut the dog into three pieces. Mr. Dong had its original corpse[21] taken, chopped up, and thrown into a stream. His wife immediately regained consciousness.

Although the wife was not, strictly speaking, a patient, from the family's standpoint she needed therapy, and Zhao duly cured her of her infatuation.

Anecdotes about women bewitched by animals are not very rare. What is interesting about this one is a layman, after an unspecified initiation by what may or may not have been a Daoist master, carrying out a great ritual that only ordained priests have the spiritual authority to perform. Not only that, but the divine general deferred to Zhao Shandao as the ritualist in charge, and even recommended that he send a memorial to the celestial bureaucracy. Even more unlikely, it was duly accepted. According to the rules of the Daoist movements that have come down to us, all this would be unthinkable, but in the real world their regulations were no more rigorously enforceable than imperial edicts were.

Zhao's rites smack of the military ones that were becoming popular at the time. This is true not only of his calling down a general in charge of "investigating and summoning (*kaozhao* 考召)" and his retinue, but his impressing a seal on a bewitched woman was also characteristic. "The Great Rites of the Divine Treasure" were an eclectic agglomeration; the version that Zhao learned contained military as well as civil rites.

In the eleventh century thunder rites were among the popular, Daoist, and Buddhist liturgies that were spreading among the elite.[22] Influenced by Tantric Buddhism and military in style, these practices involved their practitioners transforming themselves into fierce gods who "investigated and summoned" shades suspected of causing trouble among humans, and who then wielded thunder and

[19] From here on "Guo" evidently refers to the child.

[20] Shangdi 上帝, the supreme god of the celestial hierarchy, and thus the celestial counterpart of the emperor.

[21] That is, the disinterred dog's body.

[22] Reiter 2007b, 84, has suggested that the vogue of thunder rites was to some extent due to their highly influential propagators at the court of Huizong.

lightning to exorcise the guilty ones. Some popular exorcists began using rites resembling these as long as two thousand years ago. Daoists took up thunder rites around 940, and used them on a large scale beginning in the twelfth century.[23] Officials often learned them, and used them to good effect. Here is an example of official exorcism from the same compilation[24]:

> Song Anguo 宋安國 was Military Director-in-chief of the Western Circuit of Zhejiang, and was stationed in Hu prefecture 湖州. He had not abandoned his practice of Heart of Heaven rites. [Because of this,] a family of Deqing 德清that was being harassed by demons invited Song to visit its residence.[25] His remedy was unsuccessful, and the ghosts tormented them all the more.
>
> Song became enraged. He visited a Daoist abbey in a nearby hamlet, and carried out rites of self-purification for seven days, writing talismans and chanting incantations with unsurpassed concentration. Then, using his sword as a staff and with his hair unbound,[26] he took his place below a great tree in the rear of the [victims'] home. He did the Steps of Yu, whirling about. Suddenly a thunderbolt came out of the sky. Although the tree was several dozen feet high, and it would have taken ten people with arms stretched out to encircle it, it split in two from crest to root. Several more thunderbolts struck. Every tree in the grove, regardless of how thick its trunk, split like counting-rods[27] and piled up, covering the ground.
>
> Every trace of the spooks was swept away.

The Rectifying Rites of the Heart of Heaven (*tianxin zheng fa* 天心正法) began in the tenth century as Daoists adapted thunder rituals. It was one of the earliest of the new movements that eventually swept South China.[28] The anecdote gives a sketchy but identifiable picture of its practice. This official apparently needed to prepare himself to better perform the rites he had already learned. They transformed him into a wild warrior god who uses talismans and incantations in a violent thunder rite. His destruction of the family's grove of trees apparently frightened away the shades. The account passes over the officiant's examination of the demons.

Stephen Bokenkamp has made an important point about the persistence of Daoism: it "stemmed from its permeable belief system and relative lack of organizational structure. These features softened the religion's outlines and allowed for strategies of eclecticism and co-option that assured the spread of Daoist movements, although Daoists were few, throughout two millennia of Chinese history."[29]

---

[23] See, among other sources, Boltz 1993, Davis 2001, Reiter 2007a, Katz 2008, 65–66, and Chao Shin-yi 2011, 52–59.

[24] *Yijian zhi*, "Yijian ding zhi 夷堅丁志," 4: 568.

[25] Song was in charge of the circuit's military forces. This was normally the duty assignment of a civil official. He is not mentioned in the *Song History*, nor have I found a biographical notice elsewhere. In view of Song's fairly high civil service rank, an invitation of this kind would have come only from a family of notable social standing. What attracted them would have been his skills learned in the Heart of Heaven movement.

[26] These are familiar characteristics of military gods.

[27] The rods used for computation on a counting board were sometimes flat on one side and rounded on the other.

[28] Andersen 2008.

[29] Bokenkamp 2004, 198.

It is true, by the way, that there were not as many Daoists as clerics of other religions. We have government censuses from 1021 to 1077. They show that the ratio of registered Buddhist to Daoist clergy was 23 to 1 at the beginning of that interval, and 12 to 1 at the end.[30] It is likely that the ratio became even smaller during the reign of Huizong 徽宗 (r. 1101–1126), since he issued many edicts to increase the number of Daoists,[31] but we have no idea exactly which of his measures remained in effect after his reign.

The long eleventh century was a period of unprecedented change for all three of the elite religions. The state religion was affected most by the beginnings of fundamental change in the eclectic ideology on which the state based itself, by decisive changes in the composition of the office-holding elite, by the emperors' involvement in Daoist ritual, and by the state's increased attempts to choose and register certain temples and thus gods of popular religion.[32] Daoism was altered by its proximity to the throne, and by its new relation to popular worship as the government recognized the latter. Buddhism lost some of its initial dynamism, but its clergy continued to serve the populace throughout China, and its mature forms regularly attracted the devotion and the patronage of literati.[33]

In the sections on Buddhism and Daoism that follow, I will first outline the character of the religion and developments in the eleventh century that affected the character of its therapy. Then I will describe character and development as clearly as the sources permit. Because the state's religious activities differed considerably from those of the organized religions, I will discuss them in the next chapter.

Buddhist Therapy

Buddhism, which originated on the borders of India in the fifth century B.C., made its way into at least one Chinese aristocratic circle by the first century A.D. Its scriptures were translated from the second century on, and it became widespread mainly after the fifth century. Between the seventh and ninth century it became highly elaborated, well integrated in Chinese culture, and familiar to most people. In the eleventh century it remained part of widespread complexes of beliefs.[34] Patronage and

[30] See the appendix (p. 163).

[31] Chao Shin-yi 2003.

[32] Kleeman 2005 is an excellent overview of religious change in the Song; see Kuhn 2009 for political, social, and ideological change. For a detailed account of imperial patronage of Daoist movements throughout the dynasty, see Tang Daijian 2003, 1–106.

[33] For instance, Salguero 2010 and 2014.

[34] The conventional wisdom has been that in the N. Song Buddhism had largely ceased to proliferate new ideas and spiritual practices, but for evidence to the contrary see Gregory & Getz 1999, especially pp. 1–20. For textual translation and production see Salguero 2014 and Hureau 2010.

charity continued to support its large clergy—monks, nuns, and priests.[35] We know very little about the lay Buddhist organizations and Buddhist-oriented sectarian religions that existed then but only began to proliferate from the twelfth century on.

Care for Illness

The kernel of Buddhist doctrine is the Four Noble Truths: that existence is fundamentally suffering; that the cause of suffering is attachment to desires; that one can end suffering by giving up desires; and that certain spiritual disciplines of enlightenment make it possible to do so. This was the Buddha's prescription for recovery from the sickness that is human life. Illness is one—but only one—of the many forms of suffering, and suffering is inevitable. A scripture prior to the fifth century puts it eloquently: "That is why sentient beings of the ten directions possess bodies—it is exclusively to undergo pain. That is why they are born … If there were neither body nor mind, then old age, illness, death, and torments would have nothing upon which to fasten. In the same way, a bad wind can overthrow a great tree, but were it not for the tree the wind would have nothing to pull down."[36] The long-term aim of Buddhist cultivation is to attain a life free of delusion, no longer doomed to the round of rebirth and endless lifetimes of suffering. That kind of spiritual striving was beyond most Chinese laymen, who sought in Buddhist devotion ways to live a healthy life, avoid suffering and earn a better rebirth in which intensive religious cultivation would be feasible.

Early Buddhism in the Indian cultural sphere was the work of small monastic communities whose individual members strove arduously for spiritual transcendence. Medical treatment for an episode of illness was misplaced effort for monks whose concern was curing themselves once and for all of deluded consciousness. But some doctrines urged those with healing skills to help sick members of the religious community. These monks dealt with disorders that laymen did not experience, for instance, those that arose because of incorrect meditation, and "maladies of Māra (*mo* 魔)," which projected delusions into insight meditation. These could be cured only by guidance in devotional practice. Other illnesses arose because of misdeeds committed in past lives as well as the present one.[37]

The version of Buddhism that evolved in China went far beyond this all-consuming effort of ascetics to reach enlightenment. In the "Greater Vehicle (Mahāyāna)," the strivers hoped to become bodhisattvas. These perfected beings postponed their own Buddhahood, re-dedicating the merit they personally earned to the salvation of *all* sentient beings. The compassion at the heart of the Greater

[35] The distinction between priestly and monastic Buddhism (or Daoism) is less sharp than in Christianity. I use "monk" or "nun" to refer to those mainly involved in spiritual self-cultivation, and "priest" (male and female) for those mainly serving communities of believers.

[36] Demiéville 1985, 19, translated from T616, 2: 249b.

[37] Demiéville 1985, 81–82, 85.

Vehicle led Chinese clerics to reach out to everyone in whose lives Buddhist doctrines could play a part. Curing laymen proved the power of the Buddha and his devotees, and attracted support for the monastic community.

By the eleventh century, the result was monasteries famous for treating the public, and lineages of monks who passed down special medical skills for generations. Along with methods from India, they appropriated Chinese therapies, and adapted them to religious frames of legitimacy.[38] Some establishments also educated their monks in poetry, calligraphy, instrumental music, and other skills popular among literati. These accomplishments encouraged the gentry to interact with them as peers. We learn as much about medical monks and their traditions from the writings of scholar-officials as from Buddhist biographies.[39]

The ability to cure through faith is what powered the spread of Chinese Buddhism from aristocratic courts to the populace at large, accelerating from the fifth century on. Some of those who dedicated their lives to therapy did so not as monks but as priests, responsible for a community. Both groups were driven by compassion to help people in pain who could not hope to single-mindedly pursue enlightenment. Many of them eagerly learned the curative methods of popular religion.

For the poor of China, the doctrinal goals of Buddhism were beside the point. They had no prospect of release from the wheel of rebirth. What occupied their horizons were miserable conditions of life, physical suffering, and abysmal luck. Priests could strengthen their faith, and gain their support, by offering divine protection, encouraging hope, and helping them materially in simple ways. Many of the clergy added to their repertories secular methods of health care, no doubt enhancing their ability to cure and, as a result, attracting new believers.[40]

Contributions from India

The medicine that monks practiced was partly what they had learned from Indian sources, and partly the techniques of Chinese therapists in all their diversity. Their best-known contributions to elite medicine lay in ethical doctrines, but they also influenced surgical practice, which was more elaborate in India. The very diverse religious literature included much miscellaneous information on diseases and their treatment. For instance, a sutra from India on *zhi* 痔 disorders—a term that in China refers to hemorrhoids but in this text named excrescences in many parts of the body including the nose, tongue, and ears—was quoted fairly widely after translation.[41]

---

[38] Salguero 2009, 207.

[39] See the discussion with details in Huang Minzhi 2005, 74–75, and Salguero 2014.

[40] I am grateful to Lu Zhenzhen for reminding me of this point. For excellent accounts of Buddhist healing see Salguero 2014, Demiéville 1985, Birnbaum 1989, and Liu Shufen 2008a.

[41] The text lists types of *zhi* and provides a mantra for curing them. For details see Ma Jixing et al. 1998, 783–785, and Despeux 2010, II, 977–978. For the entire text see the tenth-century Japanese compilation *Ishin hō*, 7: section 15, 174a.

The ethics of compassion for all sentient beings—not just for humans—was a central doctrine. It enjoined Chinese believers to prevent suffering and relieve it wherever they found it. This encouraged a degree of altruism in doctors—although accounts of eminent physicians suggest that they rarely treated patients in social classes far below their own.[42] The first full-fledged statement of ethical ideals in medicine appears in *Formulas Worth a Thousand* (650/659), the first of Sun Simiao's two great handbooks. It is not a code of ethics in the modern sense but, as the essay's title announces, an ideal account of "the perfect integrity of the great physician."[43] Its first part is about competence, the second about compassion, and the third about personal integrity. The middle section is such an eloquent application of Buddhist ideals to therapy that it might have been written for monks rather than doctors[44]:

> From ancient times, when eminent physicians have treated illness, many of them have used living creatures to aid those in acute danger. Although one may explain this as placing small value on animals because human beings have a nobler place, man and beast are identical in their love of life. When one injures a living creature to benefit oneself, one does violence not only to it but to one's own feelings. Is this not even truer when other people [i.e., patients] are involved? In taking life for the sake of giving life, we put life even further from us. This is indeed the reason that I do not use living things in these formulas.
>
> If you find such creatures as horseflies and leeches already dead in the market, you may buy them and use them; that is an exception. As for chicken eggs in which the contents are not yet differentiated [into a visible embryo], you may hide your compassion and use them only in great emergencies where there is no choice. [Completely abstaining is a standard] even a great sage cannot measure up to.
>
> When a patient suffers from wounds or running bowels so foul that people cannot stand to look at him and he has become an object of disdain, resolve to treat him with regret, pity, and concern. [The great physician] does not hesitate at all: that is my resolve.

Most later writings on ethics in Western Europe as well as China tend to be concerned more with the relations between practitioners than that between doctors and patients.[45] Sun's concern is squarely about the physician's attitude and behavior toward the patient. This ideal also differs markedly from the conventional emphasis on the need to treat people differently depending on hierarchy, kinship, and other social relationships. Another emphasis, not peculiar to Buddhism, stands out in this document: although technical skill is essential, the key to becoming a great physician is spiritual and moral cultivation.

---

[42] See, for instance, the listings in Anonymous 1986.

[43] Fox & Swazey 1984 have pointed to differences between U.S. medical ethics and its counterpart in China, which they call "medical morality."

[44] *Qian jin fang* 千金方, 1: 1b. For the opening of this section, see above, p. 59. On Sun's Buddhist connections, see Fan Jiawei 2007, 226–229.

Historians sometimes mention "A Plea to Doctors (*Quan yi lun* 勸醫論)" of the Liang emperor Jianwen 梁簡文帝 as a precursor. But its plea is simply for learning by assiduous practice, and its model is the poet. The emperor quotes a predecessor: "if you read a thousand pieces of rhymeprose, you will be able to write rhymeprose." See *Quan Liang wen* 全梁文, 11: 8a–9a. See also Zhou Yimou's 周一谋 anthology of medical morality (1983).

[45] Berlant 1975; Wear et al. 1993.

Āyurvēda, the Indian medical tradition that historians have neglected least, evolved early, and surgery was one of its strengths. That is not to say that Indian physicians routinely performed serious procedures, although the early use of analgesics made surgery somewhat less perilous than elsewhere.[46]

In the mainstream of Chinese medicine, physicians felt no need for surgery. They knew that violent intrusion could kill. They could affect vital processes without cutting into the body. Their doctrines of pathology paid a great deal more attention to imbalances of bodily functions than to internal lesions. When they needed to restore balance and free circulation of vitalities, they relied on various techniques, including acupuncture and moxibustion, to adjust the flow of *qi*. Elite physicians generally left such unambiguously surgical problems as broken bones to bonesetters and others of low status. By the eleventh century only a few gentlemen, as military doctors, had become skilled in the treatment of wounds.[47]

There are good reasons to believe that isolated early accounts of surgery in China mostly reflect anecdotes from India rather than local practice, although after the eleventh century there were a few original Chinese surgical techniques.[48] The Indian technique that attracted most emulation in China is using a needle to couch cataracts (that is, to push the clouded lens out of the line of sight). Chinese practiced it well before the eleventh century. This procedure could not restore vision of details, since there was no way to replace the lens. The later advent of eyeglasses brought some improvement.[49]

Approaches to Therapy

The involvement of Buddhism in therapy was central to spreading the faith. The religion's emphasis on compassion was attractive to ordinary people. In a society where few were willing to care for people with infectious or other dangerous diseases, Buddhist monks set an example. Doing so became an express matter of Greater Vehicle doctrine: "The Buddha said 'From now on, you should pay attention to sick people, and observe sickness. Those who wish to serve me should first serve the sick.'"[50]

---

[46] There are very few historical studies of Indian therapy that meet critical historiographic standards, and they tend to focus on summaries of books rather than on social practice. For exceptions see Zimmerman 1978 and Wujastyk 1993 and 2001.

[47] See Zhu Kewen 朱克文 et al. 1996, 57–61. The historical record is very sparse on this topic.

[48] Chen Yinke 陳寅恪 1930 argues persuasively for Indian origins. On neglected records of surgery through history, see Li Jingwei 李经纬 1998, 227–322.

[49] The earliest known Chinese book of Indian derivation on this topic is *Longshu yan lun* 龍樹眼論 (*Nagarjuna's Discussion of the Eyes*), of the Sui or Tang period. It is lost, but is quoted in later writings, on which see Deshpande 2000, 371–372, with translation in Deshpande & Fan 2012. Deshpande 2000, 383–387, discusses Indian influence on cataract surgery. The well-known *Yin hai jing wei* 銀海精微, attributed to Sun Simiao, was almost certainly written in the sixteenth century. Eyeglasses entered China in the early 15th century; see Chiu 1936.

[50] *Si fen lü* 四分律, 22: 861.

Some historians have supposed that in the eleventh century, as the role of the state in therapy expanded, that of Buddhism became marginal. Not all Indian medical doctrines conveyed in Buddhist documents greatly appealed to Chinese, but Indian ways of thinking about spiritual and physical health became part of medical thought. The role of compassion in shaping ethics is only one example. Even more important were the curative practices of Buddhist clergy.

Despite the Song government's repeated but short-lived attempts to expand medical education and to prohibit all but classical health care (as we have seen in chapter 4), its initiatives had little lasting effect in administrative centers and practically none in the towns and the countryside. In the eleventh century, Buddhists were an important force in health care because they were everywhere. There were Buddhist temples in every town—which could not be said of Daoism over most of the eleventh century. Buddhists were sprinkled throughout rural China, in places where no one ever saw an official of the central government. Some Buddhist clerics were missionaries, serving people far from any temple who had no other source of medical care but ritual masters of the popular religion. This was not a matter of competition. Popular priests, usually part-time, poor and illiterate, were neighbors of the sick, but Buddhist clerics had a reputation for miraculous powers, derived from what seemed to Chinese the exotic origins of the religion.

Actually, what Buddhist clerics in China practiced reflected Indian therapeutic doctrines and techniques only to a small extent. Much of their medical practice (as distinct from their ritual curing) did not differ notably from that of educated physicians. Even the taboos in their formulas did not differ from those other Chinese observed in connection with ritualistic activity: "[Prepare the formula] on an auspicious day. Avoid cripples [?],[51] pregnant women, and mourners. Don't let people prone to jealousy see it. Don't let flying birds or running animals see it."[52]

It was Buddhist monasteries that first established hospitals.[53] In the seventh through ninth centuries, the government occasionally took over nominal control of them, for a total of about forty years. While it paid the expenses—otherwise mainly supported by donations—clerics continued to do the work. In some instances the state assigned functionaries to provide diagnosis and therapy. Even then, monks still prepared the medicines and nursed the patients, and so kept popular esteem.

In the Northern Song period, there were hospitals in the capital, paid for by the state, and a few in administrative cities that individual officials coping with epidemics had founded. These were hospitals in the same sense as in Europe before 1800,

[51] *Juzu ren*具足人 is corrupt, and its meaning uncertain. "Cripples" is a guess, based on a taboo common in other sources. See chapter 5, p. 109 for another list.

[52] From a roll of miscellaneous formulas excavated from Dunhuang. Its title is lost; its modern editors arbitrarily and misleadingly call it "Daoist formulas," but it is more probably Buddhist. It is published in Ma Jixing et al. 1998, p. 761, citing ll. 14–15. These taboos are in addition to monks' dietary prohibitions of alcohol, meat, and aromatic vegetables such as onions and garlic.

[53] The remainder of this subsection is largely based on the scholarship of Liu Shufen 2008a, 146–162, Huang Minzhi 2005, 36ff., and Ma Boying 1994, 368–370. For Japanese parallels to these institutions see Saunders 1968.

that is, places for the sick to rest who were too poor to rest or die at home. Therapy was not their central function, although it was more or less available.

The most important idea proper to Buddhist medicine was that of karmic disease (*yezhang bing* 業障病). It is obvious that some people lead altruistic lives and die miserably, while others do great harm to others and expire comfortably, surrounded by loving relatives and admirers. Why are good and bad conduct not visibly rewarded and punished? Any society without a persuasive answer to that question—China before Buddhism and Daoism was one of them—can count only on convention or coercion to inspire goodness. Buddhism found a powerful answer. Karma was a principle of the conservation of moral balance through rebirth. If you were good and came to a bad end, or vice versa, the balance would be spontaneously and precisely righted by your being reborn at a higher or lower level. If the good you did was not requited in this life, you would be born higher up the scale of being—that is, the scale of opportunity for spiritual cultivation. If you were immoral and did not suffer for it while you were alive, you would be born as a lower sort of being, perhaps an animal, or even a worm. You would then have to go through countless more lives before you regained the chance for perfection that you had thrown away. Eventually, through innumerable reincarnations devoted to what goodness your place in the chain of being permitted, you might become a holy adept who was able to leave the cycle of rebirth once and for all.

These principles, which theologians spent their lives defining and improving, might seem irrelevant to the lives of most Buddhists, whose opportunities were tightly limited. But, as one anthropologist has put it, "the flip side of the Karmic law—that whatever a person does, good or bad, comes round again—provides a strong motivating force for behaviour."[54]

What, then, was immoral conduct? No two people had exactly the same convictions, but to the extent that definitions were shared they depended on some commonly accepted authority. The law represented the government's attempt to define a stable socio-political order. What was desirable and undesirable in the theology of karma differed from the state's standard in many ways.

Leprosy was a particularly traumatic karmic disease, which could make you an outcast. The infractions in a previous life that caused leprosy in the present included, among many other causes, disobeying the ordinances in sutras, obstructing the spiritual progress of others, and hindering the propagation of Buddhism. An instance of the latter occurs in the story of Zhou Zong 周宗, a soldier who in A.D. 430 deserted with five of his comrades. "As they were traveling to the north of Pengcheng, they came across a deserted temple, with no monks. In it there was an image made of crystal. They stole it and, in a village, pawned it to buy food. One of the men was so haggard and unhealthy that his comrades despised him. He alone received no share of the proceeds. After each returned home, over the next three or four years, one by one five of them became ill with leprosy and died. The one who received no share

[54] Desjarlais 1992, 82.

was the only one who escaped this fate."[55] This was a case in which the infraction and its outcome happened in the same life. One might object that the one soldier who escaped the disease did not do so because of great merit. He presumably did not acquiesce in the theft, and clearly did not benefit from it.

Because of leprosy's moral etiology, it was often cured by a monk's advising the patient to memorize and repeat the text of a holy book or an incantation, and at the same time repent his sins of a former life.[56] It is obvious from many accounts of this kind that the morality of karma favored a society that revered Buddhism and respected its aims, and that acceptance of its practices and devotions was an essential step in religious therapy. By the eleventh century, the notion that one earned merit for a better rebirth by charity—above all by donations to Buddhist institutions—had long been widespread.

I have noted that monks often studied conventional medicine. Some also mastered special therapies taught within religious circles. Certain famous physicians studied such writings with them. Monks wrote widely distributed collections of formulas, books on pulse diagnosis, and other medical treatises.[57] Before printed books became widely affordable, religious foundations or patrons had some handbooks carved on steles. That made it easy to copy them one page at a time, slowly, by making rubbings (*tuoben* 拓本).[58] Some temples, with lay or even imperial patronage, stored large supplies of drugs to distribute to laymen for use in epidemics.

Three special types of therapy characterized Buddhism: incantations (*zhou shu* 咒術); rituals of repentance; and drugs energized by incantations or by invocation of divine beings.[59] Eventually these therapies became widely used outside Buddhist institutions. For instance, the palace medical schools of both the Tang and Song periods trained incantation ritualists.

This example of an influential Buddhist incantation originated in China by 1082:

Dhāraṇī of the Great Compassionate White-Robed Guanyin

… The subtle and wondrous dharma of utmost profundity
Is difficult to encounter during millions, nay, billions of eons.

---

[55] *Fa yuan zhu lin* 法苑珠林, 79: 875. *Ming xiang ji* 冥祥記 (lost), cited in *Taiping guang ji* 太平廣記, 116: 806. Several places are named Pengcheng.

[56] The fragmentary Mawangdui manuscript that its editors have named "Buddhist Formulas, type 1" prescribes both incantations and rituals of repentance; see Ma Jixing et al. 1998, 751–752.

[57] Many of these are listed in the treatises on bibliography of the Standard Histories from the Sui on (*Sui shu* 隋書, 34: 1040–1051). The Song bibliography includes formularies and monographs on disorders and on drugs (*Song shi* 宋史, 207: 5303–5320). The earliest surviving medical book by a Buddhist cleric, *Lingnan weisheng fang* 嶺南衛生方, was not written until 1283, after the end of the Song dynasty.

[58] Unlike Europeans, Chinese reproduced stone carvings not by literally rubbing, but by dabbing ink on the back of paper that had been moistened, pressed into the image, and allowed to dry almost completely.

[59] In addition to Liu Shufen 2008a, see Demiéville 1985, 83–87, almost entirely based on Indian documents. Greene 2012, 240–244, argues that the main function of such rites in early Buddhism was to get rid of karmic obstructions revealed by Chan meditation.

Now that I have heard it [with my own ears], I will take it securely to heart
And hope I can understand the true meaning of the Tathāgata Invocation:

Bowing my head to the Great Compassionate One, Bolujiedi
Practicing meditation focused on the sense of hearing, [the bodhisattva] entered samādhi
Raising the sound of the tide of the ocean,
Responding to the needs of the world.
No matter what one wishes to obtain, [she] will unfailingly grant its fulfillment.

Homage to the Original Teacher Śākyamuni Buddha
Homage to the Original Teacher Amitabha Buddha
Homage to the Sovereign Master Buddha of Precious Moon and the Light and Sound of Wisdom Peak
Homage to Great Compassionate Guanshiyin Bodhisattva
Homage to White-robed Guanshiyin Bodhisattva

Front mudra, back mudra, mudra of subduing demons, mind mudra, body mudra.

Dhāraṇī:

I now recite the divine mantra. I beseech the Compassionate One to descend and protect my thoughts. Here then is the mantra:

Namu heladana, shaolayeye, namualiye, bolujiedi, shaobolaye, putisadoboye, mohejieluni-jiaye, anduoli, duoli, duduoli, dududuoli, suopohe.[60]

When you persuade someone else to chant the dhāraṇī, the effect is the same as when you chant it yourself.

By the eleventh century, many words and phrases derived from Buddhism were embedded in the Chinese language.

Drug formulas used with Buddhist invocations turn up in non-religious literature. Here is a formula set down by the renowned man of letters Su Shi 蘇軾 (1037–1101)[61]:

[60] Translation in Chün-fang Yü 2001, 126–127, slightly abridged and revised. "Ritual gesture" is *mudrā*, a powerful hand gesture; see Ren Zongquan 任宗权 2002, Saunders 1960 and Mitamura 2002 (which takes up differences between Buddhist and Daoist forms). Guanyin 觀音, also called Guanshiyin 觀世音, is the most widely revered of the bodhisattvas.

The usual Buddhist terms for "incantation" are dhāraṇī (*tuoluoní* 陀羅尼) and mantra (*zhenyan* 真言). Both are rare in therapeutic writing, where *zhou* or *zhu* 祝 is usual. Buddhist incantations are usually Chinese transliterations of Indian chants, or imitations of them. Incantations also appear in Daoist and popular ritual, sometimes in the same forms as Buddhists use. See, for instance, the method for familial harmony in *Qianjin yi fang* 千金翼方, 30: 360a, from a Daoist master's handbook.

In this text, "Tathāgata," "Śākyamuni," and "Amitabha" are ways of referring to the Buddha, and samādhi is a state of enlightenment. Bolujiedi and the syllables at the end of the Dhāraṇī are words imitative of Indian languages, common in Chinese Buddhist spells.

[61] Cited in *Bencao gangmu* 本草綱目, 9: 68, s.v. realgar, repeated with the differences noted in square brackets in 11: 73, *s.v.* alum. Realgar is As_2S_2, and alum is more or less pure $KAl(SO_4)_2.12H_2O$. The book ascribes the formula to *Su dongpo liang fang* 蘇東坡良方 (Superior formulas of Su Shi), which must be a scribal error for *Su Shen liang fang* 蘇沈良方 (Superior formulas of Su [Shi] and Shen [Kuo], which *Bencao gangmu's* list of sources does include. On this source see Sivin 1995d, 47 (more recent evidence supports a date of 1141/1151). The formula does not occur in the extant version of *Su Shen liang fang*.

For Poisoning from *Gu* Witchcraft[62] or Vermin

Realgar and raw alum, equal parts. On the fifth day of the fifth month, grind them to powder, melt [yellow] wax, and make [the product] into pills the size of a Chinese parasol-tree seed.[63] Take seven pills per dose. Intone "Medicine King Bodhisattva" seven times, and take them with boiled water.

The use of incantations for enhancing the power of drugs died out—so far as I have been able to find out—in China, but is alive and well in modern Japan. I have bought in Yoshino吉野, Japan (a mountain stronghold of esoteric Buddhism), digestive tablets called "pills energized by an incantation (*darani suke maru* 陀羅尼助丸)." The pills were energized by a cleric in large batches as they were manufactured, so it was unnecessary for a priest to administer this medicine.

For karmic diseases, the preeminent treatment from the third century A.D. on has been rituals of repentance (*lichan* 禮懺). These were not individual confessional rites of the early Daoist type, but more elaborate ceremonies. They were originally part of monastic discipline. Before the sixth century monks began to use them for treating laymen, and by the seventh, some laymen were performing these rites by themselves.[64]

The biography of the sixth-century scholar Yu Shen 庾詵 (ca. 455–532) specifies that "in his house he installed a ritual space (*daochang*道場) in which [monks] circumambulated in rituals of repentance that did not stop for six hours. They intoned the Lotus Sutra every day." For instance, the important official Cui Kuan 漼寬 (d. 755) "was a fervent believer in the Buddhist scriptures, and was often in touch with monks, who burnt incense and carried out rituals of repentance [on his behalf]. As he grew old he became more devout."[65] By the eleventh century these rituals had become especially prevalent among the scholar-official class.

As for meditation, elite laymen practiced it widely. Here is a poem by the celebrated Bai Juyi 白居易, written in 814, when he was 42:

In my early years, reading too much, I suffered,
In later years, pain drew from me many tears.
Unaware my eyes were hurt, I took them for granted;
When they were really ill, I knew it—what could I do?
Dusk coming on: like a lamp going black;
Morning so dark: like an unpolished mirror.
A thousand medicines, a myriad formulas, can't cure it.
All that's left is to close my eyes and learn to shake off the dust.[66]

---

[62] *Gu* 蠱, in Su's time, was a poison usually associated with women of non-Han peoples on what literati considered the wild southern frontiers of China. As with witchcraft in later Europe, use of *gu* was usually an imputation. See Huang Shijie 2004 and, for a later period, Haar 2006.

[63] I.e., twice the size of a soybean and a tenth the size of an average egg yolk. See Sivin 1968, 254, on standards for pill sizes. The tree is *Firmiana simplex.*

[64] On the paramount role of such rituals in Chinese Buddhism until the early fifth century, see Greene 2012.

[65] *Tong zhi* 通志, 178: 59a; Liu Shufen 2008a, 161–162; *Jiu Tang shu* 舊唐書, 100: 3131. Devoted Buddhists in Taiwan still carry out rituals of repentance.

[66] *Toutuo* 頭陀 is a transliteration of Sanskrit *dhūta*, "shaking off," used by Buddhists for the meditation disciplines that overcome obstacles to enlightenment (and sometimes used for monks dedicated to those disciplines). For the text of the poem, see Bai's poetry collection, *Chang qing ji* 長慶集, 14: 16a.

This is one of many poems in which Bai uses the Buddhist euphemism "shaking off the dust" for meditation.

What Buddhist laymen most frequently did to prevent and cure disease when treatment by a cleric was not feasible was to pray. One could ask for health in any prayer. There were special gods to whom people could address entreaties, especially the Medicine Buddha (Yaoshifo 藥師佛), and—as we have seen—the compassionate Guanyin. Prayer also customarily involved some sort of offering, simply incense or, often, food. A request takes on the validity of a contract only when an offering (what the law calls a consideration) accompanies it.

We can see in all these types of Buddhist therapy the pattern already visible in popular religion—and, transmuted, in modern medicine. A structure of intellectual authority, legitimate because people accepted it, defined disease in a way that maximized power over it. The individual therapist, through attentive performance of the rites now called diagnosis, could convince the patient that knowledge made it possible for him to exert power over a disturbing bodily irregularity—that is, that he knew how to moderate or cure it. The meanings embedded in the ensuing ritual, using the symbology of religion in the past or that of science in the present, could then strengthen the patient's will and ability to recover. This is not psychotherapy, but use of the meaning response to back up the autonomous or (occasionally) the specific response and affect physically the state of health.

Daoist Therapy

Here I give "Daoism" the sense best stated by Stephen Bokenkamp: "Daoism is by its own account the higher religion of China, characterized by the doctrine that the primordial and eternal Dao acts in human history both directly through the agency of its hypostases, particularly Laozi, and indirectly through a pantheon of deities that include those resident in the human body."[67] The Dao was ineffable and had no form, so priests could not direct rites to it directly. What they worshipped instead were not transmogrified shades of humans, but the Dao's emanations, three gods that during rituals manifested themselves to act as intermediaries between it and the world.[68]

Like Buddhism, Daoism was not a unified, centrally organized religion, but a number of movements that varied in aim, liturgy and clientele.[69] The Heavenly Masters (*tianshi* 天師) movement, the first, which began in the second century A.D., was a pastoral religion that supplied a theocratic social order at a time when the imperial government was ineffective. In the fourth and fifth centuries, in south

---

[67] Bokenkamp 1997, 12; see also Lagerwey 2010, 7.

[68] Lai 1998, 16–17.

[69] Kohn 2000 and Pregadio 2008 are reliable sources for the various aspects of Daoism.

China, it metamorphosed into a guild of priests. Movements after the Heavenly Masters shifted their emphasis to individual cultivation, which meant that they oriented themselves primarily toward those with the leisure to indulge such practices—and many movements sought imperial patronage.

The Northern Song period marked epochal transitions in the goals of Daoist practice, in its objects, and in give and take with popular religion. The aims of ordained Daoists, which had been either administering communities or preparing individuals for transcendence, became "overwhelmingly therapeutic and exorcistic." A new focus of religious practice became "martial, humanized, and historicized deities rather than … cosmic powers, immortals, or emanations of the Dao." The liturgy adapted much from esoteric Buddhism, and, more than before, from the practices of popular ritual masters.[70]

The Daoist movements satisfied not only spiritual but medical, cultural, and political needs. These movements were among the forces that shaped the prevalent understanding of social and cosmic reality. They put the power to affect health and well-being at the disposal of those who could afford priestly services.

In the three centuries before the Song period, we know most about the Highest Purity (*shangqing* 上清) movement, which emphasized individual cultivation. It became a hierarchic, meditation-centered system largely formed to serve imperial courts and official families. We do not know when the theocratic communities of the Heavenly Masters ended, and what role their priests ("Libationers") played after that.[71] It is likely that they continued to provide for communities more elaborate liturgies than those of popular religion, and to perform rites for families who could afford it.

Direct involvement by the state in the long eleventh century changed the balance again. All of the Northern Song emperors were actively involved in the patronage of Daoist movements, which brought the latter increasingly under government control.[72] The state took on itself the prerogative to decide which priests and which temples were orthodox (as it did with popular religion and Buddhism) and, in times when it needed the income, to sell clerical registrations. The movements that rulers favored gained greatly in power and wealth. Between 1004 and 1077 the number of registered Daoist shrines, temples and monasteries increased from about twenty-

[70] Davis 2001, 31, and Kleeman 1993, 62. What Kleeman and I call popular ritual masters (*fashi* 法師) Davis defines as "an unorganized class of lay Daoist practitioners, some living within the communities or among the families they served, others traveling throughout the villages and towns of South China, performing exorcisms."

[71] Russell Kirkland has argued that from the early fourth to the eleventh century, the Heavenly Masters movement "lost its social base in most regions, and endured only in vestigial forms" (2002, 181). Kleeman (in Pregadio 2008, 986) agrees with Kirkland that the hereditary leadership disappeared and that surviving sources are few, but points out that the movement's scriptural corpus had become foundational, and its ordinations basic, for all Daoist masters.

[72] For details, see Tang Daijian 2003, 1–52. Only the "morose, passive, and withdrawn" Yingzong 英宗 had no discernible impact during his brief reign (1064–1067); McGrath 2009, 340).

five thousand to over forty thousand.[73] Since there were fewer than twenty thousand registered clerics in 1077 and fewer before that, many of the institutions were evidently staffed by unordained ones.[74]

In the last half of his reign, Huizong became convinced he was an avatar of the Great God Who Protects Life (Baosheng Dadi 保生大帝), the supreme divinity of the Divine Empyrean (*shenxiao* 神霄) movement. He used his remaining years on the throne trying to unify politics and religion by turning China into a theocracy, with himself as ruling deity. This involved using county and prefectural schools to train perhaps forty thousand Daoist clergy for a new network of Divine Empyrean temples.[75] But his reign did not continue long enough to realize his ambition.

The very end of the Northern Song period began a further transition in Daoist organization. A variety of new movements far from the capital, mostly in the south, evolved out of popular religion and spread from their places of origin, providing new foci of worship as the empire survived serious defeats and was forced to abandon the north.[76]

Religious institutions up to that time were essentially independent of each other. Families and temple associations, not priests, controlled the temples. Links with other temples, if they existed, were voluntary. Only those sponsored by the state were organized, and their number varied as imperial enthusiasm waxed and waned. The new movements, as they proliferated, aimed at ritual curing and the religious cultivation of their members more than the support of worship for the benefit of the state. This gave them potential for spontaneous growth, and led to the spread of temples over wide areas, mainly limited by the number of priests. Finally, late in the twelfth century—after the period that concerns us—the new Complete Realization (Quanzhen 全真) movement created monasteries bound together by the master-disciple relations of their abbots, a form of organization that eventually made them dominant among Daoist movements.[77]

Throughout the Northern Song period, before that transformation began, emperors followed a policy toward ritual that gave elements of Daoist liturgy a place in that of the state.[78] Rulers patronized the movements they found most attractive. Zhenzong (r. 997–1022) wrote or commissioned some of the documents used in state rituals during his reign.[79] Huizong (r. 1100–1126)) was intensely involved in a series of revelations from the newly revealed Divine Empyrean heaven—even

[73] Tang Daijian 2003, 142. An edict of 1018 even ordered maintenance of unregistered Buddhist and Daoist temples. I doubt that it had significant results.

[74] See the appendix, p. 163.

[75] Tang 2003, 35–39, Tang's estimate. I suspect that this number is based on existing temples (some Buddhist) that had been converted by edict to the worship of the movement.

[76] On the proliferation of new movements see Skar in Kohn 2000. Pregadio 2008 provides articles on a dozen new movements, listed on pp. xxxiv–xxxv.

[77] Goossaert 2001, 114–115.

[78] See Barend ter Haar in Pregadio 2008, 1015.

[79] *Song Zhenzong yuzhi yujing ji* 宋真宗御制玉京集 is a collection of such documents.

higher than that of Highest Purity. The Divine Empyrean movement that he sponsored was meant to make China a Daoist bastion against the alien regimes to the north, which tended to favor Buddhism. Nevertheless, in 1125–1126 one of those regimes, the Jin dynasty, drove the Song empire out of the north, ending Huizong's rule and that of his family.[80]

The aim of masters and their disciples in the new movements of the eleventh century was religious salvation. Therapy, whether exorcistic or pharmacological, was a way to share the power that cultivation gave them. Hindsight tells us that what they received in return was esteem and livelihood for themselves, and increased backing for their religious order.

Although a few historians have claimed that Daoists were pioneers in scientific and medical experimentation, these judgments depended entirely on vague definitions of a disembodied philosophical essence that are irrelevant to what clergy were actually doing over nearly two thousand years. Certain Daoist adepts used curative skills for their own purposes, but claims that they were more innovative than laymen have been based on faith, not evidence. Most medical innovation we know about came from the literati, who wrote almost all of the medical treatises.[81]

Liturgy

Daoists differed from everyone else in only a few of the ways they treated illness. They, Buddhists, and popular masters regularly adapted methods from each other. Here I will emphasize the methods that, according to people at the time, characterized the Daoist movements, and that were Daoist in origin.

What most obviously differentiated Daoist liturgy from that of popular religion and Buddhism was its paperwork. Imperial governments depended on the movement of written documents up and down the hierarchy.[82] As the Heavenly Masters began to organize their religious communities in the detritus of the second century A.D., they judged that the Han dynasty had failed to live up to its mandate to rule, after which that heavenly charge duly passed to the Daoist theocrats—not to the unstable, squabbling regimes that ensued. Daoist masters adopted the paraphernalia and bureaucratic forms of the imperial government—those of prior dynasties, which was not illegal.[83] The range of metaphors that formed Daoist ritual differed in many ways from that of Buddhist rites. Those based on physiology and alchemy are examples.[84]

[80] On Huizong, see Kohn & Kirkland in Kohn 2000, 339–340, and Ebrey 2014.

[81] For details see Sivin 1995c.

[82] See among other sources Ahern 1981, 16–22.

[83] Seidel 1983.

[84] See the detailed comparison of cognate Buddhist and Daoist rituals in Orzech 2002, 218–230.

In the first couple of centuries of this movement in West China, up to about 400, diseases were manifestations, not mere outcomes, of one's own sins. One could recover only by confessing them in forms prescribed by ritual, with the confession reported to the celestial civil service by a priest. In this early example, there was no room for drugs or other therapy: "As for those who were ill, they were not to use medicine, acupuncture, or moxibustion. What they did was to ingest talismans while drinking water, and to confess their transgressions from birth onward. Those whose guilt deserved death were all amnestied. Of those whose illnesses had become serious, none failed to survive."[85]

That view of health care was the norm in the theocratic communities of the Heavenly Masters in west China between the third and fifth centuries. But after the leader of this movement surrendered to the Generalissimo Cao Cao 曹操 in 215, Cao ordered communities of Daoists relocated to other parts of China. The communities of religious practice survived into the sixth century, but they no longer were socially isolated from their neighbors.[86] As they encountered the religious lives of those around them, their own gradually metamorphosed into forms that were no longer theocratic. They eventually adopted a wide range of conventional therapies that their new neighbors took seriously.[87]

Six Dynasties documents of the Three Caverns (*sandong*三洞) movement—an early offshoot of the Heavenly Masters in south China—prescribed confessional petitions for overcoming disease.[88] By the fourth or early fifth century, the same movement was using acupuncture, moxa, and drugs. Daoist masters of other traditions also adopted drug therapy. About 500, Tao Hongjing 陶弘景, the codifier of the Highest Purity movement, edited and expanded the founding canon of pharmacognosy and recommended its contents for therapeutic use.[89]

Daoist masters wielded a variety of curative rites. Perhaps the best-known was prescribing talismans, to be burnt and the ashes washed down with water. Talismans were originally exorcistic written commands, written in fantastic characters (the language of the gods, not that of humans) on strips of paper, and signed with the ritualist's seal of authority (see above, p. 109). Ca. 1100, they became part of the state cult. When Huizong opened Divine Empyrean Palaces—that is, temples of the Daoist movement of which he was head—they included "Humane

[85] *Lu Xiansheng dao men ke lue* 陸先生道門科略, 1b–2a. Written in the second half of the fifth century, this tractate claims to describe the situation in the earliest Daoist communities. There is a complete translation in Nickerson 1996.

[86] Raz 2012, 264–265. On the complicated relationship between Cao and Daoist communities, see Li Gang 2012.

[87] See Nickerson in Kohn 2000, 256–282, for Daoist movements in the south, and Kohn in the same volume, pp. 283–308, for a narrower range of northern phenomena.

[88] There is an extraordinary assortment of understandings of *sandong* in both the Kohn 2000 and Pregadio 2008 encyclopedias.

[89] *Shen zhou zhi bing kou zhang* 神咒治病口章, p. 31b; *Shen zhou jing* 神咒經, 9: 6b, discussed in Mollier 1990, 138; Tao's *Bencao jing ji zhu* 本草經集注.

Aid Stations (*renjiting* 仁濟亭," which issued "talisman water (*fushui* 符水)" to those whose medical conditions warranted it.[90]

In the early Song period, members of the new gentry elite of the southeast were attracted at the same time to the Daoist movements and to the popular worship of their localities. The encounter of the two led many members of the gentry to revere and support local gods. It also led to new uses for oral spells and written talismans. The attitude that had long led Daoists and literati to condemn popular religion as "illicit cults (*yinsi* 淫祀)" had always been in tension with involvement in folk practices. Now the government's greatly increased acceptance of popular deities and their temples tipped the balance in favor of tolerance.[91] So did the multiplication of unordained, unregistered ritual masters who drew freely on the elements of both Daoist and popular rituals.

Bureaucracy

The Daoist cleric, unlike his Buddhist counterparts, was a member of the bureaucracy of the gods. As part of his ordination, the Shangqing priest received a register (*lu* 籙) that specified his post; what deities protect him, convey petitions on his behalf, and enable him to heal others; and what precepts, and what master, he must obey in return. One might think of it as a kind of employment contract.[92]

Like terrestrial office-holders, the priest could submit documents to the top of the hierarchy. Popular priests knew their way round in the underworld government, but Daoists had the authority to order those below them in the divine hierarchy to "conform to the authority of the codes and statutes (*ru lüling* 如律令)," and to propose action to those higher up.

Like every religious movement, those of the Daoists originally evolved from popular worship. Their bureaucratization asserted their place in the center of the social order rather than the periphery, asserting an authority far beyond that of local priests. The eleventh-century Daoist priest could petition for curing. The form he used stated the identity of the supplicant, declared the malady and the sins that caused it, expressed his client's repentance, and requested help from the relevant celestial officials.

---

[90] *Song da zhaoling ji* 宋大詔令集, 219: 843; see also Chao Shin-yi 2006.

[91] It was in the Song period that Daoists positioned themselves as organizers and protectors of the popular pantheon, and incorporated popular gods in their own rituals (Kleeman 1993, 62).

[92] There were several types of registers through history. For an overview, see Amy Lynn Miller in Pregadio 2008, I, 39–42.

The Daoist knowledge that made curing possible was deep familiarity with the divine civil service. Here is a sample from a rather miscellaneous treatise of ca. 1100 on aspects of the pantheon that one must know in order to perform thunder rites.[93]

> There are the Five Thunders, namely Celestial Thunder, Divine Thunder, Dragon Thunder, Water Thunder, and Thunder ordered by the god of the locality.
>
> … The Fire Master[94] says: Now that you know the Five Thunders, you should learn about the Thunder Court. Once you understand a certain agency [in it], when you have a request for it, it will immediately respond.
>
> … At the center is the Headquarters Office for the Five Thunders, which issues its commands in accord with the seasons. There is also a Commissioner for the Five Thunders who has sole authority and jurisdiction over the Five Thunders. Below him and under his control are the North Pole Bureau, the Jade Pivot Bureau, and the Penglai Bureau.
>
> The Headquarters Office for Thunders is one of the authorized agencies in the bureaucracy of the God of the North. Its various appointees aid in the administration of the Jade Pivot.[95] When in the world there is flooding due to excessive rain, or drought demons [at work, the administrators] request the Jade Pivot Bureau to hear the case and take remedial action. [Even] with respect to thunder axes and halberds, and rewards and punishments, there are regulations [for every exigency], with no disorderliness, in the hands of the authorities. …
>
> The Fire Master says: Of the four offices mentioned above, only the Five Thunders Bureau has exclusive authority. Although all of them are subject to regulation [from above], each of the offices has its own fierce commanders, clerks and troops, with jurisdiction over the four bureaus. Their prestige is great, not at all like the troops of other organizations. Gentlemen who are studying the true methods of worship always make their requests for troops from there. The details are in the transmitted codes; it is desirable that your knowledge include them.
>
> Positions of thunderclap gods:
>
> The Celestial Imperial Lord of the Six Waves;
> The Chief Minister of the Jade Headquarters, Five Thunders Commissioner
> The Realized Lord of the Bureau of the Jade Pivot
> The Penglai Bureau Commissioner of Waterways

This list, to be memorized, continues for a total of nearly two hundred titles.

The priest's ability to call on the correct celestial agency, in other words, depended not only on his clerical standing but on a detailed familiarity with bureaucratic structure that came from being initiated into and memorizing texts like this. That was true not only for thunder rites, but for all his powers—among them, of course, many modes of healing.

---

[93] *Dao fa hui yuan* 道法會元, 56: 2a–2b, 3b, 4b–5a. The book was compiled in the fifteenth century, but Schipper & Verellen 2004, 1107, relate the section in which *juan* 56 occurs to the Shenxiao movement of Huizong's time. For an extended translation, see Reiter 2007a, especially pp. 71–72, 75–76. Nickerson 1997, 232–233, discusses bureaucratization and enumerates other new elements that Daoists added to death ritual. See also Nickerson 2006.

[94] The Thunderclap Fire Master (Leiting huo shi 雷霆火師) is the divinity who, in this treatise, reveals the institutional mysteries.

[95] I agree with Reiter that *yu ji* 玉機 should read *yu shu* 玉樞. On the legal procedures mentioned in the next sentence, see Katz 2008 and 2009.

Let us look, for instance, at an exorcistic incantation aimed at interdicting epidemic disorders of various kinds (*jin shiqi que yi fa* 禁時氣卻疫法). It comes from the famous *Canon of Interdiction* in Sun Simiao's 孫思邈 seventh-century *Supplement to Formulas Worth a Thousand*[96]:

> I am a Libationer of the Heavenly Masters, and it is fitting that I chase out [demons] on the Heavenly Master's behalf. On my head I wear the sun, moon, northern dipper, and the five planets. A hundred thousand troops with the efficacy of pure yang (*qian* 乾) accompany me, to my left and right, before and behind me. In my body are the Most High Old Lord, and the father and mother of heaven and earth. In my left hand I grasp the tally, and in my right the pendant. What ghost will not become my servant? What spirit will not flee? What malign being will not go away? What ghost will dare to stay? Conform to the authority of the codes and statutes![97]

Just as a terrestrial official, however personally unimpressive, clothes himself in the authority of imperial government, in this incantation the cleric subdues the possessing spirits by revealing the awesome entourage that he embodies and that, when he exteriorizes it, surrounds him.

As the last line of the incantation, which regularly ends interdictions, restates, his charisma is that of the celestial civil service. The Daoist master, because he had that authority, spoke on behalf of the Divine Order in his spells, incantations, and exorcisms. "Quickly, quickly, conform to the authority of the codes and statutes (*ji ji ru lü ling* 急急如律令)," "Conform to the authority of the codes and statutes of the Most High Ancient Lord (*ru Taishang Laojun lü ling* 如太上老君律令)," and so on, were set formulas. Derived from governmental phraseology of the Han period, they invoked for the priest a legitimacy which, like that of the imperial administration, was based on the authority of the law.

The level of authority implied or expressed was always high enough to command obedience. The practitioner may state in the incantation that his methods were learned from the Sovereign Father of the East (Dong wang gong 東王公) or the Sovereign Mother of the West (Xi wang mu 西王母),[98] rulers of two of the paradises of early folk belief, or from the constellations Herdboy and Weaving Maid. He may assert that he is performing a mission for Mount Tai (Taishan 太山, 30: 5b) or for Hebo 河伯, god of the Yellow River. Hebo is a dragon with three heads and nine tails who eats nothing but disease demons and who "has issued an emblem of authority requesting [me] to

[96] "Jin jing 禁經," j. 29–30 in *Qianjin yi fang* 千金翼方. Sun's two formularies are conflated in *Daozang* under the title *Sun Zhenren bei ji qianjin fang* 孫真人備急千金方. Interdiction procedures similar to Sun's appear in the manuscript "Essential Explanations to the Hidden Regulations" ("Xuanke yao jue 玄科要訣") in Archive Schipper.

[97] *Qianjin yi fang*, 29: 16a (p. 348). "Libationer" was an early name for a Daoist initiate who had achieved a rank high enough to function as a priest. *Qian is* the hard, or pure yang, principle of the *Book of Changes*. The Most High Old Lord (Taishang Laojun 太上老君) is Laozi as a divine emanation of the Way.

[98] The usual translation of the second title, "Queen Mother of the West," is misleading. She is not a queen mother.

seek them out." The priest may describe his own mouth as "Heaven's gate" or his words as "Heaven's thunder." In meditation he can visualize and call out from within his body the Imperial Spirits of the cardinal points and whole celestial armies.[99]

Curing individuals

In the eleventh century some Daoists were treating individual patients, our main concern. A liturgical text of the Tang dynasty that Song practitioners knew outlines a sequence of rites for expelling the agents of illness. I will analyze some of the main points to clarify what they would have meant, first to priests and then to patients[100]:

> For the sevenfold rite of the vital breaths, … stand facing the reigning direction.[101]
>
> Step One: First visualize yourself as a spirit bearing heaven on his head and stamping on the earth with his feet. A five-colored cloud of vapor covers your body. … [four further steps of elaborate visualization follow]
>
> Next visualize above your head the seven stars of the Dipper, with the star at the end of the handle pointing at the spot where the sufferer feels pain. Then visualize … a Realized Official wearing the nine-phoenix hat, mounted upon red vapors of the sun. Imagine that he performs the Steps of Yü with the seal in his hand, then brings it down once on the patient's heart.[102] Next he presses it once on the patient's stomach, then once again on the place where he feels pain. Visualize the toxic *qi* coming out of the patient and rushing away. … Then recite this spell:
>
> "The spirit-seal of the Monarch of Heaven:
> When you seal a mountain, it turns to a lake.
> Seal a stone and it turns to earth. …
> Seal sickness, sickness disperses.Seal demons, demons flee.
> It overcomes the symptoms and eliminates knotted breaths,
> banishes afflictions and punishes infusion by ghosts.
> May they all flee of their own volition
> and the Realized Spirits take up their abode in you.
> Swiftly, swiftly, in accordance with the Statutes and Ordinances of Lord Lao the Most High."
>
> Then bring down the seal [on the patient's body]. … Then recite:
>
> "The woman (or man) named (fill in full name), born in (fill in) year, month, day, and hour, in his present life is troubled by (fill in) ailment and has requested me, your servant, to cure it. Your servant respectfully requests the General of the Three Divisions, the General Who operates the Seal, the General Who Cures Illness, the General Who Destroys Disease-

---

[99] "Jin jing," 29: 19b; 29: 19a, 21a; 29: 16b, 17b, 18b; 29: 21a, 30: 5b; 29: 20b; 29: 15a; 30: 16a.

[100] From *Zhengyi fawen xiuzhen zhi yao* 正一法文修真旨要 (Tang period), 15b–20a. I have abridged and slightly revised this passage from Strickmann 1993, 11–20, and incorporated posthumously in Strickmann 2002, 126–131.

[101] Directions go through cycles of dominance correlated with the passage of cyclical time.

[102] The seal, carved in stone or cast in metal, embodies an official's authority; compare p. 133. On the Steps of Yu, also see p. 134.

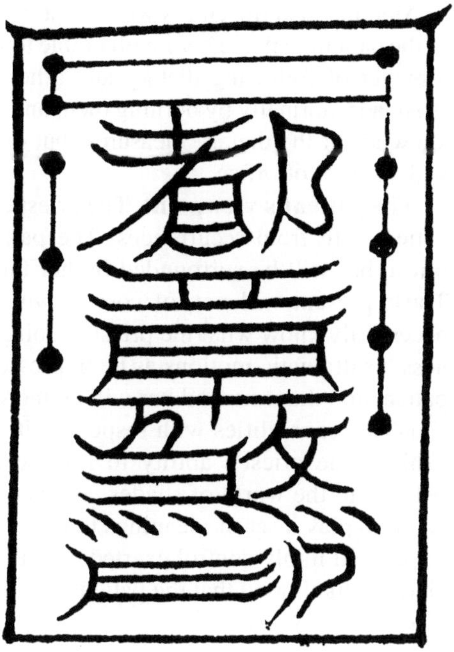

Fig. 6.1 A seal to repel demons that cause Warm Factor disorders (from *Sheng ji zong lu,* 295: 33b).

Wraiths, and the General Who Arrests Devils: all of you, accompany the seal and cure the illness, save that person from the ailment in his body."

[To invading spirits:] "Swiftly, swiftly, come out! Now, with the seal of the Yellow God's Emblem of Transcendence, I seal the heart—take it out of his heart!" … [more spells accompany the priest's application of the seal to other parts of the patient's body].

… After impressing the seal, have the sufferer swallow three or two talismans. [Note in text: A man eats three talismans, a woman two.]

In using spells to cure illness, always visualize the realized *qi* of the ten regions [as you recite the spells]. Before taking action, you should enjoin the sufferer not to consume the five aromatic vegetables for three days, or the flesh of the animals of the twelve asterisms. Indeed, all shellfish, wine, and fresh meat should be avoided. Only a very small amount of dried deer meat is acceptable. Then you may apply the seal. If the patient is unable to follow these instructions, impressing the seal will cause him harm, and do no good at all.

The priest's viewpoint. The first step of this ritual directs the priest to become a god. In that sense, based in Tantric Buddhism, it resembles thunder rites (cf. p. 198). It is nonetheless firmly Daoist in that the transmogrified master remains a bureaucrat armed with that most potent of weapons, the seal of authority (see Fig. 6.1). In the ensuing steps the priest calls forth his internal gods and arranges them around himself, orienting this array with respect to the cosmos. Thus surrounded by overwhelming power, he issues orders to end what he clearly understands as possession by malevolent spirits.

Mentioned at the end is what must begin this procedure, namely the purification of the patient to make her invulnerable to further demonic invasion. This is, as usual, a matter of following dietary and other taboos, and is reinforced by swallowing talismans, normally by burning them and putting the ashes in water. The patient may know about the dietary measures; but only a priest can provide a talisman signed with his seal of office.

The patient's viewpoint. The priest can not only cure the disorder but keep the patient safe from recurrences. The patient normally will not be alone with the priest, but will be surrounded by her family and perhaps by neighbors or others. Those present will not, of course, witness the master's visualizations, nor even necessarily know what the priest is doing; but all will hear the spells, and will witness his dramatic motions as he impresses the seal on the body of the patient. The patient and those around her will be more or less familiar with the spirit world and ritualists' capabilities with respect to it. The ritual is in effect a performance that exhibits the priest's ability to impose order on a disorderly phenomenon that belongs to the world of shades, and is out of place in that of humans. His actions call into play a set of meanings that each patient will interpret differently, but that for all will imply control exerted over the agents of sickness. Again we can appreciate the likelihood that the patient's meaning response will affect the course of the disorder.

Ancestral etiology

A particularly Daoist therapy comes from much earlier, beginning in the fourth century. Since long before that time, imperial law had held everyone in a family line responsible for misdeeds of any member. For instance, the penalty for a very serious crime could be extermination or enslavement of the culprit's entire clan. In the most severe crimes, the penalty could be destruction of his ancestors' bones—that is, wiping out the family line, past as well as future.

The new idea was that disease could result, not only from one's own sins, but from those of one's dead father or another relative. The notion of karma (see p. 210) that Buddhists brought to China strengthened this conviction. Well before Daoism, people widely believed that the dead who had not died naturally, or had not been buried with the proper rites, were doomed to long residence in a purgatory—which, with the spread of Buddhism, became a series of hells. Since as long ago as the fifth century B.C., the living saw the dead as governed by the bureaucracy of the otherworld.[103] The idea developed that resentful dead people were prone to bring suit in the sub-terrestrial courts against those responsible for their misery—people who had mistreated them or even brought about their deaths, or

[103] Nickerson 1997, 244–245, documents this view. On purgatory see also Teiser 1993.

family members who had failed to carry out the rituals (including burial rites) required to transform them into properly revered ancestors.

Daoist ritualists often explained a patient's pain and suffering as the result of an otherworldly lawsuit that a resentful shade had brought against a dead ancestor. Clergy, because of their authority in the celestial bureaucracy, could, as Michel Strickmann put it, "fight the charges, dispute the allegations, and, if possible, file a counter-suit." They could also, through ritual, annul ancestral crimes.[104]

Diagnosis meant that the priest and patient worked together to search the family's history and find the ancestor responsible for some crime. In a society that expected great devotion to parents, patients could not accuse their own ancestors of crimes, but a Daoist master had the charisma to voice such unspeakable thoughts.

This ritual, Strickmann has suggested, may have served some of the purposes of psychotherapy. Actually, the two have little in common. In early China curing normally involved families rather than isolated individuals. The modern scenario of an expert on the human mind alone in a quiet office with a patient or a group of them is beside the point. As I have argued above (chapter 5, p. 185), success in many rituals involved untwisting tangled relationships with relatives or neighbors rather than changing individual psyches.[105]

Here is a relatively simple ceremony to deal with various calamities due to a sepulchral lawsuit. This document, which has come down to us from the sixth century, is a bureaucratic form which the priest prepares by filling in the client's particulars, and then submits to the celestial administration. The source does not say anything about the preceding steps that revealed legal charges in the world of the dead, the rites that accompanied the petition, or what happened afterward. The ritual document was parallel to the forms civil servants prepared for judicial purposes.

Ursula-Angelika Cedzich has reconstructed the elaborate ritual of preparing and forwarding the petition, in which the priest read it aloud, materialized messengers from his body to deliver it, and finally visualized his own journey with it to the headquarters of the celestial bureaucracy.[106]

This petition form makes clear the profoundly bureaucratic nature of the Daoist priest's liturgy:

> Specify your priestly rank.
>
> [Petition to] send up: Now (fill in full name), of (fill in prefecture, township, and village), has submitted and endorsed a statement in correct form, in which he states that the fortunes of his house have been declining, his family has been burdened with disease, its activities have become unprofitable, and the lives of their members have become insecure.

[104] Strickmann 2002, Bokenkamp 2007; *Shen zhou zhi bing kou zhang,* pp. 32b–33a.

[105] Strickmann 2002, 13–23.

[106] Cedzich 1987; Bokenkamp 1997, 232–234.

> He has requested me to submit a memorial to resolve a sepulchral lawsuit. Now, on the basis of his statement, it is possible to determine approximately the root [of his difficulties]. I fear that [among] his seven generations of ancestors, nine generations of his forebears, and all of his relatives or kin, someone when alive committed many crimes, and after death has been subjected to various examinations and penalties. Because [the guilty person's] descendants have not redeemed him, he is left lamenting in the darkness. Or the complaint may have to do with his being buried at the site of a spring, or of [a former] temple, or at a geomantic node,[107] or someone's coffin being damaged [by the burial], or being buried at the same site as a [former] tomb, or committing a trespass against a recent burial,[108] [or] as the years and months have passed, his posterity have become oblivious [of his circumstances], or it may have to do with drowning or burning, with injury by insects or poisonous drugs, with weapons or imprisonment, with an epidemic or an abscess, or with an uncle, brother, aunt, or sister passing on an infection, with disastrous results. [In any such case,] none [of the responsible spirits] will escape punishment when [the otherwordly judiciary] judges them in the Palace of Fengdu 酆都. Because of this, I (?) will be content if the Dark Statutes extend their grace and permit the fault to be pursued.[109]
>
> Your servant [i.e., the officiating priest], consistently relying on *The Rites of the Twelve Hundred [Celestial] Officials,* as well as the teachings of the Realized Immortal of Orthodox Unity, the Ritual Master of the Three Heavens, and the rites of the Primal Ruler of the Purple Void at the Southern Peak for curing medical disorders and destroying everything noxious, respectfully sends up [this petition].[110]
>
> I request the Lord of Celestial Brightness (*Tian chang jun* 天昌君) and his hundred thousand yellow-clad troops to arrest the 120 disaster-causing demons (*yangguai* 殃怪) in [the sponsor's] house, violent presences (? *qiangyang* 強殃) inside and outside it, and the dozen murderous spooks, and order them annihilated.

The form goes on to make analogous requests of other gods, celestial generals, and their troops.

> I request that the twenty-four lords [and their subordinate] officials, commanders, clerks, and troops invited above, on this very day, come down together. In accordance with their duties, on behalf of (fill in name), let them disperse, interrogate, banish, or annihilate the disaster-causing devils. Let them also harmonize and dissolve the *qi* that infuses [the client and his family? *zhu qi* 注氣], whether [due to] a spirit deceased earlier or later, whether of the same clan or a close relative, who has acted brutally or indiscriminately caused harm to innocent people, [or who has] died far from home or who has no posterity. Whether [their circumstances] are anticipated in the eighty-one types of lawsuit mentioned earlier, or those that result from a million interrogations (*kaozhu* 考注) of spirits of every sort, let every one of them be laid to rest and made immobile, or all of them dissipated.

---

[107] The *xue* 穴 is a place in the ground crucial to the local circulation of *qi*, analogous to an acupuncture locus in a human; Bennett 1978.

[108] Here the form offers the priest an assortment of appropriate complaints to choose from.

[109] The overall meaning of this sentence is unclear. Fengdu is the seat of the otherworld's judiciary.

[110] The divinities to whom these flowery appellations belong are Zhang Daoling 張道陵 , the putative founder of the Heavenly Masters movement, and Wei Huacun 魏華存, the goddess who revealed many of the Highest Purity teachings. This petition evidently originated in the latter corpus.

The text goes on to issue threats to miscreant spirits, more invitations to gods and their entourages, requests to protect the petitioner and his family, and a promise to reward celestial officials who carry out the request. Finally, it lists the gifts that the client has pledged:

> He has turned over 30 feet of figured purple cloth, seven gallons of fate rice, 1200 coins, one set of fitted pure[111] clothing, 120 sheets of paper for documents, two sticks of ink, two writing brushes, half an ounce of cinnabar (*or* vermilion), a scholar's knife, a pure sitting-mat, and a pure turban.[112] These are to recompense the [celestial] officials, lords, generals or clerks for their assiduous, effective grace.
>
> To the Most High, etc., etc. I respectfully [petition] respecting (fill in)—himself, his abode, his illness—[requesting] that [the culprits,] whether they died earlier or later, be interrogated and taken into custody (? *kao qi zhu dai* 考氣注逮). With obeisances, I submit one petition re a great sepulchral lawsuit, etc., etc.[113]

The handbook from which this document comes gives forms for a gamut of petitions. Especially striking are the long lists of possible causes that may have been responsible for the lawsuit, designed to cover every exigency.

In a sense, a priest had greater power than a terrestrial civil servant. The latter could only beg for his memorial to be taken seriously. He could be savagely punished for a small error—or if he unwittingly offended an irritable superior. The cleric could confidently invite specific godly help, offering rewards if and when it materialized and succeeded. Such proceedings were to a large extent what priests did.

To understand the content of petitions like this one, it is important to recognize the profound ambiguity of death. Remembering the ancestors, maintaining the ancestral line, was a central activity of families. But death can also make a relative a ghost rather than an ancestor. This calls for explanation.

"Death (*si* 死)" was a much more complicated idea in ancient Chinese than in modern English. *Si* meant simply that the soul *qi* responsible for someone's consciousness had departed her body.[114] This happens all the time in sleep, fainting, and so on. Chinese today, like English speakers, often say "I was frightened to death (*wo xiaosile* 我嚇死了)," a distinctly temporary condition. People expect the consciousness of a healthy person to return in due course.

---

[111] "Pure" in this list implies suitable for use in ritual. The form actually lists twenty-three lords, not twenty-four, but discrepancies like this are not unusual. "Fate rice (*mingmi* 命米)" may be analogous to *mingzeng* 命繒, "fate silk," silk offered to the gods when praying for increased length of life.

[112] Or *jin* 巾 may refer to any finished length of cloth from a napkin to a turban.

[113] See the full translation by Nickerson in Bokenkamp 1997, 261–271, from "Da zhong song zhang 大塚訟章," in *Chisongzi zhang li* 赤松子章曆 , 5: 19a–23b. "Etc. (*deng* 等)" indicates standard features of petitions.

[114] See chapter 5, note 228.

The ancient Chinese death rituals first called the soul *qi* back. If it did not reenter the body on its own, and did not respond to the ceremonial pleas of the family, death moved to the next phase of ritual, which aims to keep the soul *qi*—now recognized as free-floating and dangerous—away. Death ritual from then on strives to settle the person's *qi* along with the body in the tomb, where it will be separated once and for all from the living. A family and its dead ancestors thus remain *only* spiritually connected. The ancestors, once ritually settled, remain benevolent, a force entirely for good. Life proceeds with the blessings of the dead, and without interference from them.

From well before this rite was performed, in a long period of political and social turmoil, members of the gentry had learned to find ghostly interference endemic, and to explain many of their troubles by it. Because such clients could afford the ministrations of Daoists, priests developed rituals (or, in many cases, they mutated rites of popular origin into their own liturgical forms). They thus restored order by re-separating the dead from the living. Their purpose is simple: to make up for the lack of the death ritual that should have been carried out, or that failed to settle the deceased due to his or his family's fault.

Peter Nickerson has nicely described the priest's aim toward the ghostly source of his client's troubles: "the invocation of the power of a heavenly ruler in order to effect the installation of the deceased securely in the afterlife, free from punishment or demonic harassment. The accomplishment of this goal would in turn prevent the return of the wandering spirit to vex the living. … Prior to Daoism, the indigenous solution to this problem had been (outside, perhaps, of the sacrificial cult of ancestors) rites of exorcism. Daoists transformed these into rites of salvation."[115] The document I have quoted shows how a priest saves a shade by massing the forces of the celestial government against the demonic figures ultimately responsible.

Great rituals

Ordained priests' main demonstrations of ceremonial authority to cure illness came in their great collective rituals. The *jiao* 醮, or offering rituals, customarily took a week or more, involved several priests, and were performed on behalf of a community or a patron to renew a quasi-contractual relationship with tutelary gods.[116] Most offering rituals were either periodic or were meant to prevent or end calamities such as epidemics or crop failures.[117]

[115] Nickerson 1997, 247.

[116] For an important study of the origins of the *jiao* in imperial ritual, see Raz 2007.

[117] See Poul Andersen in Pregadio 2008, 538–544, on the transition in the tenth and eleventh centuries from the grand purification ritual (*zhai* 齋) to the offering ritual as the main liturgical program. There are no general studies of Song *jiao*, but see the detailed analysis of modern ones, with some discussion of historical change, in Lagerwey 1987, and the documentation in Liu Zhiwan 劉枝萬 1967 and 1974.

The large-scale ceremonies were expanded forms of the petitioning rituals that marked Daoism from its beginning. Here too, the formal bureaucratic document, the practices used to forward it, and the priest's surroundings and conduct were parallel—although not identical—to those of the civil servant of an earlier time.

The medical purpose of great offering rituals was ordinarily to prevent or cure the infection of a collectivity. The priest who conducted the ceremony, as a member of the celestial bureaucracy, petitioned directly for divine action against the epidemic demons. Because of the power and elaborateness of these grand ceremonies, they were usually the most expensive form of religious therapy, and therefore were never common. Only the state, a wealthy community, or an exceptionally wealthy family could afford them. The lavish rituals of offering ordered by the emperor were, of course, carried out on behalf of the entire realm.[118] This excerpt outlines the structure of a rite from a collection of 1116:

> To expel spirits (*guishen* 鬼神) assigned to the Ministry of Epidemics (*Wenbu* 瘟部)[119]: For Cold Damage Disorders, eruptive disorders, reddened eyes, mouth sores, various ague disorders,[120] alternating hot and cold sensations, spells of madness, dysentery, and other diseases, when taking medicine has not made them abate and exorcism has had no effect. First collect information about the patient. When submitting it in proper form has resulted in an order to do so, you may submit an express memorial to Heaven above, carrying out an offering ritual [for the patient] to apologize [on his behalf], show [his] repentance, and wipe away his crime. Afterwards, give him talisman water so that he can swallow as well as wear copies of the form. The kings of the twelve years[121] will take charge. Toxic drugs and toxic *qi* will be unable to transmit [disease] to his family. You can also use a numinous talisman as well as a "covering method"[122] to [ensure that] he will never [again?] suffer from a Warm Factor Disorder.
>
> It is also essential to make a food offering to the spirit soldiers to thank them for sending the spirits of the Ministry of Epidemics far away. On the same day the problem abates, perform an offering ritual to thank heaven above and acknowledge its grace.[123]

While various Daoist movements were making their bids for imperial sponsorship, the proportion of unordained priests increased because preparing for and

---

[118] See the discussion in Little & Eichmann 2000, 189–225. Figure 44, p. 190, a painting of an imperial palace ritual in the 1720's, includes fifteen priests. For a detailed, illustrated description of ritual spaces and the objects used in them, see Huang 2012, 196–199, and elsewhere in part 2.

[119] Malignant spirits are classified here by the office in the celestial bureaucracy responsible for them. *Wen* 溫, 瘟, "Warm Factor Disorders," is a group of epidemic febrile diseases documented in *Shanghan zabing lun*. See Hanson 2011.

[120] *Nue* 瘧 is a group of disorders that result in autumn, if in summer the body and mind were unable to adjust to the seasonal rhythms.

[121] Gods responsible in turn for each year of the 12-year Grand Year (or Counter-Jupiter) cycle. See Sivin 2010, 95–96.

[122] *Gan'gaifa* (贛<with 匚 radical>蓋法) is evidently a technical term. I have no idea what it means.

[123] *Taishang zhu guo jiu min zong zhen mi yao* 太上助國救民總真祕要, 1: 5a. This source is the earliest comprehensive summary of large-scale rituals used by the Heart of Heaven movement (tianxin zheng fa 天心正法). As the book's title implies ("for assisting the country and saving the people"), it was written to attract imperial patronage. See Andersen in Pregadio 2008, 951–952.

certifying ordination was so expensive (see pp. 131–132). This was bound to blur the line between Daoist and popular practitioners. Unordained Daoists performed rituals for individuals and communities who could not afford the much more expensive liturgy of their registered counterparts. They even offered rites for farm animals; a procedure for a bovine epidemic disorder survives in the Daoist Canon.[124]

The role of Daoists with respect to popular religion

As Daoist movements evolved from popular cults, they defined themselves in opposition to them. They repeatedly condemned them (and sometimes other Daoist movements) as "illicit cults" that worshiped false gods, thus betraying their believers. But once the Heavenly Masters ceased to live in closed communities, anathematizing the beliefs of their neighbors was no longer a productive way to spread their own. Since they lacked a central organization, individual clerics had to decide on whether and how to accommodate. For the sake of acceptance and livelihood, although they never approved of popular religion, they coexisted with it.

From the eleventh century on, when the state began its large-scale authentication and registration of popular temples and their deities, Daoists could hardly refuse to accept them as respectable (see p. 103). They offered great rites to ordinary gods when that was what their clients demanded; reciprocally, popular priests offered rites to specifically Daoist gods such as the Three Pure Ones (*san qing* 三清, direct emanations of the ineffable Way.[125]

Much earlier, Daoist clergy had begun transforming especially prominent local deities into Daoist gods, "reforming" them ritually and enrolling them among guardians of the Way. This process resembles to some extent the early Christian conversion of local deities into saints. Eventually Daoists took on a stance of empire-wide oversight, arranging orthodox local gods into neat pantheons, performing rituals in popular temples, organizing temple construction and renovation, and carrying local cults beyond their original ambits. They became the "highest religious professionals tending to the common pantheon." But this new role did not develop far in the Northern Song period.[126]

The efficacy of Daoist therapy, some of it characteristic, some shared with other religious curers, and some with physicians, cannot be dismissed as useless. Nor can we validate it by the specific response on which evidence-based medicine is solely based. The value of the rituals, which their high esteem by intelligent people in the eleventh century suggests can be taken seriously, to some extent came from their ability to motivate the patient's own will to recover, which was bound to

---

[124] *Taishang shuo niuhuang miao jing* 太上說牛癀妙經, in classical sutra form. The biomedical counterpart of the disease is uncertain. For a talisman used against animal epidemics, see Ch'en 1942, 50–51.

[125] Katz 1995, 108, 175–176.

[126] Kleeman 2005, 98; Brown 1981 on Christian saints.

affect the autonomous response. But its main component was no doubt the meaning response. The charisma of the Ritual Master of High Merit (Gao gong fashi 高功法師)—that is, the ordained Daoist priest—was extraordinarily high, comparable in popular and gentry esteem only to that of high-ranking government officials and senior Buddhist clerics. (Some of the gentry despised them nonetheless.) The priest's ability to command a multitude of celestial beings against the demonic causes of illness vastly decreased people's terror. So did his ability to intervene in the law courts of the otherworld, and to metamorphose himself into a powerful god ready to interrogate and punish troublesome shades. People usually called upon him only when the popular priest's rites had failed. Because he was an outsider, and more powerful, and his ceremonies grander in scope, his services were considerably more expensive. The talismans he used were empowered by his seal of authority in the divine bureaucracy.

A thousand years after the Northern Song period, we cannot hope to measure the therapeutic success of elite clerical curers—or of any other kind. But their ability to support the autonomous response and invoke the meaning response is worth thinking about. There is something that we can learn from them not only about Chinese culture but about how physicians today can make better use of long-established strengths that evidence-based practice, as a matter of high-minded principle, ignores.

Appendix. Ratio of Buddhist and Daoist Clergy

Essential Documents and Regulations of the Song Period contains several censuses by province of government-registered clergy.[127] This table aggregates the figures:

A	B	C	D	E	F	G	H
960	Taizu			[67403]			
1021	Zhenzong	19606	731	397615	61239	479191	23:1
1034	Renzong	19538	588	385520	48742	454389	22:1
1042	Renzong	19680	582	348108	48417	416787	20:1
1068	Shenzong	18746	638	227061	34037	280482	13:1
[128]1075	Shenzong			203512			
[129]1077	Shenzong	18513	708	202872	29692	251785	12:1

A = year; B = ruler; C= Daoist priests; D = Daoist nuns; E = Buddhist priests; F = Buddhist nuns; G = Total clergy; H = Ratio of Buddhists to Daoists

---

[127] *Song hui yao ji gao. Dao shi* 宋會要輯稿.道釋, "Daoshi 1, appendix": 618–619. This document also gives regional numbers. The figure for 960, the first year of the N. Song, is a combined count of Buddhist priests and nuns. At this time many areas of what later became Northern Song lands were not yet under government control.

[128] This figure is given separately on p. 621.

[129] This figure is confirmed by a report on p. 621, but the latter is not necessarily independent.

These figures include only clergy recognized by the government and included in required periodic reports from the localities. They provide no information at all about unordained clergy or popular priests.

The table reveals two facts that have not played a role in previous scholarship on the Northern Song dynasty: first, registered Buddhist clergy greatly outnumbered Daoists; second, the ratio shrank from 23 : 1 in 1021 to 12 : 1 in 1077. It is disappointing that we do not have comparable figures for the reign of Huizong, whose involvement in Daoism was even deeper than that of his forbears. Since he established government schools to train Daoists on a large scale for the new temples he established, converted some Buddhist priests and returned others to the laity, the proportion no doubt changed even more—but this happened too late in his reign to last. Another intriguing datum has survived for the years 1075–1077. In those three years, the bureau in charge of registering clergy distributed (in some cases, sold) an empire-wide total of 26,865 ordination certificates for Daoist and Buddhist priests and nuns. This figure is not comparable to those in the table, which come from local censuses.[130]

References

Abbreviations

DZ = Volume number in *Daozang*
ES = *Ersishi shi* 二十四史 of Zhonghua Shuju, 1959–1977.
HY = text in Harvard-Yenching Concordance series
j. = *juan* 卷 (chapter)
RW = published by Renmin Weisheng Chubanshe 人民衛生出版社, Beijing
S = Title number in Schipper 1975
SQ = Siku quanshu 四庫全書
SV = Schipper & Verellen 2004
T = *Taishō shinshū Daizōkyō* 大正新修大藏經
UP = University Press
YZ = Yi tong zheng mai quan shu 醫統正脈全書
ZD = Volume, item, *juan,* and page numbers in *Zhonghua daozang* 中华道藏
ZS = published by Zhonghua shuju 中華書局, Beijing
ZZ = Zhongyi zhenben congshu 中醫珍本叢書 ed.

[130] Pp. 636–637. There were 9108 in 1075, 8364 in 1076, and 9393 in 1077. At the same time, the government was periodically returning clergy, largely Buddhist, to secular life (pp. 621–648).

Classical Chinese Sources

Bei ji qian jin yao fang 備急千金要方 (Revised formulas worth a thousand, for every urgent need). Sun Simiao 孫思邈. 650/659. Taipei: Guoli Zhongyao Yanjiusuo reproduction of Edo Igaku ed. of 1849.

Bencao gangmu 本草綱目 (Systematic materia medica). Li Shizhen 李時珍. Compiled 1552–1593, printed 1596. Commercial Press reprint, 1959.

Chang qing ji 長慶集 (Collected poems). Bai Juyi 白居易. 825. SQ.

Chisongzi zhang li 赤松子章曆 (Petition almanac of the Red Pine Master). Anonymous. Early fourth/sixth century. S615, DZ335–336. A manual of petitions for use by Heavenly Masters clerics.

Dao fa hui yuan 道法會元 (Daoist methods: the principles collected). Compiled by Zhao Yizhen 趙宜真. Ca. 1450. S1220, DZ 884–941. A large collection of Qingwei rituals. On probable time of compilation, see SV 1106.

Fa yuan zhu lin 法苑珠林 (Grove of Jewels in the Garden of the Law). Daoshi 道世. 668. T2122.

Jin jing 禁經 (Canon of interdiction). Anonymous. Before late seventh century. In *Qian jin yi fang*, j. 29–30.

Jiu Tang shu 舊唐書 (Old history of the Tang period). Liu Xu 劉昫. 945. ES.

Lingbao da fa 靈寶大法. See *Lingbao wuliang duren shangjing dafa.*

Lingbao wuliang duren shangjing dafa 靈寶無量度人上經大法 (Lingbao upper scripture: Great method for limitlessly saving people). Anonymous. Ca. 1200. S219, DZ 85–99. See SV 1028.

Longshu yan lun 龍樹眼論 (Nagarjuna's discussions of the eyes). Anonymous. Sui or Tang period. Lost. See Okanishi 1958, 448–449. See Deshpande 2000 and Deshpande & Fan 2012.

Lu Xiansheng dao men ke lue 陸先生道門科略 (Abridged codes of Master Lu for Daoist communities). Attributed to Lu Xiujing 陸修靜. Late fifth century. S761, DZ1127.

Qian jin fang 千金方. See *Bei ji qian jin yao fang.*

Shen zhou zhi bing kou zhang 神咒治病口章. See *Taishang dongshen dongyuan shen zhou zhi bing kou zhang.*

Sifen lü 四分律 (Dharmaguptaka Vinaya, lit., Four-part community regulations). Anonymous Indian author, translated in early 5th century by Buddhayaśas. T1428.

Song da zhaoling ji 宋大詔令集 (Unabridged collection of edicts and commands of the Song period). Anonymous. 1131–1162. ZS 1962 ed. Medical data collected in Han Yi 韓毅 2007.

Song hui yao ji gao. Dao shi 宋會要輯稿.道釋 (Draft reconstituted edition of the *Essential Documents and Regulations of the Song Period.* Section on Daoists and Buddhists). Xu Song 徐松. Early Ming period. In *Song hui yao ji gao. Fanyi dao shi* 宋會要輯稿.蕃夷道釋. Chengdu: Sichuan Daxue Chubanshe, 2010. Gathered from various Song compilations covering up to 1220.

Song Zhenzong yuzhi yujing ji 宋真宗御制玉京集 (Jade capital collection, by emperor Zhenzong of the Song period). Before 1022. S315, DZ 163, ZD, 44/060, 5: 581. Collected statements of intention (*yi* 意) for use in Daoist rituals.

Su Shen liang fang 蘇沈良方 (Superior formulas by Su & Shen). Su Shi 蘇軾 & Shen Kuo 沈括. Anonymously compiled, 1141/1151. Combines Shen's *Liang fang* with some unpublished medical writings by Su. In *Zhi buzu zhai congshu* 知不足齋叢書.

Taishang dongshen dongyuan shen zhou zhi bing kou zhang 太上洞神洞淵神咒治病口章 (Oral petitions for the healing of medical disorders, a scripture of the Divine Incantations of the Cavern Spirit and the Cavern Abyss of the Most High). Anonymous. Probably early fifth century A.D. S 1290, DZ 1008.

Taishang shuo niuhuang miao jing 太上說牛黃妙經 (Wondrous sutra of the Most High on *niuhuang*). Anonymous. Date unknown. S366, DZ 180. See SV 960. Not cited in Despeux 2010.

Taishang zhu guo jiu min zong zhen mi yao 太上助國救民總真祕要 (Secret essentials, comprehensive and realized, of the Most High, for assisting the country and saving the people). Yuan Miaozong 元妙宗. 1116. S1227, DZ 986–987.

Tong zhi 通志 (General history). Zheng Qiao 鄭樵. Presented to throne 1161. Sibu congkan ed.

Yijian zhi 夷堅志 (Records of the listener). By Hong Mai 洪邁. Written over the period 1157–1202. 4 vols. ZS, 1981. Only 207 of the original 420 j. survive.

Zhengyi fawen xiuzhen zhi yao 正一法文修真旨要 (Essentials of the Practice of Realization, from the Correct Unity Ritual Canon). Anonymous. Tang period. S1270, DZ1003. On diagnosis and exorcistic therapy using a carved seal.

Other Sources

Ahern, Emily M. 1981. *Chinese Ritual and Politics.* Cambridge Studies in Social Anthropology, 34. Cambridge UP.

Andersen, Poul. 2008. Tianxin zhengfa 天心正法. In Pregadio 2008, 2:989–993.

Anonymous. 1986. *Ershiliushi yijia zhuanji xin zhu* 二十六史医家传纪新注 (New annotations to the biographies of physicians in the 26 Histories). Shenyang: Liaoning Daxue Chubanshe.

Baldrian-Hussein, Farzeen. 2008. *Hun* and *Po.* In Pregadio 2008, 521–523.

Bennett, Steven J. 1978. Patterns of the Sky and Earth: A Chinese Science of Applied Cosmology. *Chinese Science* 3: 1–26.

Berlant, Jeffrey. 1975. *Profession and Monopoly: A Study of Medicine in the United States and Great Britain.* Berkeley: University of California Press.

Birnbaum, Raoul. 1989. Chinese Buddhist Traditions of Healing and the Life Cycle. In *Healing and Restoring: Health and Medicine in the World's Religious Traditions,* ed. Lawrence E. Sullivan, 33–57. New York: Macmillan.

Bokenkamp, Stephen R. 1997. *Early Daoist Scriptures.* Taoist Classics, 1. Berkeley: University of California Press.

Bokenkamp, Stephen R. 2004. Daoism and Buddhism. In *Encyclopedia of Buddhism,* ed. Robert E. Buswell, Jr., 197–201. New York : Macmillan Reference USA/Thomson/Gale.

Bokenkamp, Stephen R. 2007. *Ancestors and Anxiety: Daoism and the Birth of Rebirth in China.* Berkeley: University of California Press.

Boltz, Judith Magee. 1993. Not by the Seal of Office Alone. New Weapons in Battles with the Supernatural. In Ebrey & Gregory 1993, 241–305.

Boltz, Judith M[agee]. 2008. Pudu. 2. The Ritual. In Pregadio 2008, 2:794.

Brown, Peter. 1981. *The Cult of the Saints. Its Rise and Function in Latin Christianity.* University of Chicago Press.

Campany, Robert Ford. 2005. Two Religious Thinkers of the Early Eastern Jin: Gan Bao and Ge Hong in Multiple Contexts. *Asia Major,* ser. 3, 18.1: 175–224.

Cedzich, Ursula-Angelika. 1987. *Das Ritual der Himmelsmeister im Spiegel früher Quellen. Übersetzung und Untersuchung des liturgischen Materials im dritten chüan des Teng-chen yin-chüeh.* Würzburg: The author.

Chao, Shin-yi. 2003. Daoist Examinations and Daoist Schools during the Northern Song Dynasty. *Journal of Chinese Religions* 31: 1–37.

Chao, Shin-yi. 2006. Huizong and the Divine Empyrean Palace Temple Network. In Ebrey & Bickford 2006, 324–358.

Chao, Shin-yi. 2011. *Daoist Ritual, State Religion, and Popular Practices: Zhenwu Worship from Song to Ming (960–1644).* Routledge Studies in Daoism. New York: Routledge.

Ch'en Hsiang-ch'un. 1942. Examples of Charm against Epidemics with Short Explanations. *Folklore Studies,* 1: 37–54.

Chen Yinke 陳寅恪. 1930. *Sanguo zhi* Cao Chong Hua Tuo yu Fojiao gushi 三國志曹沖華佗與佛教故事 (The biographies of Cao Chong and Hua Tuo in the *History of the Three Kingdoms*, and Buddhist legends). *Qinghua xuebao* 清華學報 6. 1: 17–20.

Chiu, Kaiming (Qiu Kaiming). 1936. The Introduction of Spectacles into China. *Harvard Journal of Asiatic Studies* 1: 186–193.

Davis, Edward L. 2001. *Society and the Supernatural in Song China.* Honolulu. University of Hawai'i Press.

Demiéville, Paul. 1985. *Buddhism and healing: Demiéville's article Byô from Hôbôgirin,* trans. Mark Tatz. Lanham, MD: University Press of America.

Deshpande, Vijaya. 2000. Ophthalmic Surgery: a Chapter in the History of Sino-Indian Medical Contacts. *Bulletin of the School of Oriental and African Studies* 63. 3: 370–388.

Deshpande, Vijaya, & Fan Ka Wai. 2012. *Restoring the Dragon's Vision (Nagarjuna and Medieval Chinese Opthalmology).* Hong Kong: Chinese Civilization Centre, City University of Hong Kong. Translates three ophthalmic texts related to India, with indexes.

Desjarlais, Robert R. 1992. *Body and Emotion. The Aesthetics of Illness and Healing in the Nepal Himalayas.* Series in Contemporary Ethnology, 2. Philadelphia: University of Pennsylvania Press.

Despeux, Catherine, ed. 2010. *Médecine, religion et société dans la Chine médiévale. Étude de manuscripts chinois de Dunhuang et de Turfan.* 3 vols. Paris: Institute des Hautes Études Chinoises.

Ebrey, Patricia Buckley. 2014. *Emperor Huizong.* Harvard UP.

Ebrey, Patricia Buckley, & Maggie Bickford. 2006. *Emperor Huizong and Late Northern Song China. The Politics of Culture and the Culture of Politics.* Harvard East Asian Monographs, 266. Harvard University Press.

Ebrey, Patricia Buckley, & Peter N. Gregory, eds. 1993. *Religion and Society in T'ang and Sung China.* Honolulu: University of Hawaii Press.

Fan Jiawei 范家偉. 2007. *Da yi jing cheng. Tangdai guojia, xinyang yu yixue* 大醫精誠. 唐代國家, 信仰與醫學 (The perfect integrity of the great physician. State, belief, and medicine in the Tang dynasty). Yangsheng fangji congshu 養生方技叢書. Taipei: Dong Da Tushu Gongsi.

Fitzgerald, C. P. 1965. *Barbarian Beds: The Origin of the Chair in China.* London: Cresset Press.

Fox, Renée, & Judith P. Swazey. 1984. Medical Morality is not Bioethics—Medical Ethics in China and the United States. *Perspectives in Biology and Medicine* 27. 3: 336–360.

Goossaert, Vincent. 2001. The Invention of an Order: Collective Identity in Thirteenth-century Quanzhen Taoism. *Journal of Chinese Religions* 29: 111–138.

Greene, Eric. 2012. Meditation, Repentance, and Visionary Experience in Early Medieval Chinese Buddhism. Ph. D. dissertation, Buddhist Studies, University of California, Berkeley.

Gregory, Peter N., & Daniel A. Getz, Jr., eds. 1999. *Buddhism in the Sung.* Studies in East Asian Buddhism, 13. Honolulu: University of Hawai'i Press

Haar, Barend J. ter. 2006. *Telling Stories. Witchcraft and Scapegoating in Chinese History.* Leiden: E. J. Brill.

Hansen, Valerie. 1990. *Changing Gods in Medieval China, 1127–1276.* Princeton UP.

Hanson, Marta. 2011. *Speaking of Epidemics in Chinese Medicine. Disease and the Geographic Imagination in Late Imperial China.* Needham Research Institute Series, 9. London: Routledge.

Huang Minzhi 黄敏枝. 2005. Songdai de sengren yu yiliao 宋代的僧人與醫療 (Buddhist monks and medical therapy in the Song period). In Zhang Xueming & Liang Yuansheng 2005, 26–78.

Huang, Shih-shan Susan. 2012. *Picturing the True Form. Daoist Visual Culture in Traditional China.* Harvard East Asian Monographs, 342. Cambridge, MA: Harvard University Asia Center.

Huang Shijie 黄世杰. 2004. *Gu du. Caifu yu quanli de huanjue. Nanfang minzu shiyong chuantong duyao yu jieyao de renleixue yanjiu* 蠱毒: 财富与权利的幻学. 南方民族使用传统毒药与解药的人类学研究 *(Gu* poisoning: The magic of wealth and power. An anthropological study of the use of poisons and antidotes by southern Chinese peoples). Nanning: Guangxi Minzu Chubanshe.

Hureau, Sylvie. 2010. Translations, Apocrypha, and the Emergence of the Buddhist Canon. In Lagerwey & Lü 2010, 741–774.

Katz, Paul R. 1995. *Demon Hordes and Burning Boats. The Cult of Marshal Wen in Late Imperial Chekiang.* Albany: State University of New York Press.
Katz, Paul R. 2008. Trial by Power: Some Preliminary Observations on the Judicial Roles of Taoist Martial Deities. *Journal of Chinese Religions* 36: 54–83.
Kirkland, Russell. 2002. The History of Taoism: A New Outline. Research Note. *Journal of Song–Yuan Studies* 30: 177–193.
Kleeman, Terry F. 1993. The Expansion of the Wen-ch'ang Cult. In Ebrey & Gregory 1993, 45–73.
Kleeman, Terry. 2005. The Evolution of Daoist Cosmology and the Construction of the Common Sacred Realm. *Taiwan Journal of East Asian Studies* 2. 1: 89–110.
Kohn, Livia. 2000. *Daoism Handbook.* Handbook of Oriental Studies, section 4, vol. 14. Leiden: Brill.
Kohn, Livia, & Harold D. Roth, eds. 2002. *Daoist Identity: History, Lineage and Ritual.* Honolulu: University of Hawai'i Press.
Kuhn, Dieter. 2009. *The Age of Confucian Rule. The Song Transformation of China.* History of Imperial China. Belknap Press of Harvard UP.
Lagerwey, John. 1987. *Taoist Ritual in Chinese Society and History.* New York: Macmillan.
Lagerwey, John. 2010. *China. A Religious State.* Hong Kong UP. Four lectures.
Lagerwey, John, & Lü Pengzhi, eds. 2010. Early Chinese Religion. Part Two: The Period of Disunion (220–589 AD). Handbook of Oriental Studies, section 4, vols. 21–22. Leiden: Brill.
Lai, Chi Tim [Li Chih-t'ien 黎志添]. 1998. The Opposition of Celestial-master Taoism to Popular Cults during the Six Dynasties. *Asia Major* (Taipei), ser. 3, 11. 1: 1–20.
Li Gang. 2012. Cao Cao and Taoism. In Mou Zhongjian 2012, 101–117.
Li Jingwei 李经纬. 1998. Shi lun Zhongguo gudai waike shoushu 试论中国古代之外科手术 (Essay on surgery in ancient China). In Li Jingwei 李经纬, *Zhongguo yixue zhi huihuang. Li Jingwei wen ji* 中国医学之辉煌. 李经纬文集 (The glory of Chinese medicine. Collected essays of Li Jingwei), 298–301. Beijing: Zhongguo Zhongyiyao Chubanshe.
Liang Jun 梁峻. 1995. Zhongguo gudai yizheng shi lue 中国古代医政史略 (Outline history of ancient Chinese medical administration). Hohhot: Neimenggu Renmin Chubanshe.
Little, Stephen, & Shawn Eichmann. 2000. *Taoism and the Arts of China.* The Art Institute of Chicago. Catalogue of exhibition, Nov. 2000–Jan 2001, with essays by specialists.
Liu Shufen 劉淑芬. 2008a. Tang Song shi sengren, guojia he yiliao de guanxi: Cong Yaofang dong dao Huimin ju 唐宋時僧人國家和醫療的關係: 從藥方洞到惠民局 (Buddhist monks, the state, and medical therapy in the Tang and Song periods. From Formulary Cave to the Bureau for Benefiting the People). In Li Jianmin 2008, 145–202.
Liu Zhiwan 劉枝萬. 1967. *Taibei Songshan qi an jian jiao jidian* 臺北松山祈安建醮祭典 (Great propitiatory rites of petition for beneficence at Songshan, Taipei, Taiwan). Institute of Ethnology, Academia Sinica, Monographs, 14. Nankang: Academia Sinica.
Liu Zhiwan 劉枝萬. 1974a. *Zhongguo minjian xinyang lun ji* 中國民間信仰論集 (Essays on Chinese Folk Belief and Folk Cults). Institute of Ethnology, Academia Sinica, Monographs, 22. Nankang: Academia Sinica.
Lopez, Donald S., Jr. 1996. Religions of China in Practice. Princeton Readings in Religions. Princeton UP.
Ma Boying 马伯英. 1994/2010. *Zhongguo yixue wenhua shi* 中国医学文化史 (A history of medicine in Chinese culture). 2d ed. 2 vols. Shanghai Renmin Chubanshe.
Ma Jixing 馬繼興 et al. 1998. *Dunhuang yiyao wenxian ji jiao* 敦煌醫藥文獻輯校 (Collected collations of the medical texts from Dunhuang). Dunhuang wenxian fen lei lu jiao congkan 敦煌文獻分類錄校叢刊. Nanjing: Jiangsu Guji Chubanshe.
McGrath, Michael. 2009. The Reigns of Jen-tsung (1022–1063) and Ying-tsung (1063–1067). In *The Cambridge History of China.* Vol. 5, part 1. *The Sung Dynasty and its Precursors,* 279–346. Cambridge UP.
Mitamura, Keiko. 2002. Daoist Hand Signs and Buddhist Mudras. In Kohn & Roth 2002, 235–255. On symbolic gestures.
Mollier, Christine. 1990. *Une apocalypse taoïste du Ve siècle. Le livre des incantations divines des grottes abyssales.* Mémoires de l'Institut des Hautes Études Chinoises, 31. Paris: L'Institut.

Mou Zhongjian, ed. 2012. Taoism, ed. and tr. Pan Junliang & Simone Normand, Religious Studies in Contemporary China Collection, 2. Boston: Brill, 2012. Surveys and research papers from Chinese scholars.
Nickerson, Peter. 1996. Abridged Codes of Master Lu for the Daoist Community. In Lopez 1996, 347–359.
Nickerson, Peter. 1997. The Great Petition for Sepulchral Plaints. In *Early Daoist Scriptures,* ed. Stephen R. Bokenkamp, 230–74. Berkeley: University of California Press.
Nickerson, Peter. 2006. 'Let Living and Dead Take Separate Paths.' Bureaucratisation and Textualisation in Early Chinese Mortuary Ritual. In Penny 2006, 10–40.
Orzech, Charles D. 2002. *Fang yankou* and *Pudu:* Translation, Metaphor, and Religious Identity. In Kohn & Roth 2002, 213–234.
Penny, Benjamin, ed. 2006. Daoism in History. Essays in Honour of Liu Ts'un-yan. London: Routledge.
Pregadio, Fabrizio, ed. 2008. *The Encyclopedia Of Taoism*. 2 vols. New York: Routledge.
Raz, Gil. 2007. Imperial Efficacy: Debates on Imperial Ritual in Early Medieval China and the Emergence of Daoist Ritual Schemata. In Reiter 2007b, 83–109.
Raz, Gil. 2012. *The Emergence of Daoism. Creation of Tradition.* Routledge Studies in Taoism. London: Routledge.
Reiter, Florian C., ed. 2007a. *Basic Conditions of Taoist Thunder Magic.* Abhandlungen für die Kunde des Morgenlandes, 61. Wiesbaden: Harrassowitz.
Reiter, Florian C., ed. 2007b. *Purposes, Means and Convictions in Daoism. A Berlin Symposium.* Humboldt Universiteit Asien- und Afrika-Studien, 29. Wiesbaden: Harrassowitz.
Ren Zongquan 任宗权. 2002. *Daojiao shouyin yanjiu* 道教手印研究 (Studies of Daoist symbolic gestures). Beijing: Daojiao Wenhua Chubanshe.
Salguero, C. Pierce. 2009. The Buddhist Medicine King in Literary Context: Reconsidering an Early Medieval Example of Indian Influence on Chinese Medicine and Surgery. *History of Religions* 48. 3: 183–210.
Salguero, C. Pierce. 2010. 'A Flock of Ghosts Bursting Forth and Scattering': Healing Narratives in a Sixth-century Chinese Buddhist Hagiography. EASTM 32: 89–120.
Salguero, C. Pierce. 2014. *Translating Buddhist Medicine in Medieval China.* Encounters with Asia. Philadelphia: University of Pennsylvania Press.
Saunders, E. Dale. 1960. *Mudrā. A Study of Symbolic Gestures in Japanese Buddhist Sculpture.* Bollingen series, 58. New York: Pantheon Books.
Saunders, E. Dale. 1968. Notions of Medicine in Early Japan. In *Symposium on Chinese Studies Commemorating the Golden Jubilee of the University of Hong Kong,* 3:82–109.
Schipper, Kristofer, & Franciscus Verellen, eds. 2004. *The Taoist Canon. A Historical Companion to the* Daozang. 3 vols. University of Chicago Press.
Seidel, Anna. 1983. Imperial Treasures and Taoist Sacraments. Taoist Roots in the Apocrypha. In Strickmann 1981–1985, 2:291–371.
Sivin, Nathan. 1968. *Chinese Alchemy: Preliminary Studies.* Harvard Monographs in the History of Science, 1. Harvard UP.
Sivin, Nathan. 1978. On the Word Taoism as a Source of Perplexity. With Special Reference to the Relations of Science and Religion in Traditional China. *History of Religions* 17: 303–330.
Sivin, Nathan. 1995a. *Medicine, Philosophy and Religion in Ancient China. Researches and Reflections.* Variorum Collected Studies Series. Aldershot: Variorum.
Sivin, Nathan. 1995c. Taoism and Science. In Sivin 1995a, chapter 7.
Sivin, Nathan. 1995d. Shen Kua (1031–1095). In *Science in Ancient China. Researches and Reflections,* chapter 3, 1–53. Variorum Collected Studies Series. Aldershot, Hants: Variorum.
Sivin, Nathan. 2010. Old and New Daoisms. *Religious Studies Review* 36. 1: 31–50.
Skar, Lowell. 2008. Lingbao dafa 靈寶大法. In Pregadio 2008, 671–672.
Strickmann, Michel, ed. 1981–1985. *Tantric and Taoist Studies in Honour of R. A. Stein.* 3 vols. Brussels: Institut Belge des Hautes Études Chinoises.
Strickmann, Michel. 1993. The Seal of the Law: a Ritual Implement and the Origins of Printing. *Asia Major,* ser. 3, 6. 2: 1–83.

Strickmann, Michel. 2002. *Chinese Magical Medicine*, ed. Bernard Faure. Asian Religions and Cultures. Stanford: Stanford UP. Posthumous.

Tang Daijian 唐代劍. 2003. *Songdai daojiao guanli zhidu yanjiu* 宋代道教管理制度研究 (A study of regulation of the Daoist religion in the Song period). Beijing: Xianzhuang shuju.

Teiser, Stephen F. 1993. The Growth of Purgatory. In Ebrey & Gregory 1993, 115–145.

Wear, Andrew, Johanna Geyer-Kordesch, & Roger French, eds. 1993. *Doctors and Ethics: The Earlier Historical Setting of Professional Ethics.* Wellcome Institute Series in the History of Medicine. Amsterdam: Rodopi.

Wujastyk, Dominik. 1993. Indian medicine. In *Companion Encyclopedia of the History of Medicine*, ed. W.F. Bynum & Roy Porter, 755–778. London: Routledge.

Wujastyk, Dominik. 2001. *The Roots of Āyurveda: Selections from Sanskrit Medical Writings.* Penguin classics. New Delhi: Penguin Books.

Yu, Anthony C. 2006. *State and Religion in China: Historical and Textual Perspectives.* Chicago: Open Court Books.

Yü, Chün-fang (Yu Junfang). 2001. *Kuan-yin. The Chinese Transformation of Avalokitesvara.* Institute for Advanced Studies of World Religions Books, 11. New York: Columbia UP.

Zhu Kewen 朱克文, Gao Sixian 高思显, & Gong Chun 龚纯. 1996. *Zhongguo junshi yixue shi* 中国军事医学史 (History of Chinese military medicine). Beijing: Renmin Junyi Chubanshe.

Zhuang Hongyi 莊宏誼. 1999. Songdai daojiao yiliao. Yi Hong Mai *Yijian zhi* wei zhu zhi yanjiu 宋代道教醫療—以洪邁夷堅志為主之研究 (Daoist therapy in the Song. A study based mainly on Hong Mai's *Records of the Listener). Furen zongjiao yanjiu* 輔仁宗教研究 12: 73–147.

Zimmerman, Francis. 1978. From Classic Texts to Learned Practice: Methodological Remarks on the Study of Indian Medicine. *Social Science and Medicine* 12: 97–103.

Chapter 7
Therapy in the State Religion

Abstract The state religion was the system of rituals that underlay imperial rule. Imperial religion, ritual and politics were never separable. Nor were religion and health. Since the state religion has regularly been confused with Confucianism, this chapter first explains what the religious part of its rituals actually comprised in the eleventh century, and then examines the part that health care played in it.

The most indispensable task of the emperor was a priestly one. In dynastic ideology, only he could provide the link between the cosmos and human society essential to maintaining a harmonious political order. His spiritual duties were broader and deeper than they are usually depicted as being. The ritual manual of emperor Huizong 徽宗 (1101–1126) devotes sixty-two chapters to his worship (and his officials') of a remarkably large array of, among others, the gods of sky and earth.[1] In other words, the main difference between popular and palace liturgy was that the former responded to the gods of the locality, and the latter mainly (but not only) to the gods of the whole empire.

High court officials, when spiritual intervention was essential, were assigned the duty of praying to whatever gods might be helpful for the given task. For instance, late in February of 978, the emperor "ordered the officials close to him to pray for rain in the Buddhist, Daoist, and popular temples of the capitals." These included, of course, only those edifices acknowledged and registered by the government. Two days, we are told, was enough to solicit adequate rain.[2] On top of all this, there were occasional ceremonies on a still grander scale, some of which I will discuss below. First, let me examine the ideological basis of state ritual.

[1] *Zhenghe wuli xin yi* 政和五禮新儀, j. 38–96. Cf. Zito 1996, 73, writing about the eighteenth century.

[2] *Xu zizhi tongjian chang bian* 續資治通鑑長編, 19: 42.

© Springer International Publishing Switzerland 2015

N. Sivin, *Health Care in Eleventh-Century China*, Archimedes 43,
DOI 10.1007/978-3-319-20427-7_7

State Ideology

In Chinese thought there were two microcosms, the socio-political order and the order of the human body. Curing illness and keeping the public peace were two species of maintaining order.[3] This ancient way of thinking was the basis for the idea that being an excellent doctor was in a sense equivalent to being a good prime minister (chapter 4, p. 78).

Early governments frequently expressed concern about epidemics. When a dynasty's governance was inadequate, they were among the omens—symptoms of social disorder—by which Heaven warned a dynasty that it risked losing its mandate to rule. Epidemics were fearsomely frequent in the early years of the Northern Song period. This was one of numerous reasons that its administration became the first to involve itself substantially and more or less continuously in what is now called public health.

A remarkable document explains the synapse between the emperor as cosmic priest and as medical policy-maker. The *Canon of Sagely Benefaction* (*Sheng ji jing* 聖濟經, 1118) was the last of the classics (*jing* 經) of medicine, and the only one written expressly for canonization. Its author was the emperor Huizong 徽宗 (r. 1100–1126).[4] Of the several emperors of the Northern Song period who were active in forming medical policy, Huizong was the most innovative in changing institutions. Recall that he markedly raised the status of the palace medical school to attract students of higher social status than before (see chapter 4, p. 64). One of the goals of his short book is to explain why members of the literate elite were bound to be better curers than the rank and file of doctors.

Here is part of its preface:

> One yin and one yang [i.e., their constant alternation] are called the Way; an imbalance toward yin or toward yang is called disease. Those who fail to clearly understand the Way have never been able to cure man's diseases. Yin and yang illuminate each other, cover (*gai* 蓋) each other, order each other; the four seasons succeed each other, give rise to each other, kill each other; the five phases take turns as sovereign, are unthroned, then serve as minister.[5]
>
> Human beings, born and living in the midst [of this constant change], conform to yin and yang, are attentive to the four seasons, and are regulated by the five phases. With the median comes felicity; with excess comes calamity; with license comes disease. Themselves not subject to control by the [cosmic] regularities,[6] [the sages] stand alone above the myriad forms [in the cosmos]; not subject to regulation by things, they circulate among the myriad

[3] See chapter 2, p. 10. On microcosms see Lloyd & Sivin 2002, 214–226.

[4] It is impossible to be certain what writings attributed to an emperor he himself wrote. Huizong was a prolific writer, and it is extremely likely that at least the preface translated below was his.

[5] This is a concise statement of the dynamic alternation of yin-yang and the five phases.

[6] Although the modern dictionary definition of *shu* 數 is "number," ancient authors often used it for qualitative as well as quantitative regularities. Here the word obviously refers to quality. It is well, when thinking about this statement of the sages' paramount position in the universe, to recall that emperors were conventionally considered sages.

contents of the universe. Thus they are able to use the Way to master the seasons, to apply their consciousness (*shen* 神) to make use of the regularities. Their forms intact and their seminal vitality made whole (? *fu*復), they are one with heaven and earth.

In archaic times, the Yellow Emperor, it seems, was one of those who embodied the divine and was illuminated in the Way. He asked Master Guangcheng about the Way, and went to see Dawei at Mt. Quzi.[7] He personally carried out the work [of governance] in the Palace of the Standard [i.e., the hall of audience], letting his robes hang down.[8] He created writing, invented a notation for time, and established the pitch-pipes and the calendar.

Thus he became the most tireless of all under heaven. Even [his high officials], who never rested when carrying out his commands, could not hope to keep up with him. At the same time he was saddened by how traditions of virtue had weakened, and pitied the loss of simplicity among his people.

With respect to what is above them, they defied the light of sun and moon; with respect to what is below them, they wasted the finest products of mountain and stream; with respect to what is in between, they let slip the bounty of the four seasons. Thus it happens that, in pursuit of what is improper, they wasted their authentic vitalities. They failed to live out the years that heaven had allotted them, dying in the midst of their paths through life.

That led him to make his inquiries of [his minister and teacher] Qibo and to write the *Inner Canon of the Yellow Emperor.* It transmitted the virtues of the spirits, and classified the realities of the myriad things. What it said complemented the archaic classics, but its transmission was unable to continue through the generations.[9] Thus it came about that calling someone a physician signifies no more than claiming that a diviner embodies the *Book of Changes.*

I felt much grief at this. Since my succession to the throne I have been ceaselessly busy, never daring to be free of concerns day or night. Whenever a moment is left over from a myriad emergencies, I take the opportunity to make inquiries. I have been determined to take high antiquity as my model, fathom the profundities of heaven and man, and trace to their source the principles of man's nature and the will of heaven as embodied in him (*xingming* 性命). …

I have created a book in ten chapters, with a total of forty-two sections, and have named it *Canon of Sagely Benefaction.* My aim is that gentlemen of the superior sort, when they hear [of its content], will agree with it and find that it reinforces the Way, and that gentlemen of the middling sort, as they study it, will improve themselves [? *zi hua* 自華] and act in accordance with what is actual. [With its help] one can nourish the vital *qi,* can establish heaven's will within oneself, and can help the world's people toward the longevity [that comes from cultivating] benevolence. Thus [this book] may broaden the transmission of the Yellow Emperor['s teachings]. How can that not be pleasing?

[At this point the author recapitulates some of the most general doctrines of medicine.]

Even a divine physician cannot succeed by dosing patients after the disease has become full-blown. In order to pursue the arts of the Way, reinforcing the body's own vitalities and driving out the pathological *qi,* I have established schools and offices to increase the number of [medical] scholars and nurture and educate them. We feed those who have nowhere else to turn, we save the ill, and we bury the dead.

This I have promulgated in governmental orders and deposited with the proper authorities. Nothing further remains to be said [in this preface].

---

[7] These are allusions to stories about the Yellow Emperor seeking enlightenment from teachers in *Zhuangzi* 莊子, 27/11/29 and 65/24/25.

[8] This odd metaphor describes a ruler who governs without perceptible effort.

[9] Most of this medical classic is in the form of initiation dialogues between the emperor and his ministers, Qibo and others. Its circulation remained limited until the mid eleventh century.

The *Canon* was recognized as a classic because an emperor—a sage *ex officio*—wrote it, and because in form, diction, and rhetoric it was redolent of earlier classics.[10] The book, as this preface indicates, was not addressed primarily to rank and file physicians, but to "gentlemen of the superior sort." Huizong believed that the fundamentals of medicine should be part of their educations. His new classic was obviously oriented toward the new-style literatus doctor (*ruyi* 儒醫), who he believed would be superior to the old hereditary sort.

The point of this preface is that health is the spontaneous dynamic balance of the bodily microcosm, and healing is the restoration of that balance when it is lost. The sage, who has attained that balance within himself, is thus is at the same time the ideal ruler and the ideal therapist. It is natural for the emperor who wrote this preface to picture the archaic sages as emperors themselves. The sage maintains and restores the health as well as the political order of the empire by dispensing wisdom that his civil servants—not he—apply pragmatically to form policies.[11]

This document outlines the religious character of Huizong's medical activities as he envisioned them. They are, although not a formal part of the state cult, at one with it. Precisely because he was the Son of Heaven, his worship of sky and earth guaranteed the link between the spontaneous dynamic harmony of the natural order and hard-won social stability. That made him the supreme authority on what cures human disorders, medical and social. This relationship with the state cult was abstract, but it had great practical consequences. Huizong was explaining why he involved himself in medicine and inspired many innovations in its institutions and practices.

State Rites

Civil servants, as we have seen, were customarily involved in popular and Daoist rituals. The large-scale registration of popular temples in the eleventh century obligated local officials to perform rites in each.[12] Consider, for instance, Wang Anshi 王安石 (1021–1086), primarily remembered as the boldest reformer of the century, and as the first scholar whose classical commentaries were required for study in his lifetime by candidates preparing for the imperial examinations.[13] As a local official, he too performed popular as well as Daoist rites.

[10] The conventional classics varied a great deal in all three respects; it was not hard to read into this new one a generic whiff of the archaic.

[11] This was not the only prevalent view. Many emperors and their ministers believed that the ruler should make most or all decisions. In practice, Huizong was highly activist.

[12] Iiyama 2010 shows that even in the Yuan period local officials followed Song precedents for worship in popular temples.

[13] Biography in Liu 1959.

Popular rituals

We can read a prayer to a popular god, Lord Bao (Bao Jun 鮑君), in Wang Anshi's collected prose[14]:

> (Fill in the year, month, and day.) The official (fill in name) dares make an announcement to the god Lord Bao 鮑君. The travails of agriculture are well known to the god. Among the four seasons of the year, it is winter when [farmers] have most time to rest. Still, they must pound [the earth to harden it in] the threshing spaces, put their dwellings in order, paint the storehouses, and fertilize the fields. They never have a single day to rest contentedly.
>
> And now the official has had to order them, in addition, to use their "spare time" in repairing the ditches and streams.[15] Compared to a normal year, this would seem to have increased the travails of agriculture. It would be fitting for the god to pity them and to find some way [for me] to lead them.
>
> Before they had done many repairs, it rained. When the rain had almost ended, the able-bodied, the old, and the weak were [mobilized] to set the water moving [outside the normal channels] and to dry up [the watercourses]. Before this was done it rained yet again. Nor is it only the people who are troubled by this; the official worries about it day and night. If only the god would aid them with clear weather, ending this duty soon!
>
> Now exactly what makes the official worry is that he imposes duties on the people. But for a very long time the god has been fed by the people. Your worry should not be less than the official's.
>
> Respectfully announced.

In 1048, the year he prayed this curious prayer, Wang Anshi was twenty-nine years old, and magistrate of Yin district 鄞縣 (present-day Zhejiang). As a young local official, Wang focused on pragmatic solutions to problems. He was less apt than more conventional civil servants to filter his experiences through conventional expectations and principles. This document reflects that trait. He acknowledges the ability of this deity to control the weather, and asks that it not let changeable weather add to the onerous obligations of the local farmers. There was no typical content for this kind of document, and Wang was not a typical official. At the same time that he shows reverence for the god, he is not in the least obsequious. In fact, he is respectfully lecturing it.

Daoist rituals

Officials not only performed popular rituals as part of their duties in local posts, but those in the palace contributed to Daoist ceremonies. The Song government sponsored great rituals on an increasingly lavish scale, extended in time, elaborate in

---

[14] *Wang Jinggong wenji jianzhu* 王荊公文集箋注, 49: 1684. Lord Bao was Bao Gai 鮑蓋 of the Later Han period, a low-level official who became a local god. His temple was registered by the Song government as Yongtai wang miao 永泰王廟 and promoted in 1103 to Lingying miao 靈應廟. See note 1 of Li Zhiliang 李之亮 in the source cited.

[15] This apparently refers to a kind of local labor duty. Wang, offering this prayer, was the leading local official and thus most likely responsible for the order.

liturgy, carried out by unprecedented numbers of clergy. Under emperors who were particularly enthusiastic patrons, these took place not only in temples established by government order in the capital, but also in those of prefectural capitals. Huizong designated a temple in each prefecture for rituals on his birthday and, from 1104 on, on his six Personal Destiny Days each year.[16]

By 1016, forty-nine great rituals were being performed per year. Shortly before that year, in a time of heavy military expenses as well as less tax income due to a plague of locusts, a meritorious official, Shi Pu 石普, proposed "discontinuing the offering rituals throughout the empire, which will save the equivalent of 700,000 strings of cash a year as a contribution to the empire's expenses." This proposal elicited a firestorm of wrath from the emperor and his closest officials, and led to prosecution of Shi on an unrelated charge. The high level of patronage for lavish state Daoist ceremonies continued after the Northern Song period.[17]

Not only did emperors participate in Daoist rituals, but they also commissioned (and wrote) documents for them. Here is a prayer of Shenzong 神宗 (r. 1067–1085) written for a ritual addressed to the three emanations of the Way (*Sanqing* 三清) against a plague of locusts[18]:

> I pray:
>
> Because the Way that can be given only makeshift names came into being along with the Grand Inception,[19] it is the spirit that exercises no authority but excels all others, and brings order to them all. I venture to reflect that I have respectfully received the Mandate—trembling, mindful that with grace I am to nurture the black-haired people, so that this will be a time of good government, peace, and happiness. But along the borders of the capital region, where agricultural work has just begun, suddenly swarms of locusts have come to life that are gradually destroying much of our crops. Truly we look up in the hope of aid from attentive Heaven[20] so that when we look down we can see an end to this catastrophe for humans.
>
> This is why I pray to heaven with all my heart for a positive response. I humbly hope that blessings will descend from the Pure Capital, that good fortune will accumulate [for us] at the Golden Gate-towers,[21] so that all of the natural calamities will cease, and tranquility

[16] Ebrey 2014, 150–151. The Personal Destiny Day (*benmingri* 本命日) was the one with the same sexagenary day number as the year of the person's—here, the emperor's—birth. The liturgy amounted to worshipping the god of the corresponding star in the constellation Northern Dipper.

[17] For Shi's rather offhand proposal, see *Xu zi zhi tong jian chang bian*, 88: 2027–2028, and for his biography, *Song shi* 宋史, 324: 10471–10475. For a catalogue of the most significant Daoist rituals and imperial participation in them, see *Song shi*, j. 104. Cheng Minsheng 程民生 2008, 444–446, has gathered data on the cost of rites in the Song.

[18] *Song Shenzong yuzhi yujing ji* 宋神宗御製玉京集, 5: 8a; also in ZD 44/060, 5: 581. This is a large collection of prayers written by the emperor for use in imperial offering rituals.

[19] The coming into being of the cosmos. "The Way that can be given only makeshift names" alludes to the Way's ineffability as described in the *Laozi*, 1.

[20] I take *tian jian* 天鑒 tentatively as equivalent to the homophonous 天監. It also implies the mirroring of the celestial and terrestrial palaces.

[21] The Pure Capital is the celestial palace. The Golden Gate-towers, in Daoist ritual, are usually the entrance to it, but here the phrase apparently refers to the gates of the imperial palace.

will spread throughout the realm. Your resplendent blessings: I receive them only to support our future perfection. My anxious heart adds increasing cares to my thoughts.[22]

Your servant, with the ultimate in earnestness, respectfully indites this document.

As in other prayers written for Daoist offering rituals, the emperor uses language that clearly expresses his hierarchic inferiority to the gods for whom he writes it. In fact, he uses forms that his officials use when they address memorials to him.

In addition to prayers of this kind, three Northern Song emperors wrote substantial numbers of hymns for use in Daoist liturgy.[23] Here is one of ten hymns by Huizong. It clearly states that such imperial rituals were intended, among other aims, to prevent epidemics[24]:

The precious registers, a model for cultivating realization;
With sincere hearts we memorialize Heaven.
We approach it like thin ice or a deep abyss,[25] [on behalf of] our innumerable people;
[Dressing before] daylight, [eating after] dark, we bring about peace and prosperity.[26]
For the myriad creatures we allay catastrophes and epidemics[27];
From the three luminaries we verify good omens.
The sound of Pacing the Void is clear and penetrating;
Then we intone the Cavern Mystery verses.

This is the seventh of ten hymns that Huizong wrote for Pacing the Void, the rite in which, after the officiant first enters the sacred space, the other priests circumambulate him, symbolically voyaging round the cosmos. As the words indicate, the rite that follows is that of the Cavern Mystery. The Golden Register Retreat of which both are part (the "precious registers" of the first line) was the main ceremony of the Lingbao tradition and its successors.[28]

Huizong went even further, incorporating many Daoist rites, and specifying Daoist temples for some ceremonies, in the comprehensive manual of government rituals that was compiled to his specifications and published in 1113. He was also responsible for assembling a new Daoist Canon, the first to be printed.[29]

---

[22] This figure of speech alludes to the *Book of Songs* (*Mao shi* 毛詩, 248/1), and the *Book of Changes* (*Zhou yi* 周易, hexagram 1, 9 in the 3rd place).

[23] Daoist hymns by Taizong, Zhenzong, and Huizong are gathered in *Jinlu zhai sandong zanyong yi* 金籙齋三洞讚詠儀 "Pacing the Void" hymns by Huizong are included in the Ming collection *Yuyin fashi* 玉音法事 (1: 5a–6b, 3: 23b).

[24] *Jinlu zhai sandong zanyong yi,* 3: 6b; ZD 43/010, 3: 41.

[25] An allusion to Mao *shi,* 195/6, where it expresses trepidation.

[26] The first half of this line is a proverbial assertion of the government's dedication and assiduity. *Kang* 康 implies health as well as prosperity.

[27] Alludes to *Zhuangzi,* 1/30, a story about a spiritual immortal (*shenren* 神人) whose power is so great that, with no effort, he allays catastrophes and epidemics and brings about good harvests. This implies a comparable spiritual potency for the officiant. The next line refers to observing the sun, moon, and northern dipper for good astrological portents.

[28] See Maruyama Hiroshi in Pregadio 2008, 580. Schipper 1989 transcribes the melody used in late twentieth century Taiwan offering rituals for this hymn. See also Kaltenmark 1960.

[29] On the *Zhenghe wan shou daozang* 政和萬壽道藏 (or *Zhenghe wan shou zang jing* 政和萬壽藏經), see Van der Loon 1984, 29–63, and Ebrey 2014, 252–254. The ritual manual was *Zhenghe wuli xin yi* 政和五禮新儀. On the latter see Ebrey 2014, 243–252.

Distinguished officials wrote "green documents." These were originally prayers written on strips of green paper in vermilion ink. Emperors ordered Academicians—palace dignitaries—to prepare them, to be performed by the officiant as part of a great ritual.[30] Such documents often show up in their authors' literary collections and elsewhere. Twenty-six by Wang Anshi 王安石 survive, as do twenty-seven by Xia Song 夏竦 (985–1051), a zealous persecutor of popular priests[31]; a hundred and twenty-five by Hu Su 胡宿 (996–1067), celebrated as a local and palace official; a hundred and forty-one by Wang Gui 王珪 (1019–1085), who became prime minister; and seventeen by Su Shi 蘇軾 (or Dongpo 東坡, 1037–1101) , the leading literary figure of his time.[32]

These short Daoist documents were written for the whole range of governmental purposes that motivated rituals: to celebrate festivals and birthdays of emperors and their families and of gods, to pray for imperial offspring, and to end epidemics and other disasters. Here is an example from among the "green documents" written by Su Shi. Although ritual documents are generally bureaucratic in diction as well as form, this one makes it clear that the genre left room for personal expression[33]:

> **Green Document for an Offering Ritual to the Northern Peak 醮北嶽**
>
> When, as a young man, I became a civil servant, my hopes were set on saving people [who need help]. In old age, tired out by official travel,[34] I have no patience at all left for give and take with others. Benighted and with much guilt, through adversity and suffering, wandering aimlessly with no place to go, I stopped, gazing upward at the carriage of a realized immortal as it alit on the south side of the lofty peak.
>
> I kowtowed and made a sincere commitment, purifying my mind and regretting my misdeeds. I hope that the immaculateness of this one thought will wash away the worldly distractions of a thousand ages, its power limitless. [Let me] first loosen the web in which I am entangled, [so that] I will be lit by the divine light. With good fortune I will meet with an outstanding teacher. I swear that, for the rest of my life, I will always conform to the perfect Way.

Literati also wrote such documents for whatever purposes the gentry who sponsored private rituals could afford. It was in this context that we find "green documents" that were devoted to curing individuals. Wang Shang 王賞 was a Presented Scholar of 1103, whose promising subsequent career as a civil servant was cut short by the fierce partisan battles of his generation. He was also a well-known littérateur of his time.[35] He wrote three surviving "green documents" for offering rituals meant to cure diseases of parents. This, like the other two, is conventional in form and diction.

---

[30] *Qingci* 青詞, 青辭, *qingzhang* 青章, *lüzhang* 綠章. For further specifications, see *Zhenghe wuli xin yi,* 4: 1a.

[31] See chapter 4, p. 145, footnote.

[32] Zhang Zehong 张泽洪 1999, 75, provides data for eight Song figures. Many esteemed officials also wrote parts of the liturgy for great rituals not performed under imperial auspices. Zhang also discusses the rites that authors were required to perform *when writing* such documents (p. 145).

[33] *Dongpo quan ji* 東坡全集 98: 19b. Mt. Tai, the Northern Peak, was the seat of the otherworldly judiciary, Fengdu.

[34] Some of it to and from exile due to political infighting.

[35] Chang Bide 昌彼得 1974–1976, 1:214.

Green Document for an Offering Ritual to Overcome a Catastrophic [Illness] on Behalf of One's Mother

That parents will live long lives is the human heart's strongest wish. Those [offspring] who are not selfish toward others hope that heaven's oversight will not turn against [their parents]. They fully express their sincerity, earnestly praying for heavenly protection.

I respectfully think about my mother, of the (fill in name) fief, who has been harassed by a disease that has caused great concern. Although she has been helped by drugs, I am still anxious, day and night. Perhaps, because of some infraction long ago, she has been unable to escape a hidden penalty.[36] I hopefully seek your abundant grace. I pray that you will grant her the boon of good health, so that together [with her family] she can attain a ripe old age, and her household can all look forward to her longevity and well-being.

Conclusion

I have discussed a number of state rituals, which are only loosely tied to the state ideology conventionally confused with Confucianism. Officials both wrote prayers and performed them. Although when literati spoke for the state they tended to be intolerant of other religions, in the eleventh century rites of popular, Daoist and Buddhist origin found their way into the state's official liturgy. Buddhist rituals were meant to be conducted by Buddhist clergy, but we have already glimpsed their influence on popular and Daoist liturgy.[37]

The central government dealt with therapy for individuals primarily through its public health initiatives, and also by the support of temples largely chosen for official registration because of their gods' demonstrated curative efficacy. State ceremony, carried out with a grandeur impossible for individuals, was more often aimed at the health of the populace than at individual curing. The main exception was for illnesses of the emperor or his immediate family.

Can such rituals be taken seriously as therapy, or was this a collective delusion? Curative rites written or performed by civil servants, like those used by clergy, obviously sometimes were followed by recovery. Had this been untrue, we would have to believe that no one at all was shrewd enough to detect a sham. The aim of Daoist rituals was clearly to go beyond the body's autonomous efforts to recover good health. They could only have done so by eliciting the meaning response. After all, they brought to bear the majesty of the imperial government to overcome threats against which, up to that point, patients had been defenseless.

We live in a world in which biomedicine can neither explain the origins of, nor cure, alcoholism and many other diseases—but in which everyone thinks of them as diseases nevertheless. Perhaps when we understand the social dynamics of that failure-proof enthusiasm we will be better prepared to grasp the confidence in religious curing long ago—or for that matter today, when it is still strong worldwide.

---

[36] Literally, "a yin penalty," exacted by the otherworld judiciary and unknown to others.

[37] See chapter 6, p. 133.

References

Abbreviations

DZ = Volume number in *Daozang*
ES = *Ersishi shi* 二十四史 of Zhonghua Shuju, 1959–1977.
HY = text in Harvard-Yenching Concordance series
j. = *juan* 卷 (chapter)
RW = published by Renmin Weisheng Chubanshe 人民衛生出版社, Beijing
S = Title number in Schipper 1975
SQ = Siku quanshu 四庫全書
SV = Schipper & Verellen 2004
T = *Taishō shinshū Daizōkyō* 大正新修大藏經
UP = University Press
YZ = Yi tong zheng mai quan shu 醫統正脈全書
ZD = Volume, item, *juan,* and page numbers in *Zhonghua daozang* 中华道藏
ZS = published by Zhonghua shuju 中華書局, Beijing
ZZ = Zhongyi zhenben congshu 中醫珍本叢書 ed.

Classical Chinese Sources

Dongpo quan ji 東坡全集 (Complete collected writings of Su Shi). SQ.

Jinlu zhai sandong zanyong yi 金籙齋三洞讚詠儀 (Hymns for Golden Register Purification rituals of the Three Caverns). Compiled by Zhang Shangying 張商英. 1104/1123. S310, DZ 161, ZD 43/010. See SV 1039.

Mao Shi 毛詩 (Mao recension of the *Book of Songs*). Anonymous. In final form by late sixth century B.C.? HY.

Song shi 宋史 (History of the Song period). Tuotuo 脫脫. 1345. ES.

Song Zhenzong yuzhi yujing ji 宋真宗御制玉京集 (Jade capital collection, by emperor Zhenzong of the Song period). Before 1022. S315, DZ 163, ZD 44/060, 5: 581. Collected statements of intention (*yi* 意) for use in Daoist rituals.

Wang Jinggong wenji jianzhu 王荊公文集箋注 (Annotated short prose writings of Wang Anshi), with notes by Li Zhiliang 李之亮. Date of compilation unknown. Chengdu: Ba-Shu Shushe, 2005.

Xu zizhi tongjian chang bian 續資治通鑑長編 (Long draft of the Continuation of the Comprehensive Mirror for Aid in Government). Li Tao 李燾. 1183. ZS reprint, 2004.

Yuyin fashi 玉音法事 (Liturgy of precious music). Anonymous. Ming period? S607, DZ 333. Major hymns of Lingbao liturgy, elaborately annotated.

Zhenghe wuli xin yi 政和五禮新儀 (New forms of the five categories of rites of the Regnant Harmony era). Edited by Zheng Juzhong 鄭居中. 1113. In SQ *zhenben chu ji* 珍本初集.

Zhonghua daozang 中华道藏 (Chinese Daoist canon). 49 vols. Beijing: Huaxia Chubanshe. Digital edition of *Daozang*, in simplified characters, with some revisions and added texts.

Zhou yi 周易 (Changes of the Zhou dynasty; usually referred to as Book of Changes). Anonymous. Original text late ninth century B.C.; Ten Wings between third and second century, except that "Xu gua" is Later Han. HY.

Zhuangzi 莊子 (The Book of Master Zhuang). Partly by Zhuang Zhou 莊周? Ca. 320 to late second century. Partial translation: Graham 1981; on authorship see also Graham 1990, 283–321.

Other Sources

Chang Bide 昌彼得 et al. 1974–1976. *Song ren zhuanji ziliao suoyin* 宋人傳記資料索引 (Index to biographical sources on Sung personages). 6 vols. Taipei: Dingwen Shuju.

Cheng Minsheng 程民生. 2008. *Songdai wujia yanjiu* 宋代物价研究 (A study of commodity prices in the Song period). Beijing Renmin Chubanshe. Gathers prices from a wide range of sources, argues that they cannot be reduced to a common measure.

Ebrey, Patricia Buckley. 2014. *Emperor Huizong*. Harvard UP.

Graham, A. C. 1981. *Chuang-tzu. The Seven Inner Chapters and Other Writings from the Book Chuang-tzu.* London: Allen & Unwin.

Graham, A. C. 1990. *Studies in Chinese Philosophy and Philosophical Literature.* SUNY Series in Chinese Philosophy and Culture. Albany: State University of New York Press.

Iiyama, Tomoyasu. 2010. Maintaining Gods in Medieval China: Temple Worship and Local Governance in North China under the Jin and Yuan. *Journal of Song–Yuan Studies* 40: 71–102.

Kaltenmark, Max. 1960. Ling-pao 靈寶: Note sur un terme du Taoïsme religieux. *Mélanges de l'Institut des Hautes Études Chinoises* 2: 559–588.

Liu, James T. C. 1959. *Reform in Song China. Wang An-shih (1021–1086) and his New Policies.* Harvard East Asian Studies, 3. Harvard UP.

Lloyd, G. E. R., & Nathan Sivin. 2002. *The Way and the Word. Science and Medicine in Early China and Greece.* New Haven: Yale UP.

Pregadio, Fabrizio, ed. 2008. *The Encyclopedia Of Taoism*. 2 vols. New York: Routledge.

Schipper, Kristofer. 1989. A study of Buxu: Taoist Liturgical Hymn and Dance. In *Studies of Taoist Rituals and Music of Today,* ed. Pen-yeh Tsao & Daniel P. L. Law, 110–120. Hong Kong: Society of Ethnomusicologica.

van der Loon, Piet. 1984. *Taoist Books in the Libraries of the Sung Period. A Critical Study and Index.* Oxford Oriental Institute Monographs, 7. London: Ithaca Press.

Zhang Zehong. 1999. *Daojiao zhaijiao keyi yanjiu* 道教斋醮科仪研究 (Studies in the liturgy of Daoist offering rituals). Ru Dao Shi boshi lunwen congshu 儒道释博士论文丛书. Chengdu: Ba-Shu Shushe.

Zito, Angela. 1996. City Gods and their Magistrates. In Lopez 1996, 72–81.

Chapter 8
Conclusions

Abstract This chapter summarizes the main conclusions of the study: classical medicine played a very small direct role in the ailments of the population as a whole; there is a remarkable extent of overlap between therapies that originated in different religious milieux; the classical view of the body, its processes, and its disorders in the eleventh century was strikingly different from that of both pre-modern European medicine and biomedicine; the health-care initiatives of the time were compromised by officials' persecution of popular ritualists in the south and elsewhere, and by the inconsistency with which medical policies were applied. With respect to the social and political setting, despite the considerable sharing and appropriation of therapeutic methods, one cannot speak of a health care system, for there was no integration; and one cannot assume that state edicts were obeyed or even enforced throughout the empire. The chapter finally outlines several desirable next steps in understanding ancient health care.

This book has described, in a first crude fashion, a range of the kinds of health care available in eleventh-century China. In addition to physicians, it has identified a wide variety of other therapists: popular priests, Daoists, Buddhists and, to a smaller but notable extent, officials. I have argued that all of them were capable of helping the sick, mainly because the ritual circumstances of their curing motivated and supported the patient's meaning and autonomous responses. Curing was a family matter. Even rural families with very limited cash could get help from local or itinerant herbalists and curers. When these were inadequate, priests could often untangle knotted social relationships that burdened the patient. We know too few details of individual cases, and of their familial and cultural settings, to compare the roles of the autonomous and meaning responses. But the biomedical standard—exclusive reliance on scientifically tested specific remedies—can yield very little trustworthy information on the value of therapies before very recent times.

Below I will summarize my main conclusions.

© Springer International Publishing Switzerland 2015

N. Sivin, *Health Care in Eleventh-Century China*, Archimedes 43,
DOI 10.1007/978-3-319-20427-7_8

Classical Medicine and Public Health

Overall, classical medicine played a very small role in treating the ailments of the whole population. This is a matter of who had access to it. There seem to have been enough classical doctors, along with hereditary physicians, to treat urban, literate gentry and wealthy commoners, as well as an unknown number of the same sorts of people who still lived in the countryside. Case records of the time provide no evidence that the patients of physicians included a significant number of the poor peasants and laborers who made up most of the population. Even in the voluminous case-record compilations that began gathering momentum about 1600, although the indigent and uneducated were still the overwhelming majority of the population, and there were a great many more physicians, the latter still concentrated on treating the gentry and the well-off.

Therapeutic Distinctions

My second finding, based on the recent research of others as well as my own, is that there is a remarkable extent of overlap between the therapies that different kinds of non-medical curers used to care for their patients. Around the end of the long eleventh century, for instance, the thunder rites that began in esoteric Buddhism, and that popular *fashi* had long been performing in their own way, became the basis of new Daoist movements, and some officials also found it useful to learn them. The state's registration procedures, without intending to do so, had greatly blurred the distinction—never sharp—between popular gods and those that Daoist and Buddhist clerics originally worshiped. As a result of those procedures, local officials also were required to carry out rites of worship in the state-approved temples of their constituencies. The gods of those temples, their efficacy thus publicly recognized, gained in charisma. That, we are told, added to their power to cure.

In the Northern Song period, local temples, unlike monasteries, were not ordinarily the property of Daoist or Buddhist movements. They were places of public resort, available for ceremonial use by any cleric. That mixing encouraged the appropriation of methods that originated in one movement by liturgists of another. Such appropriation began early, as the first Daoist movements adapted popular rites. By the early fifth century Buddhists were molding their rites to fit Chinese customs (see chapter 6, p. 133).

I will sum up below the other main conclusions of this book, first those that have to do with understanding the body and its processes, physiological and pathological; then those that bear on religious curing; then those related to the social and political dimensions of health care; and finally, what are likely to be fruitful next steps in exploring the history of health care.

The Body and Its Processes

Westerners are used to thinking of the body in terms of anatomy and physiology, where the latter, as taught in medical schools, is concerned with the organic, chemical, and physical functions of anatomical parts, tissues, and other components of the body. Chinese physicians were interested in body functions and their dynamics to an extent that minimized their concern for anatomy; their understanding of the body was built much more on vital processes than structures. The contents of the abdomen were integrated systems of functions that (like government bureaus) regulated the body's spontaneous vital functions.

No society before 1800 could reliably connect the signs and symptoms of a sick patient with the pathology revealed by dissecting a cadaver. This was the primary limit on the effectiveness of therapy. That is why in European medicine bleeding and purging were common for such a long time. These methods could not necessarily alter the course of disease, but they could at least show the patient that the physician could control body processes as the patient experienced them. Chinese therapies were on the whole less drastic, and left more scope for the body to heal itself, backed by the curative power of symbol and rite.

Because *qi* was not a purely medical concept but one of the universal bases of Chinese thought, religious curing also drew on it. Popular notions of vitality were a great deal less abstract than those of the doctors. Religious ritual focused on the battle between the body's vitalities and the shades, themselves *qi,* that invaded it from outside.

Diseases, syndromes, symptoms

In chapter 3, pp. 68ff, I argued that not only the diseases, but even the syndromes and symptoms, of classical medicine sliced up the spectrum of suffering in ways quite different from those prevalent in early Europe—and more different still from those of biomedicine. People in their subcultures negotiated nosologies on the basis of patients' and therapists' perceptions.

An additional problem of nomenclature arises because therapy is local. China was an enormous and highly diverse country, in which there were innumerable dialects, with a range nearly as wide as that of Western Europe's languages. The names of diseases accordingly varied from one region to another. That largely accounts for the enormous diversity of diseases identified in handbooks of etiology and symptomatology. One of the things that made such handbooks valuable was that they attempted to separate mere synonyms from terms for different disorders. One could carry such work of disentangling only so far, since it was often impossible to be certain that a disease common in the north was the same as one called by the same name in the deep south that had a dissimilar balance of symptoms.

Religious Setting

Ideologues had only contempt for popular curing, and careerists got ahead by opposing it. We saw in chapter 5 that even in the eleventh century certain officials ran brutal campaigns on their own to wipe out what they called wizardry, and that occasionally they attracted imperial backing to persecute popular priests in unregistered temples of the south. This seems to have been a matter of prejudice rather than ignorance; some, at least, of the officials most active in such campaigns were southerners themselves.

In China as elsewhere, curing was religion's most potent source of support. Sick people depended on popular priests, Buddhists, and Daoists for therapy, and patronage depended on how well they met those needs. Local officials performed popular and Daoist rituals as part of their duties, and learned that doing so strengthened their authority. An official's performing a thunder rite was not part of his duties. From the modern point of view it may seem a lapse into irrationality, but the result of its symbolism, at least part of the time, was recorded as therapeutic success.

Social and Political Setting

Was there a health care system?

The notion that a list of the varieties of health care in a given time and place adds up to a system is common currency among people who write about such matters. "Health care system" is an organizational cliché. In recent years bureaucrats have tried to update it to "health system." That is a corollary of the World Health Organization's 1946 definition of "health" as "a state of complete physical, mental, and social well-being and not merely the absence of disease or infirmity." In that light, looking at the care of medical disorders alone seems myopic.

The aims of the imperial Chinese state, however, were more modest than those of the World Health Organization. Most dynasties were concerned quite irregularly, and seldom urgently, with doing what little they could to minimize death and physical suffering from disease. The Northern Song government, as we have seen, gave public health exceptionally high priority, but again in an on-and-off fashion. Even when officials were most involved, a number of them did harm to public health by attacking popular religious curing, the only activity outside the family capable of reaching the great majority of the population. Although the central government chose temples for registration according to reports of their efficacy, such reports were prompted as consistently by pressure from the local elite as by the therapeutic experience of commoners.

The sum of local therapy of all kinds, classical medicine, and the many species of religious curing was in no sense an integrated system.[1] If "system" meant nothing more

[1] This is not an original point. Zimmerman 1978, 97, asserts in a study of medicine in Kerala that "the idea that there is a system is pure assumption."

than the sum of all activities of a given kind, the word would have no explanatory value. Rather than a stable synthesis of many dynamic elements, what we see in the eleventh century is curers of all sorts endlessly competing and appropriating each other's methods. Literati physicians strove against their peers, whom they freely labeled incompetent, and spoke of doctors further down the social scale and other curers as incapable to the point of manslaughter. At the same time, the more enterprising of them eagerly borrowed the medicaments of herbalists, and learned thunder rites when such skills promised to help their reputations. So did local officials when epidemics or demoniac outbreaks prompted them to become involved.

The notion of a system implies that the choice between curers depended on rational principles. Actually the main constraints were where one was born and lived, and what one could afford. There might or might not be a herbalist of some sort in the neighborhood. A local family might or might not follow its own tradition of providing a formulation to anyone who might benefit, as a charitable act that earned its members merit for a better rebirth. There might or might not be a physician or a Daoist or Buddhist cleric nearby. If one lived in a poor village or neighborhood, one might not be able to pay for anything but the simplest therapy; it was possible that one or another local ritual master or herb-gatherer would accept food or something else in place of money.

Fluctuations in state involvement

There were metamorphoses in every aspect of health care in the long eleventh century, and in other kinds of technical enterprise as well.[2] A main cause was government policy. The state defined, edited, and distributed a canon of medical classics, and tried to replace the hereditary medical servitors to the elite by training "literati physicians" who came from the governing class. For economic reasons it processed drugs, established drug stores, and published a manual that enabled self-therapy using the packaged formulas that it sold. It sought to register the popular, Buddhist, and Daoist ritualists who actually met most of the therapeutic needs of the population. The main criterion for the registration of popular temples (not of clerics) was efficacy. The ability of gods to consistently answer prayers for the cure of suffering—among other goals—very frequently proved it. Thus the state was involved in one way or another in all the main dimensions of health care. But it did nothing to regulate unregistered clerics, aside from occasional persecution.

Health care policies were not consistent. Most were the products of two periods of reform. The reforms of the 1040s were largely abortive, but some of the ideas behind them remained alive. The "New Policies" initiatives of the 1070s (see chapter 4, p. 65) were soon reversed, but Zhezong 哲宗 and Huizong revived some of them from 1086 on. The fall of the Northern Song government in 1127 meant that, while some changes continued, many ended once and for all. The registration of

[2] Sun Xiaochun 孫小淳 2007 surveys change in physical science, with additional studies in Sun & Zeng Xiongsheng 曾雄生 2007.

temples and clerics continued into the Southern Song period; the drug store system shifted its focus to epidemic relief; and the attempts to operate local medical schools were, so far as the evidence goes, abortive.

Historical myths

As usual in trying to gauge the achievements of the imperial state, it is a bad idea to assume that an edict establishing new institutions in the provinces means that they soon could be found there, or that making a law meant that the law was obeyed or even enforced. To the contrary, official correspondence regularly reveals that the building for a new prefectural medical school was never erected, or was standing empty, or that drugs that the government bought for epidemic relief had been adulterated or had vanished.

Given the enormous size and the social and ethnic diversity of China, and the isolation of local officials assigned by the central government, it is likely that an official assertion about government and its operations is trustworthy *at best* for a couple of hundred miles around the capital.[3]

Next Steps

Popular curing

In popular curing lies the most flagrant blank in our understanding. There is ample documentation of what ritual masters did, and why. Most Sinologists ignore popular religion, unaware of its importance. That is not their fault. Specialists in Chinese religion, who write almost entirely for fellow specialists, and for whom nothing but Daoism or Buddhism is worth knowing about, teach them to ignore it. The few specialists in popular religion cannot even agree on what to call it (see chapter 5, p. 94).

The fact remains that popular religion continued to shape and energize Buddhism and Daoism through their history; its borders with them have always been fluid. We saw that in the eleventh century the state's sharpening of criteria for registration of clergy and temples actually increased the number of unregistered (and thus illegal) curers, for whom doctrinal distinctions important to ordained priests carried no weight. Officials who tried to get rid of unregistered curers did not care whether a local priest was originally trained as a Daoist; all of them were wizards, and all deserved flogging. This was likely to encourage unrecognized curers of various

[3] Skinner 1985 enunciated this important principle.

kinds to cooperate with each other (and learn each other's methods) for the sake of survival.

This is more than a health care issue. It can cast light on the political history of center vs. locality, and on the resistance of the latter to coercion by the former. It can also help us to better understand local officials, who on the one hand were skewered between the government they represented and the people whose folkways and values they had to learn about as they ruled. On the other, while carrying out duties in some periphery of the empire, they were at the same time concerned with the next steps in a career that could advance toward greater responsibility, and service in the palace.[4]

In the private sphere, there remains the intriguing question of the divided consciousness of elite officeholders. As children they were exposed to local ceremonial life, organized round the family on the one hand and the gods of the community on the other. If they joined the civil service and became local officials, they were expected to worship at local temples in the name of the state. If they rose to the high rank of Academician they were often assigned to write parts of the liturgy for imperially sponsored Daoist rituals. Temples that did not merit official registration were quite another matter, to be torn down or burnt down, or their ritualists threatened or brutalized, as the latest government campaign or the local magistrate's bias decreed.

We have no idea how difficult it was for individual civil servants to reconcile their intellectual and moral formations with what their superiors expected of them as policies toward "wizardry" came and went. I noted in chapter 5 (p. 96) that many of the most ostentatious opponents of southern "wizardry" came from the south themselves. That opens the possibility that they felt impelled to prove they did not conform to old-fashioned northerners' stereotype of superstitious southerners. A longitudinal study of the careers of a number of wizard-baiters can determine whether this was true and significant.

The economic dimension

Economic studies of ancient China have been restricted to a few topics, mostly fiscal. Some aspects of the role of money in religion, such as patronage, are obvious, but I cannot think of any generalization that we might make with confidence. Many wider themes are worth exploring, for which there are ample local sources once we look for them:

- Clerics did not subsist on wages; we have no idea how their income varied. The incomes of temples and monasteries depended on the initiative of those who ran them, but what were the variables?

[4] For a general introduction to Song society and politics, see Hymes & Schirokauer 1993 or Kuhn 2009.

- How were drugs distributed, and what set their prices? To what extent were the gatherers and growers of medicinal plants involved in trade networks outside their locality? How did the unification of China (and the splits that preceded and followed the Northern Song period) affect markets?

Local variation

There have been a very few studies of the effects of local variation on health care in later periods, such as Marta Hanson's book (2011) on the part that Warm Factor Disorders played in the formation of south Chinese identity. There have been none for imperial China before 1400, and none for non-medical aspects of health care. This is an exceptionally promising area for study. It is clear that popular ritual masters in eleventh-century south China were predominantly spirit mediums, but how predominantly? And to what extent was this true in the north, and in the distinctive culture of Sichuan?

We are also quite ignorant of the distribution of clerics in the eleventh century. This is not an easy question to answer, but the surviving gazetteers published in the Song dynasty offer a relatively trustworthy source of data to begin with. Vincent Goossaert has recently estimated that the number of Daoist clerics in China in the eighteenth century was so small they could not have served the whole population. As I have noted above (chapter 6, p. 148), this was equally true in the eleventh century. In the appendix I provide data from part of that century that shows registered Buddhist clerics greatly outnumbered Daoists, despite the Daoist enthusiasms of emperors. It is already clear that imperial patronage in the Northern Song period was generous and more or less steady, but how this affected the population of monks in various parts of the empire after 1077 (the last year for which we have data) is not a matter to be guessed at.

The history of the hospital has not received the attention it deserves. We have a fair number of sources about both privately funded foundations such as that of Su Shi 蘇軾 (1089) and state hospitals from 1102 to the end of the dynasty (see chapter 6, p. 142). For reasons I have already given, we cannot assume that all, or even most, of those ordered up by imperial edict actually came into being. A thorough study of reports to the throne from officials should let us see for this important example how realistic the issuance of edicts was.

A Last Word

One useful outcome of this book should be more realism about the scientific status of biomedicine. Spokesmen for medicine assume that public esteem depends on its cleaving as close as possible to the model of the physical sciences. Over the past century that has led to a narrowing of the scope of clinical practice, to the point that training is being restricted increasingly to what the gold standard of clinical research has technologically validated. The result is more attention to the quantitative outcomes of tests, and less to closely and thoughtfully observing and listening to patients. Medical schools do not teach students to maximize the curative power of empathy and of symbolism (what used to be called the "bedside manner"). Unfledged doctors are learning to respond to patients as if the latter were laboratory animals rather than complicated individuals. This is unlikely to change, so that the ability of doctors to deliver care as well as medicaments will depend on their own initiative in learning the humanistic rudiments of symbolic anthropology, medical sociology, and the history of medicine.

Most educated people are aware that the opposition of mind and body, from the time of Plato on, has been a weak point of European philosophy. Its effect on medicine has been to dichotomize it and hand all its parts over to distinct specialists. What used to be the general practitioner has become the primary care or family care specialist, who, at best, has been only perfunctorily educated to grasp how the physical and emotional needs of the patient are related. The gamut of early curing practices discussed in this book, including classical medicine, are generally holistic, in the sense that they saw the physical and the emotional as a single entity. Learning about them can be of some help to people who want to learn how to overcome the mind-body gap. Early physicians, but not ritual curers, conceived illness as a process that needs to be tracked step by step. They also learned to listen attentively to what the patient said, and to pay close attention to signs and symptoms.

Finally, if used sensibly, current clinical knowledge can be useful in reconstructing the medicine of earlier times. I have argued that applying biomedicine to diagnose past ailments for which the evidence is scanty and vague is a waste of time. There is no basis for the assumption that modern medicine is a universal model whose nosology contains every disease found in another culture or another time. On the other hand, biomedicine is a most useful tool when applied *after* one has used the categories of the time and place to comprehend what the data mean.

There are, to sum up, a number of ways in which the study of curing in other times and places can uncover a wider range of possibilities for modern medicine. This, I believe, is salutary in a time when the dominant trend has been toward increasing narrowness, toward more management and less care.

References

Abbreviations

DZ = Volume number in *Daozang*
ES = *Ersishi shi* 二十四史 of Zhonghua Shuju, 1959–1977.
HY = text in Harvard-Yenching Concordance series
j. = *juan* 卷 (chapter)
RW = published by Renmin Weisheng Chubanshe 人民衛生出版社, Beijing

S = Title number in Schipper 1975
SQ = Siku quanshu 四庫全書
SV = Schipper & Verellen 2004
T = *Taishō shinshū Daizōkyō* 大正新修大藏經
UP = University Press
YZ = Yi tong zheng mai quan shu 醫統正脈全書
ZD = Volume, item, *juan,* and page numbers in *Zhonghua daozang* 中华道藏
ZS = published by Zhonghua shuju 中華書局, Beijing
ZZ = Zhongyi zhenben congshu 中醫珍本叢書 ed.

Hanson, Marta. 2011. *Speaking of Epidemics in Chinese Medicine. Disease and the Geographic Imagination in Late Imperial China.* Needham Research Institute Series, 9. London: Routledge.

Hymes, Robert, & Conrad Schirokauer, eds. 1993. *Ordering the World: Approaches to State and Society in Sung Dynasty China.* Berkeley: University of California Press.

Kuhn, Dieter. 2009. *The Age of Confucian Rule. The Song Transformation of China.* History of Imperial China. Belknap Press of Harvard UP.

Skinner, G. William. 1985. Presidential Address: The Structure of Chinese History. *Journal of Asian Studies* 44. 2: 271–292.

Sun, Xiaochun 孫小淳. 2007. State and Science: Scientific Innovations in Northern Song China, 960–1127. Ph.D. dissertation, History and Sociology of Science, University of Pennsylvania.

Sun, Xiaochun & Zeng Xiongsheng 曾雄生, eds. 2007. *Songdai guojia wenhua zhong de kexue* 宋代国家文化中的科学 (Science and the State in the Song Dynasty). Beijing: Zhongguo Kexue Jishu Chubanshe.

Zimmerman, Francis. 1978. From Classic Texts to Learned Practice: Methodological Remarks on the Study of Indian Medicine. *Social Science and Medicine* 12: 97–103.

References

Abbreviations

DZ = Volume number in *Daozang*
ES = *Ersishi shi* 二十四史 of ZS, 1959–1977.
HY = text in Harvard-Yenching Concordance series
j. = *juan* 卷 (chapter)
RW = published by Renmin Weisheng Chubanshe 人民衛生出版社, Beijing
S = Title number in Schipper 1975
SQ = Siku quanshu 四庫全書
SV = Schipper & Verellen 2004
T = *Taishō shinshū Daizōkyō* 大正新修大藏經
UP = University Press
YZ = Yi tong zheng mai quan shu 醫統正脈全書
ZD = Volume, item, *juan,* and page numbers in *Zhonghua daozang* 中华道藏
ZS = published by Zhonghua shuju 中華書局, Beijing
ZZ = Zhongyi zhenben congshu 中醫珍本叢書 ed.

Classical Chinese Sources

Baopuzi neipian 抱樸子內篇 (The inner chapters of the Master who Keeps to Simplicity). Ge Hong 葛洪. Ca. A.D. 320. Pingjinguan congshu 平津館叢書 ed. of 1885. See also emendations in Wang Ming 王明 1980.

Bei ji qian jin yao fang 備急千金要方 (Revised formulas worth a thousand, for every urgent need). Sun Simiao 孫思邈. 650/659. Taipei: Guoli Zhongyao Yanjiusuo reproduction of Edo Igaku ed. of 1849.

Bencao gangmu 本草綱目 (Systematic materia medica). Li Shizhen 李時珍. Compiled 1552–1593, printed 1596. Commercial Press reprint, 1959.

Bencao jing ji zhu 本草經集注 (The canon of materia medica, with collected annotations). Tao Hongjing 陶弘景. Ca. 500. Lost. Partial reconstruction in Okanishi 1972.

Bi shu lu hua 避暑錄話 (Anecdotes set down while avoiding the summer heat). By Ye Mengde 葉夢得. Completed 1135. In *Quan Song biji* 全宋筆記 (Complete jottings of the Song period; Zhengzhou: Da Xiang Chubanshe), series 2, vol. 10, 1: 239.

© Springer International Publishing Switzerland 2015

N. Sivin, *Health Care in Eleventh-Century China*, Archimedes 43,
DOI 10.1007/978-3-319-20427-7

Boji fang 博濟方 (Broadly helpful formulas). Wang Gun 王袞. Author's preface 1047. Preface in Yan Shiyun 严世芸 1990–1994, 2180–2181, s.v. *Wang shi boji fang* 王氏博濟方. Lost, quoted in *Yongle da dian* 永樂大典.

Chang qing ji 長慶集 (Collected poems). Bai Juyi 白居易. 825. SQ.

Chisongzi zhang li 赤松子章曆 (Petition almanac of the Red Pine Master). Anonymous. Early fourth/sixth century. S615, DZ335–336. A manual of petitions for use by Heavenly Masters clerics.

Chisongzi zhou hou yao jue 赤松子肘後藥訣 (Handy oral instructions for medicines by the Red Pine Master). Anonymous. eighth or ninth century? S883B, DZ 583, pp. 4b–15b. Omitted from all *Daozang* indexes.

Chuan ya 串雅 (The Penetrator Improved). Zhao Boyun 趙柏雲, ed. Zhao Xuemin 趙學敏. Completed 1759. Reprint, Hong Kong, 1957.

Daguan bencao 大觀本草. See *Jing shi zheng lei Daguan bencao.*

Dao fa hui yuan 道法會元 (Daoist methods: the principles collected). Compiled by Zhao Yizhen 趙宜真. Ca. 1450. S1220, DZ 884–941. A large collection of Qingwei rituals. On probable time of compilation, see SV 1106.

Dao men ke lue 道門科略. See *Lu Xiansheng dao men ke lue.*

Daozang 道藏 (Daoist canon). Anonymous. Compiled 1406–1445, printed 1447. 1120 vols. Reprint, Shanghai: Commercial Press, 1923–1926.

Dongpo quan ji 東坡全集 (Complete collected writings of Su Shi). SQ.

Fa yuan zhu lin 法苑珠林 (Grove of Jewels in the Garden of the Law). Daoshi 道世. 668. T2122.

Fan Wenzheng Gong ji 范文正公集 (Collected writings of Fan Zhongyan). Fan Zhongyan 范仲淹. Compiled 1053? In Sibu congkan 四部叢刊 (Taibei: Taiwan Shangwu Yinshuguan, 1979).

Gu jin lu yan fang 古今錄驗方 (Register of Effective Medical Formulas Old and New). Chen Quan 陳權 & Chen Liyan 陳立言 (?). Ca. 620. Lost. Reconstituted version, ed. Xie Pangen 谢盘根. Beijing: Zhongguo Yiyao Keji Chubanshe 中国医药科技出版社, 1996.

Henan Shao shi wen jian hou lu 河南邵氏聞見後錄 (Sequel to Things Heard and Seen by Mr. Shao of Honan). Shao Bo 邵博. Posthumously compiled 1157. ZS, 1983. Sequel to Shao's father's *Wen chien lu.*

Huangdi jiayi jing 黃帝甲乙經 (A–B Canon of the Yellow Emperor). Huangfu Mi 皇甫謐. Compiled 256/282. In YZ under title *Zhenjiu jiayi jing* 鍼灸甲乙經.

Huangdi bashiyi nan jing 黃帝八十一難經 (Canon of Eighty-one Problems in the Inner Canon of the Yellow Emperor). Anonymous. Probably 2nd C. A.D. In YZ under title *Nan jing.*

Huangdi jiu ding shen dan jing jue 黃帝九鼎神丹經訣 (Canon and oral instructions for the divine elixir of the Yellow Emperor's nine ritual cauldrons). Anonymous, j. 1 probably of Han period, remainder probably of seventh century. S885, DZ584–585.

Huangdi neijing. See *Huangdi neijing su wen, Huangdi neijing ling shu,* and *Huangdi neijing tai su.*

Huangdi neijing ling shu 黃帝內經靈樞 (Inner canon of the Yellow Emperor: Divine pivot). Anonymous. First century B.C. or first century A.D. In *Ling shu jiao shi* 靈樞校釋 (2 vols.; RW, 1982).

Huangdi neijing su wen 黃帝內經素問 (Inner canon of the Yellow Emperor: Basic questions). Anonymous. First century B.C. or first century A.D. Taipei: Xuanfeng Chubanshe, 1973.

Huangdi neijing tai su 黃帝內徑太素 (Inner canon of the Yellow Emperor: Grand basis). Yang Shangshan 楊上善. 666/683. In *Tōyō igaku zempon sōsho* 東洋醫學善本叢書 (Collected rare books on Oriental medicine). Osaka: Tōyō Igaku Kenkyūkai.

Ishin hō (Chinese: *Yi xin fang)* 醫心方 (Formulas at the heart of medicine). Tamba no Yasuyori 丹波康賴. Completed 982. RW reprint of 1310 MS.

Jiayou bu zhu Shennong bencao 嘉祐補注神農本草I (The Divine Farmer's materia medica, with supplementary annotations, of the Excellent Protection era). Compiled by imperial order. 1061. Lost, but incorporated in later imperially sponsored materia medica collections such as *Zhenghe bencao.*

Jin gui yao lue 金櫃要略 (Essentials in the Golden Casket). Attributed to Zhang Ji. In present form by 1057. YZ.

Jin jing 禁經 (Canon of interdiction). Anonymous. Before late seventh century. In *Qian jin yi fang*, j. 29–30.

Jinlu zhai sandong zanyong yi 金籙齋三洞讚詠儀 (Hymns for Golden Register purification rituals of the Three Caverns). Compiled by Zhang Shangying 張商英. 1104/1123. S310, DZ 161, ZD 43/010. See SV 1039.

Jing shi zheng lei Daguan bencao 經史正類大觀本草 (Materia medica of the Great Prospect era, classified and verified from the classics and histories). Tang Shenwei 唐慎微. 1108. Tokyo: Hirokawa Shoten, 1970.

Jiu Tang shu 舊唐書 (Old history of the Tang period). Liu Xu 劉昫. 945. ES.

Li ji 禮記 (Record of rites). Anonymous. Early second century A.D. HY.

Lingbao da fa 靈寶大法. See *Lingbao wuliang duren shangjing da fa.*

Lingbao wuliang duren shangjing da fa 靈寶無量度人上經大法 (Lingbao upper scripture: Great method for limitlessly saving people). Anonymous. Ca. 1200. S219, DZ 85–99. See SV 1028.

Lingnan weisheng fang 嶺南衛生方 (Formulas for health in the deep south). Jihong 繼洪 (Buddhist cleric). Author's preface 1283. ZZ.

Longshu yan lun 龍樹眼論 (Nagarjuna's discussions of the eyes). Anonymous. Sui or Tang period. Lost. See Okanishi 1958, 448–449, Deshpande 2000 and Deshpande & Fan 2012.

Lu Xiansheng dao men ke lue 陸先生道門科略 (Abridged codes of Master Lu for Daoist communities). Attributed to Lu Xiujing 陸修靜. Late fifth century. S761, DZ1127.

Lun yu 論語 (Analects). Successors of Confucius. 479/249 B.C. HY. Translation and notes in Leys & Nylan 2014. For tentative dating, see Brooks & Brooks 1998.

Mai jing 脈經 (Canon of pulsating vessels). Wang Xi 王熙 (or Shuhe 叔和). Third century A.D. YZ.

Mao Shi 毛詩 (Mao recension of the *Book of Songs*). Anonymous. In final form by late sixth century B.C.? HY.

Mengzi 孟子 (Mencius). Anonymous. Chapters written between ca. 320 and the first century B.C. HY.

Mo jing. See *Mai jing*

Neng gai zhai man lu 能改齋漫錄 (Desultory records from the Studio of Corrigibility). Wu Zeng 吳曾. 1157. SQ.

Pingzhou ke tan 平洲可談 (Acceptable chats from Pingzhou). Zhu Yu 朱彧. Author's preface 1119. Critical ed. in Tang Song shiliao biji 唐宋史料筆記, ZS, 2007.

Qian jin fang 千金方. See *Bei ji qian jin yao fang.*

Qian jin yi fang 千金翼方 (Revised formulas worth a thousand). Sun Simiao. Late 7th century. RW, 1955, reproduction of 1307 ed.

Quan Liang wen 全梁文 (Complete short prose of the Liang period). See *Quan Shang gu San dai Qin Han San guo Liu chao wen.*

Quan Shang gu San dai Qin Han San guo Liu chao wen 全上古三代秦漢三國六朝文 (Complete short prose from antiquity to the Six Dynasties). Yan Kejun 嚴可均. Completed 1836, printed 1893. Taipei 1963 ed.

San yin ji yi bing yuan lun cui 三因極一病源論粹 (The three causes epitomized and unified: the quintessence of doctrine on the origins of medical disorders). Chen Yan 陳言. 1174 or shortly after. Beijing, 1957 ed., under the title *San yin ji yi ping zheng fang lun* 三因極一病證方論. Commonly referred to as *San yin fang* 三因方.

Shan hai jing 山海經 (Classic of mountains and seas). Anonymous. 290/240 B.C.? SQ. The layers in this work and their dates are contentious. See Riccardo Fracasso in Loewe 1993, 357–367.

Shanghan jiushi lun 傷寒九十論 (Ninety Discussions Based on the Treatise on Cold Damage Disorders). Hsu Shuwei 徐叔微. 1132. In *Zhongguo yixue dacheng* 中國醫學大成 (6 vols., Changsha, 1990), vol. 3.

Shanghan lun 傷寒論. See *Shanghan zabing lun*. In YZ.

Shanghan zabing lun 傷寒雜病論 (Treatise on Cold Damage and miscellaneous disorders). Attributed to Zhang Ji 張機. 198–220. Divided into *Shanghan lun* and *Jin gui yao lue* 金櫃要略 by 1057.

Shen zhou jing 神咒經. See *Taishang dongyuan shen zhou jing.*

Shen zhou zhi bing kou zhang 神咒治病口章. See *Taishang dongshen dongyuan shen zhou zhi bing kou zhang.*

Shen yi pu jiu fang 神醫普救方 (The divine physician's formulary for universal relief). Jia Huangzhong 賈黃中 et al. Compiled and promulgated by imperial order, 986. A mammoth compilation, in 1010 *juan.* Lost.

Sheng ji jing 聖濟經 (*Canon of Sagely Benefaction*). Compiled by order of Emperor Huizong. Promulgated 1118. In Zhenben yishu jicheng 珍本醫書集成, vol. 9.

Sheng ji zong lu 聖濟總錄 *(General Record of Sagely Benefaction).* Shen Fu 申甫 et al., compiled by order of Emperor Huizong. 1117. RW ed. of 1952, reprint of 1982.

Shennong bencao 神農本草 (The Divine Farmer's materia medica). Anonymous. Late first or second century A.D. Lost; of the many reconstructions, that in Ma Jixing 1995 is superior.

Shi Zaizhi fang 史載之方. See *Zhinan fang.*

Sifen lü 四分律 (Dharmaguptaka Vinaya, lit., Four-part community regulations). Anonymous Indian author, translated in early 5th century by Buddhayaśas. T1428.

Song da zhaoling ji 宋大詔令集 (Unabridged collection of edicts and commands of the Song period). Anonymous. 1131–1162. ZS 1962 ed. Medical data collected in Han Yi 韓毅 2007.

Song hui yao ji gao. Dao shi 宋會要輯稿. 道釋 (Draft reconstituted edition of the *Essential Documents and Regulations of the Song Period.* Section on Daoists and Buddhists). Xu Song 徐松. Early Ming period. In *Song hui yao ji gao. Fanyi dao shi* 宋會要輯稿. 蕃夷道釋. Chengdu: Sichuan Daxue Chubanshe, 2010. Gathered from various Song compilations covering up to 1220.

Song shi 宋史 (History of the Song period). Tuotuo 脫脫. 1345. ES.

Song Zhenzong yuzhi yujing ji 宋真宗御制玉京集 (Jade capital collection, by emperor Zhenzong of the Song period). Before 1022. S315, DZ 163, ZD, 44/060, 5: 581. Collected statements of intention *(yi* 意) for use in Daoist rituals.

Su Shen liang fang 蘇沈良方 (Superior formulas by Su & Shen). Su Shi 蘇軾 & Shen Kuo 沈括. Anonymously compiled, 1141/1151; combines Shen's *Liang fang* with some unpublished medical writings by Su. In *Zhi buzu zhai congshu* 知不足齋叢書.

Sui shu 隋書 (History of the Sui period). Wei Zheng 魏徵. 636. ES.

Sun Zhenren bei ji qian jin fang 孫真人備急千金方 (Formulas worth a thousand for urgent need, by Sun the Realized Immortal). Compiled anonymously. Date unknown. S1162–1163, DZ 799–820. A conflated version of Sun Simiao's *Beiji qianjin yao fang* and *Qianjin yi fang.*

Taiping guang ji 太平廣記 (Extensive records compiled in the Great Peace and Prosperous State era). Li Fang 李昉, by imperial order. 978. ZS, 1961.

Taiqing dan jing yao jue 太清丹經要訣 (Essential formulas for oral transmission from the alchemical canons). Sun Simiao, late 7C? Critical ed. and translation in Sivin 1968.

Taiping sheng hui fang 太平聖惠方 (Imperial grace formulary of the Great Peace and Prosperous State era). Compiled by Wang Huaiyin 王懷隱, printed, and promulgated by imperial order. 992. RW, 1958.

Taiqing shi bi ji 太清石壁記 (Records from the stone wall, a Great Purity canon). Anonymous. 758/759. S882, DZ582–583. Alchemical formulary. See SV 381.

Taishang dongshen dongyuan shen zhou zhi bing kou zhang 太上洞神洞淵神咒治病口章 (Oral petitions for the healing of medical disorders, a scripture of the Divine Incantations of the Cavern Spirit and the Cavern Abyss of the Most High). Anonymous. Probably early fifth century A.D. S 1290, DZ 1008.

Taishang dongyuan shen zhou jing 太上洞淵神咒經 (or *shen zhu jing* 神祝經; Scripture of Divine Incantations of the Cavern Abyss of the Most High). Anonymous. Accreted between the early fifth century and 900. S335, DZ 170–173.

Taishang lingbao wufu xu 太上靈寶五符序 (The five talismans, divine treasure of the Most High). Anonymous, 317/420. Anthology of the Taiqing 太清 Daoist tradition. Despite *xu* in the title, not a preface. S388, DZ 183.

Taishang shuo niuhuang miao jing 太上說牛黃妙經 (Wondrous sutra of the Most High on *niuhuang*). Anonymous. Date unknown. S366, DZ 180. See SV 960. Not cited in Despeux 2010.

Taishang zhu guo jiu min zong zhen mi yao 太上助國救民總真祕要 (Secret essentials, comprehensive and realized, of the Most High, for assisting the country and saving the people). Yuan Miaozong 元妙宗. 1116. S1227, DZ 986–987.

Taishō shinshū Daizōkyō 大正新修大藏經 (Newly edited Great Buddhist canon of the Taishō period). 85 vols. Tokyo: Issaikyō Kankōkai, 1924–1932.

Tong zhi 通志 (General history). Zheng Qiao 鄭樵. Presented to throne 1161. Sibu congkan ed.

Waitai mi yao 外臺祕要 (Arcane essentials from the Imperial Library). Wang Tao 王燾. 762. RW.

Wang Jinggong wenji jianzhu 王荊公文集箋注 (Annotated short prose writings of Wang Anshi), with notes by Li Zhiliang 李之亮. Date of compilation unknown. Chengdu: Ba-Shu Shushe, 2005.

Wu li xiao zhi 物理小識 (Notes on the Patterns of the Phenomena). Fang Yizhi 方以智. Preface 1643, printed 1664. Ningjingtang ed. of 1884.

Xin Tang shu 新唐書 (New history of the Tang period). Ouyang Xiu 歐陽修 et al. 1060. ES.

Xu zizhi tongjian chang bian 續資治通鑑長編 (Long draft of the Continuation of the Comprehensive Mirror for Aid in Government). Li Tao 李燾. 1183. ZS reprint, 2004.

Xuandu lü wen 玄都律文 (Regulations of the dark capital[, the seat of the Ancient Lord]). Anonymous. Ca. 700? S188, DZ 78. Fragments, mainly of an early Heavenly Masters document.

Yao xing lun 藥性論 (On the characteristics of drugs). Attributed to Zhen Quan 甄權. Ca. 620. Lost, but richly quoted in *Jiayou bu zhu Shennong bencao* 嘉祐補注神農本草.

Yijian zhi 夷堅志 (Records of the listener). By Hong Mai 洪邁. Written over the period 1157–1202. 4 vols. ZS, 1981. Only 207 of the original 420 j. survive.

Yin hai jing wei 銀海精微 (Essential Subtleties on the Silver Sea). Anonymous. Sixteenth century, attributed to Sun Simiao. Jinzhang Shuju reprint, 1954. Translated in Kovacs & Unschuld 1998.

Yixue ru men 醫學入門 (Introduction to medical studies). Li Chan 李梴. Preface 1575. Tailian Guofeng Chubanshe reprint of 1973.

Yixue yuanliu lun 醫學源流論 (Topical discussions of the history of medicine). Xu Dachun 徐大椿. 1757. In *Xu Dachun yishu quanji* 徐大椿醫書全集 (Complete collected medical writings of Xu Dachun), RW, 1988).

Yuyin fashi 玉音法事 (Liturgy of precious music). Anonymous. Ming period? S607, DZ 333. Major hymns of Lingbao liturgy, elaborately annotated.

Zhen gao 真誥 (Declarations of the Realized Immortals). Compiled by Tao Hongjing 陶弘景. 499. S1016, DZ 637–640. Collected revelations of 364–370.

Zhenghe bencao 政和本草. See *Zhenghe xin xiu jing shi zheng lei bei yong bencao.*

Zhenghe wan shou daozang 政和萬壽道藏 (Longevity Daoist Canon of the Regnant Harmony era). Compiled by imperial order. Printed 1119–1122. Lost. Table of contents partly reconstructed in van der Loon 1984.

Zhenghe wuli xin yi 政和五禮新儀 (New forms of the five categories of rites of the Regnant Harmony era). Edited by Zheng Juzhong 鄭居中. 1113. In SQ *zhenben chu ji* 珍本初集.

Zhenghe xin xiu jing shi zheng lei bei yong bencao 政和新修經史證類備用本草 (Revised materia medica of the Regnant Harmony Era, classified and verified from the classics and histories, for every use). Cao Xiaozhong 曹孝忠. 1116. Extant only in the slightly revised *Chong xiu Zhenghe jing shi zheng lei bei yong bencao* 重修政和新修經史證類備用本草 of 1249, Beijing reproduction of 1957. For differences see Unschuld 1986, 77–82.

Zhengtong daozang 正統道藏 (Daoist canon of the Correct Concordance reign period). See *Daozang.*

Zhengyi fawen xiuzhen zhi yao 正一法文修真旨要 (Essentials of the Practice of Realization, from the Correct Unity Ritual Canon). Anonymous. Tang period. S1270, DZ1003. On diagnosis and exorcistic therapy using a carved seal.

Zhi bing kouzhang 治病口章. See *Taishang dongyuan shen zhou jing.*
Zhinan fang 指南方 (Compass formulary). Shi Kan 史堪. Early twelfth century. Also called *Shi Zaizhi fang* 史載之方; under that title in Liang Song ming jia fangshu jing xuan 两宋名家方书精选 collection (2003).
Zhonghua daozang 中华道藏 (Chinese Daoist canon). 49 vols. Beijing: Huaxia Chubanshe. Digital edition of *Daozang*, in simplified characters, with some revisions and added texts.
Zhouhou jiu zu fang 肘後救卒方 (Emergency remedies ready to hand). Ge Hong. Ca. A.D. 340. Survives only in form revised by Tao Hongjing 陶弘景 as *Zhouhou beiji fang* 肘後備急方. RW reprint of 1574 ed., 1956.
Zhou yi 周易 (Changes of the Zhou dynasty; usually referred to as Book of Changes). Anonymous. Original text late ninth century B.C.; Ten Wings between third and second century, except that "Xu gua" is Later Han. HY.
Zhu bing yuan hou lun 諸病源候論 (Origins and symptoms of medical disorders). Chao Yuanfang 巢元方. Completed 610. RW, 1955.
Zhuangzi 莊子 (The Book of Master Zhuang). Partly by Zhuang Zhou 莊周? Ca. 320 to late second century. Partial translation: Graham 1981; on authorship see also Graham 1990, 283–321.

Other Sources

Ackerknecht, Erwin H. 1971. *Medicine and Ethnology. Selected Essays,* ed. H. H. Walser & H. M. Koelbing. Baltimore: Johns Hopkins UP.
Agazzi, Evandro. 2014. *Scientific Objectivity and its Contexts.* Cham: Springer.
Ahern, Emily M. 1981. *Chinese Ritual and Politics.* Cambridge Studies in Social Anthropology, 34. Cambridge UP.
Albrecht, Gary L., Ray Fitzpatrick, & Susan Scrimshaw, eds. 2000. *Handbook of Social Studies in Health and Medicine.* London: Sage Publications.
Als, C., et al. 2002. Visible Signs of Illness from the 14th to the 20th Century. Systematic Review of Portraits. *British Medical Journal* 325: 1499–1502.
Andersen, Poul. 2008. Tianxin zhengfa 天心正法. In Pregadio 2008, 2:989–993.
Anonymous. 1986. *Ershiliushi yijia zhuanji xin zhu* 二十六史医家传纪新注 (New annotations to the biographies of physicians in the 26 Histories). Shenyang: Liaoning Daxue Chubanshe.
Anonymous, ed. 1994. *Minjian xinyang yu Zhongguo wenhua guoji yantaohui lunwen ji* 民間信仰與中國文化研討會論文集 (Proceedings of an international conference on popular beliefs and Chinese culture). Center for Chinese Studies Research Series, 4. 2 vols. Taipei: Hanxue Yanjiu Zhongxin 漢學研究中心.
Aronowitz, Robert A. 1998. *Making Sense of Illness. Science, Society, and Disease.* Cambridge History of Medicine. Cambridge UP.
Baldrian-Hussein, Farzeen. 2008. *Hun* and *Po.* In Pregadio 2008, 521–523.
Becker, Howard S. 1986. Culture: A Sociological View. In Becker, *Doing Things Together: Selected Papers.* Evanston: Northwestern UP.
Beier, Lucinda McCray. 2008. *For Their Own Good: The Transformation of English Working-Class Health Culture, 1880–1970.* Columbus: Ohio State UP.
Bell, Catherine. 1989. Religion and Chinese Culture: Toward an Assessment of 'Popular Religion,' *History of Religions* 29: 35–57.
Bell, Catherine. 1992. *Ritual Theory, Ritual Practice.* New York: Oxford UP.
Bell, Catherine. 2006. Paradigms Behind (and Before) the Modern Concept of Religion. *History and Theory: Studies in the Philosophy of History* 45. 4: 27–46.
Bennett, Steven J. 1978. Patterns of the Sky and Earth: A Chinese Science of Applied Cosmology. *Chinese Science* 3: 1–26.

Berlant, Jeffrey. 1975. *Profession and Monopoly: A Study of Medicine in the United States and Great Britain.* Berkeley: University of California Press.

Birnbaum, Raoul. 1989. Chinese Buddhist Traditions of Healing and the Life Cycle. In *Healing and Restoring: Health and Medicine in the World's Religious Traditions,* ed. Lawrence E. Sullivan, 33–57. New York: Macmillan.

Blacker, Carmen. 1975. *The Catalpa Bow.* London: Allen & Unwin.

Boileau, Gilles. 2002. Wu and Shaman. *Bulletin of the School of Oriental and African Studies* 65. 2: 350–378.

Bokenkamp, Stephen R. 1997. *Early Daoist Scriptures.* Taoist Classics, 1. Berkeley: University of California Press.

Bokenkamp, Stephen R. 2004. Daoism and Buddhism. In *Encyclopedia of Buddhism,* ed. Robert E. Buswell, Jr., 197–201. New York : Macmillan Reference USA/Thomson/Gale.

Bokenkamp, Stephen R. 2007. *Ancestors and Anxiety: Daoism and the Birth of Rebirth in China.* Berkeley: University of California Press.

Bokenkamp, Stephen R. 2008. *Fu* 符. In Pregadio 2008, 35–38.

Bokenkamp, Stephen R. 2010. Daoist Pantheons. In Lagerwey & Lü 2010, 1169–1203.

Bol, Peter K. 1992. *"This Culture of Ours." Intellectual Transitions in T'ang and Sung China.* Stanford UP.

Boltz, Judith Magee. 1993. Not by the Seal of Office Alone. New Weapons in Battles with the Supernatural. In Ebrey & Gregory 1993, 241–305.

Boltz, Judith M[agee]. 2008. Pudu. 2. The Ritual. In Pregadio 2008, 2:794.

Brockliss, Laurence, & Colin Jones. 1997. *The Medical World of Early Modern France.* Oxford UP.

Brooks, E. Bruce, & A. Taeko Brooks. 1998. *The Original Analects. Sayings of Confucius and his Successors.* Translations from the Asian Classics. New York: Columbia UP.

Brown, Peter. 1981. *The Cult of the Saints. Its Rise and Function in Latin Christianity.* University of Chicago Press.

Burnham, John C. 1996. Garrison Lecture: How the Concept of Profession Evolved in the Work of Historians of Medicine. *Bulletin of the History of Medicine* 70. 1: 1–24.

Cai Xianghui 蔡相煇. 1994. Yi Mazu xinyang wei li, lun zhengfu yu minjian xinyang de guanxi 以媽祖信仰為例論政府與民間信仰的關係 (The relation between government and popular beliefs, using belief in Mazu as an example). In Anonymous 1994, 437–454.

Campany, Robert Ford. 2003. On the Very Idea of Religions (in the Modern West and in Early Medieval China). *History of Religions* 42. 4: 287–319.

Campany, Robert Ford. 2005. Two Religious Thinkers of the Early Eastern Jin: Gan Bao and Ge Hong in Multiple Contexts. *Asia Major,* ser. 3, 18.1: 175–224.

Cedzich, Ursula-Angelika. 1987. *Das Ritual der Himmelsmeister im Spiegel früher Quellen. Übersetzung und Untersuchung des liturgischen Materials im dritten chüan des Teng-chen yin-chüeh.* Würzburg: The author.

Cedzich, Ursula-Angelika. 1995. The Cult of the Wu-t'ung/Wu-hsien in History and Fiction. The Roots of the *Journey to the South.* In David Johnson 1995, 137–218.

Chang Bide 昌彼得 et al. 1974–1976. *Song ren zhuanji ziliao suoyin* 宋人傳記資料索引 (Index to biographical sources on Sung personages). 6 vols. Taipei: Dingwen Shuju.

Chang, Che-chia. 1998. The Therapeutic Tug of War. The Imperial Physician-Patient Relationship in the Era of Empress Dowager Cixi (1874–1908). Ph.D. dissertation, Asian and Middle Eastern Studies, University of Pennsylvania.

Cao, Emily. 1999. The Maoist Shaman and the Madman: Ritual Bricolage, Failed Ritual, and Failed Ritual Theory. *Cultural Anthropology* 14. 4: 505–534.

Chao, Shin-yi. 2003. Daoist Examinations and Daoist Schools during the Northern Song Dynasty. *Journal of Chinese Religions* 31: 1–37.

Chao, Shin-yi. 2006. Huizong and the Divine Empyrean Palace Temple Network. In Ebrey & Bickford 2006, 324–358.

Chao, Shin-yi. 2011. *Daoist Ritual, State Religion, and Popular Practices: Zhenwu Worship from Song to Ming (960–1644)*. Routledge Studies in Daoism. New York: Routledge.

Chao Wei-pang. 1942. The Origin and Growth of the Fu Chi 扶乩. *Folklore Studies,* 1: 9–27. On the planchette.

Chao, Yuan-ling. 2000. The Ideal Physician in Late Imperial China: The Question of *San-shih* 三世. *East Asian Science, Technology, and Medicine* 17: 66–93.

Ch'en Hsiang-ch'un. 1942. Examples of Charm against Epidemics with Short Explanations. *Folklore Studies,* 1: 37–54.

Chen Keji 陳可冀 et al. 1990. *Qing gong yian yanjiu* 清宮醫案研究 (A study of the Qing medical archives). Beijing: Zhongyi Guji Chubanshe.

Chen Yinke 陳寅恪. 1930. *Sanguo zhi* Cao Chong Hua Tuo yu Fojiao gushi 三國志曹沖華佗與佛教故事 (The biographies of Cao Chong and Hua Tuo in the *History of the Three Kingdoms*, and Buddhist legends). *Qinghua xuebao* 清華學報 6. 1: 17–20.

Chen Yuanpeng 陳元朋. 1997. *Liang Sung de "shang yi shi ren" yu "ruyi." Jian lun qi zai Jin Yuan de liubian* 兩宋的「尚醫士人」與「儒醫」. 兼論其在金元的流變 ("Elite enthusiasts of medicine" and "literati physicians" in the Northern and Southern Song, with a discussion of changes in the Jin and Yuan periods). *Guoli Taiwan Daxue wen shi congkan* 國立臺灣大學文史叢刊, 104.

Cheng Minsheng 程民生. 2008. *Songdai wujia yanjiu* 宋代物价研究 (A study of commodity prices in the Song period). Beijing Renmin Chubanshe. Gathers prices from a wide range of sources, argues that they cannot be reduced to a common measure.

Chiu, Kaiming (Qiu Kaiming). 1936. The Introduction of Spectacles into China. *Harvard Journal of Asiatic Studies* 1: 186–193.

Cho, Philip S. 2006. Ritual and the Occult in Chinese Medicine and Religious Healing: The Development of Zhuyou Exorcism. Ph.D. dissertation, History and Sociology of Science, University of Pennsylvania.

Christakis, Nicholas A. 1999. *Death Foretold. Prophecy and Prognosis in Medical Care.* University of Chicago Press.

Clarke, Peter B., ed. 2000. *Japanese New Religions: In Global Perspective.* Curzon Studies in New Religious Movements. Richmond: Curzon.

Colp, Ralph, Jr. 1977. *To Be an Invalid: The Illness of Charles Darwin.* University of Chicago Press.

Crile, George, Jr. 1955. *Cancer and Common Sense.* New York: Viking Press.

Csikszentmihalyi, Mark. 2002. Traditional Taxonomies and Revealed Texts in the Han. In Kohn & Roth 2002, 81–101.

Csordas, Thomas J., & Arthur Kleinman. 1996. The Therapeutic Process. In Sargent & Johnson 1996, 3–20.

Cullen, Christopher. 2001. From Case Records to Case Histories: The Modernisation of a Chinese Medical Genre, 1912–49. In Hsu 2001: 324–336.

Cunningham, Andrew. 2002. Identifying Disease in the Past: Cutting the Gordian Knot. *Asclepio* 54, 1: 13–34.

Dale, Philip Marshall. 1952. *Medical Biographies: The Ailments of Thirty-three Famous Persons.* Norman: University of Oklahoma Press.

Daston, Lorraine, & Peter Galison. 2007. *Objectivity.* New York: Zone Books.

Davis, Deborah. 2005. Urban Consumer Culture. *The China Quarterly* 183: 692–709.

Davis, Edward L. 2001. *Society and the Supernatural in Song China.* Honolulu. University of Hawai'i Press.

Demiéville, Paul. 1985. *Buddhism and healing: Demiéville's article Byô from Hôbôgirin,* trans. Mark Tatz. Lanham, MD: University Press of America.

Deshpande, Vijaya. 2000. Ophthalmic Surgery: a Chapter in the History of Sino-Indian Medical Contacts. *Bulletin of the School of Oriental and African Studies* 63. 3: 370–388.

Deshpande, Vijaya, & Fan Ka Wai. 2012. *Restoring the Dragon's Vision (Nagarjuna and Medieval Chinese Opthalmology).* Hong Kong: Chinese Civilization Centre, City University of Hong Kong. Translates three ophthalmic texts related to India, with indexes.

Desjarlais, Robert R. 1992. *Body and Emotion. The Aesthetics of Illness and Healing in the Nepal Himalayas.* Series in Contemporary Ethnology, 2. Philadelphia: University of Pennsylvania Press.

Despeux, Catherine. 2001. The System of the Five Circulatory Phases and the Six Seasonal Influences *(wuyun liuqi)*, a Source of Innovation in Medicine under the Song (960–1279). In Hsu 2001, 121–165.

Despeux, Catherine, ed. 2010. *Médecine, religion et société dans la Chine médiévale. Étude de manuscripts chinois de Dunhuang et de Turfan.* 3 vols. Paris: Institute des Hautes Études Chinoises.

Douglas, Mary. 1966. *Purity and Danger.* London: Routledge & Kegan Paul.

Douglas, Mary. 1970. *Natural Symbols.* New York: Vintage.

Douglas, Mary, ed. 1982. *Essays in the Sociology of Perception.* London: Routledge & Kegan Paul.

Dunglison, Robley. 1839/1874. *Medical Lexicon: A Dictionary of Medical Science: Containing a Concise Explanation of the Various Subjects and Terms.* Revised ed. Philadelphia: Henry C. Lea.

Ebrey, Patricia Buckley. 2014. *Emperor Huizong.* Harvard UP.

Ebrey, Patricia Buckley, & Maggie Bickford. 2006. *Emperor Huizong and Late Northern Song China. The Politics of Culture and the Culture of Politics.* Harvard East Asian Monographs, 266. Harvard University Press.

Ebrey, Patricia Buckley, & Peter N. Gregory, eds. 1993. *Religion and Society in T'ang and Sung China.* Honolulu: University of Hawaii Press.

Eisenberg, David M., Ronald C. Kessler, Cindy Foster, et al. 1993. Unconventional Medicine in the United States—Prevalence, Costs, and Patterns of Use. *New England Journal of Medicine* 328: 246–252.

Eisenberg, Leon. 1977. Disease and Illness. Distinctions between Professional and Popular Ideas of Sickness. *Culture, Medicine, and Psychiatry* 1. 1: 9–23.

Eliade, Mircea. 1962. *The Forge and the Crucible,* tr. Stephen Corrin. New York.

Eliade, Mircea. 1968. The Forge and the Crucible: A Postscript. *History of Religions* 8: 74–88. New York: Harper & Row.

Elliott, Alan J. A. 1955. *Chinese Spirit Medium Cults in Singapore.* London: Royal Anthropological Institute.

Fan Jiawei 范家偉. 2007. *Da yi jing cheng. Tangdai guojia, xinyang yu yixue* 大醫精誠. 唐代國家, 信仰與醫學 (The perfect integrity of the great physician. State, belief, and medicine in the Tang dynasty). Yangsheng fangji congshu 養生方技叢書. Taipei: Dong Da Tushu Gongsi.

Fang Xiaoyang 方晓阳 & Chen Tianjia 陈天嘉, eds. 2009. *Zhongguo chuantong keji wenhua yanjiu* 中国传统科技文化研究 (Cultural Studies of traditional Chinese science and technology). Beijing: Kexue Chubanshe.

Farquhar, Judith. 1994. *Knowing Practice. The Clinical Encounter of Chinese Medicine.* Studies in the Ethnographic Imagination, 4. Boulder: Westview Press.

Fitzgerald, C. P. 1965. *Barbarian Beds: The Origin of the Chair in China.* London: Cresset Press.

Fox, Renée, & Judith P. Swazey. 1984. Medical Morality is not Bioethics—Medical Ethics in China and the United States. *Perspectives in Biology and Medicine* 27. 3: 336–360.

Freidson, Eliot. 1970. *Profession of Medicine. A Study of the Sociology of Applied Knowledge.* New York: Dodd, Mead and Company.

Freidson, Eliot. 2001. *Professionalism: The Third Logic.* University of Chicago Press.

Furth, Charlotte. 1999. *A Flourishing Yin: Gender in China's Medical History, 960–1665.* Berkeley: University of California Press.

Furth, Charlotte, Judith T. Zeitlin, & Ping-chen Hsiung, eds. 2007. *Thinking with Cases. Specialist Knowledge in Chinese Cultural History.* Honolulu: University of Hawai'i Press. Cases in law, medicine, religion and philosophy.

Gai Jianmin. 2012. Study of the Medical Elements in Taoist Healing: The Use of Talismans and Incantations. In Mou Zhongjian 2012, 293–308. Condescending, poorly informed.

Geertz, Clifford. 1973a. *The Interpretation of Cultures. Selected Essays.* New York: Basic Books, 1973.

Geertz, Clifford. 1966/1973b. Religion as a Cultural System. In Geertz 1973a, 87–125.

Geertz, Clifford. 2000a. *Available Light. Anthropological Reflections on Philosophical Topics.* Princeton UP.

Geertz, Clifford. 2000b. The Pinch of Destiny: Religion as Experience, Meaning, Identity, Power. In Geertz 2000a, 167–186.

Geertz, Clifford. 2000c. Anti Anti-Relativism. In Geertz 2000a, 42–67.

Gentilcore, David. 2004. Was There a 'Popular Medicine' in Early Modern Europe? *Folklore* 115: 151–166.

Giele, Enno. 1998–1999. Early Chinese Manuscripts. Including Addenda and Corrigenda to New Sources of Early Chinese History: An Introduction to the Reading of Inscriptions and Manuscripts. *Early China* 23–24: 247–337. Published 2001. Introduction to online database.

von Glahn, Richard. 2004. *The Sinister Way. The Divine and the Demonic in Chinese Religious Culture*: University of California Press.

Goldschmidt, Asaf. 2009. *The Evolution of Chinese Medicine. Northern Song Dynasty (960–1127).* Needham Research Institute Series, 8. London: Routledge.

Goossaert, Vincent. 2001. The Invention of an Order: Collective Identity in Thirteenth-century Quanzhen Taoism. *Journal of Chinese Religions* 29: 111–138.

Graham, A. C. 1981. *Chuang-tzu. The Seven Inner Chapters and Other Writings from the Book Chuang-tzu.* London: Allen & Unwin.

Graham, A. C. 1990. *Studies in Chinese Philosophy and Philosophical Literature.* SUNY Series in Chinese Philosophy and Culture. Albany: State University of New York Press.

Grant, Alicia, & Bo-Ying Ma. 2013. The Safe Use of Difficult and Dangerous Acupuncture Points. *Journal of Chinese Medicine in the UK* 2 (Supplementary issue): 47–51.

Grant, Joanna. 2003. *A Chinese Physician. Wang Ji and the 'Stone Mountain Medical Case Histories.'* Needham Research Institute Series, 2. London: RoutledgeCurzon.

Green, Monica H. 1994. Documenting Medieval Women's Medical Practice. In *Practical Medicine from Salerno to the Black Death,* ed. Luis Garcia Ballester, 322–352. Cambridge UP.

Greene, Eric. 2012. Meditation, Repentance, and Visionary Experience in Early Medieval Chinese Buddhism. Ph. D. dissertation, Buddhist Studies, University of California, Berkeley.

Gregory, Peter N., & Daniel A. Getz, Jr., eds. 1999. *Buddhism in the Sung.* Studies in East Asian Buddhism, 13. Honolulu: University of Hawai'i Press

Haar, Barend J. ter. 2006. *Telling Stories. Witchcraft and Scapegoating in Chinese History.* Leiden: E. J. Brill.

Haar, Barend J. ter. 2007. Review of von Glahn 2004. *Journal of Sung–Yuan Studies* 37: 250–258.

Han Yi 韓毅. 2007. *Songdai yixue zhaoling nianbiao yu ziliao huibian* 宋代医学诏令年表与资料汇编 (Chronology and compilation of Song imperial edicts on medicine). Beijing: Zhongguo Kexueyuan, Ziran kexueshi yanjiusuo.

Han Yi 韩毅. 2011. Bei Song zhengfu dui wuyi de kongzhi yu gaizao 北宋政府对巫医的控制与改造 (The Northern Song government's control and reform of wizard curers). *Zhongguo kejishi zazhi* 中国科技史杂志 (Studies in the history of natural sciences) 32 (supplement): 106–130.

Hansen, Valerie. 1990. *Changing Gods in Medieval China, 1127–1276.* Princeton UP.

Hanson, Marta. 2011. *Speaking of Epidemics in Chinese Medicine. Disease and the Geographic Imagination in Late Imperial China.* Needham Research Institute Series, 9. London: Routledge.

Harper, Donald J. 1998. *Early Chinese Medical Literature: The Mawangdui Medical Manuscripts.* Sir Henry Wellcome Asian Series. London: Royal Asiatic Society.

Harrell, C. Stevan. 1974. When a Ghost Becomes a God. In Wolf 1974a, 193–206.

Harrington, Anne, ed. 1997. *The Placebo Effect. An Interdisciplinary Exploration.* Harvard UP. Nine papers from a 1994 conference.

Harrington, Anne. 2008. *The Cure Within. A History of Mind-Body Medicine.* New York: W. W. Norton.

Hartwell, Robert M. 1982. Demographic, Political and Social Transformations in China, 750–1550. *Harvard Journal of Asiatic Studies* 42. 2: 365–442.

Hinrichs, TJ. 2003. The Medical Transforming of Governance and Southern Customs in Song Dynasty China (960–1279 C.E.). Ph.D. dissertation, East Asian Languages, Harvard University.

Hinrichs, TJ, & Linda L. Barnes, eds. 2013. *Chinese Medicine and Healing. An Illustrated History.* Cambridge: Belknap Press of Harvard UP.

Hinshaw, Stephen P., & Richard M. Scheffeler. 2014. *The ADHD Explosion. Myths, Medication, and Today's Push for Performance.* New York: Oxford UP.

Ho Peng Yoke (= Ping-yü, He Bingyu 何丙郁). 2003. *Chinese Mathematical Astrology. Reaching out to the Stars.* Needham Research Institute series, 3. London: RoutledgeCurzon.

Ho Ping-yü & Joseph Needham. 1959. Elixir Poisoning in Mediaeval China. *Janus* 48. 4: 221–251, reprinted in Needham 1970, 316–339.

Horton, Robin. 1973. Lévy-Bruhl, Durkheim and the Scientific Revolution. In Horton & Finnegan 1973, 249–305.

Horton, Robin, & Ruth Finnegan, eds. 1973. *Modes of Thought. Essays on Thinking in Western and Non-Western Societies.* London: Faber and Faber.

Hsu, Elisabeth, ed. 2001. *Innovation in Chinese Medicine.* Needham Research Institute Studies, 3. Cambridge UP. Papers, varying in quality, from a memorial conference in honor of Lu Gwei-djen.

Hu Daojing 胡道靜. 1963. Shen Kuo de nongxue zhuzuo *Mengxi wang huai lu* 沈括的農學著作夢溪忘懷錄 (Shen Kuo's agricultural book *Record of Longings Forgotten). Wen shi* 文史, 1963, 3: 221–225.

Hu Daojing. 1980. *Su Shen neihan liang fang* Chu Shu pan 蘇沈內翰良方楚蜀判 (Attribution of the medicinal formulas in *Superior Formulas by Su & Shen). Shehui zhanxian* 社会战线, 3: 195–210. The title is a pun.

Hu Daojing. 1981. *Mengxi wang huai lu* gouchen—Shen Cunzhung yizhu gouchen zhi yi 夢溪忘懷錄鈎沉—沈存中佚著鈎沉之一 *(Record of Longings Forgotten* reconstituted. Shen Kuo's lost works reconstituted, 1). *Hangzhou daxue xuebao* 1981, 11. 1: 1–16.

Huang Minzhi 黃敏枝. 2005. Songdai de sengren yu yiliao 宋代的僧人與醫療 (Buddhist monks and medical therapy in the Song period). In Zhang Xueming & Liang Yuansheng 2005, 26–78.

Huang, Shih-shan Susan. 2012. *Picturing the True Form. Daoist Visual Culture in Traditional China.* Harvard East Asian Monographs, 342. Cambridge, MA: Harvard University Asia Center.

Huang Shijie 黃世杰. 2004. *Gu du. Caifu yu quanli de huanjue. Nanfang minzu shiyong chuantong duyao yu jieyao de renleixue yanjiu* 蠱毒: 财富与权利的幻学. 南方民族使用传统毒药与解药的人类学研究 *(Gu* poisoning: The magic of wealth and power. An anthropological study of the use of poisons and antidotes by southern Chinese peoples). Nanning: Guangxi Minzu Chubanshe.

Hucker, Charles O. 1985. *A Dictionary of Official Titles in Imperial China.* Stanford UP.

Hureau, Sylvie. 2010. Translations, Apocrypha, and the Emergence of the Buddhist Canon. In Lagerwey & Lü 2010, 741–774.

Hymes, Robert P. 1987. Not Quite Gentlemen? Doctors in Sung and Yuan. *Chinese Science* 8: 9–76.

Hymes, Robert, & Conrad Schirokauer, eds. 1993. *Ordering the World: Approaches to State and Society in Sung Dynasty China.* Berkeley: University of California Press.

Iiyama, Tomoyasu. 2010. Maintaining Gods in Medieval China: Temple Worship and Local Governance in North China under the Jin and Yuan. *Journal of Song–Yuan Studies* 40: 71–102.

Ikels, Charlotte. 1998. The Experience of Dementia in China. *Culture, Medicine and Psychiatry* 22: 257–283.

Inglis, Alister D. 2007. *Hong Mai's Record of the Listener and its Song Dynasty Context.* Albany: SUNY Press.

Ishii Masako 石井昌子. 1968. *Shinkō* no seiritsu o meguru shiryōteki kentō 真誥の成立をめぐる史料的檢討. (Documentary investigation of the formation of the *Declarations of the Realized Immortals*). *Dōkyō kenkyū* 道教研究 (Études taoistes) 3: 79–195.

James, William. 1902/1929. *The Varieties of Human Experience. A Study in Human Nature.* New York: Modern Library.

Johnson, David, ed. 1995. *Ritual and Scripture in Chinese Popular Religion. Five Studies.* China Popular Culture Project, 3. Berkeley: The Project.

Jordan, David K. 1972. *Gods, Ghosts, and Ancestors.* Berkeley: University of California Press.

Kalinowski, Marc, ed. 2003. *Divination et société dans la Chine médiévale. Étude des manuscripts de Dunhuang de la Bibliothèque nationale de France et de la British Library.* Paris: Bibliothèque nationale.

Kaltenmark, Max. 1960. Ling-pao 靈寶: Note sur un terme du Taoïsme religieux. *Mélanges de l'Institut des Hautes Études Chinoises* 2: 559–588.

Kaltenmark, Max. 1968. Notions sur quelques grands sutras Taoïstes (sommaire). Unpublished paper read at 1st International Conference on Taoism, Bellagio, Italy.

Kaptchuk, Ted J. 1998a. Intentional Ignorance: A History of Blind Assessment and Placebo Controls in Medicine. *Bulletin of the History of Medicine* 72. 3: 389–433.

Kaptchuk, Ted J. 1998b. Powerful Placebo: The Dark Side of the Randomised Controlled Trial. *The Lancet* 351: 1722–1725.

Kaptchuk, Ted J., et al. 2009. 'Maybe I Made Up the Whole Thing': Placebos and Patients' Experiences in a Randomized Controlled Trial. *Culture, Medicine and Psychiatry* 33: 382–411.

Kaptchuk, Ted J., et al. 2010. Placebos without Deception: A Randomized Controlled Trial in Irritable Bowel Syndrome. *Plos ONE* 5. 12: 1–7 (e15591).

Kaptchuk, Ted J. 2013. Placebo-controlled Randomized Trials and Chinese Medicine. In Hinrichs & Barnes 2013, 329–331.

Katz, Paul R. 1995. *Demon Hordes and Burning Boats. The Cult of Marshal Wen in Late Imperial Chekiang.* Albany: State University of New York Press.

Katz, Paul R. 2008. Trial by Power: Some Preliminary Observations on the Judicial Roles of Taoist Martial Deities. *Journal of Chinese Religions* 36: 54–83.

Katz, Paul R. 2009. *Divine Justice: Religion and the Development of Chinese Legal Culture.* Academia Sinica on East Asia. London: Routledge.

Katz, Pearl. 1981. Ritual in the Operating Room. *Ethnology* 20. 4: 335–350.

Keightley, David N. 1998. Shamanism, Death, and the Ancestors: Religious Mediation in Practice in Neolithic and Shang China (ca. 5000–1000 B.C.). *Asiatische Studien* 52. 3: 763–828.

Kirkland, Russell. 2002. The History of Taoism: A New Outline. Research Note. *Journal of Song–Yuan Studies* 30: 177–193.

Kirkland, Russell. 2009. The Taoist Priest *(Daoshi)* in Comparative Historical Perspective: A Critical Analysis. *Pacific World: Journal of the Institute of Buddhist Studies,* series 3, 11: 307–349.

Kleeman, Terry F. 1993. The Expansion of the Wen-ch'ang Cult. In Ebrey & Gregory 1993, 45–73.

Kleeman, Terry F. 1994. *A God's Own Tale. The* Book of Transformations of Wenchang, the Divine Lord of Zitong. SUNY Series in Chinese Philosophy and Culture. Albany: State University of New York Press.

Kleeman, Terry. 2005. The Evolution of Daoist Cosmology and the Construction of the Common Sacred Realm. *Taiwan Journal of East Asian Studies* 2. 1: 89–110.

Kleinman, Arthur. 1980. *Patients and Healers in the Context of Culture: An Exploration of the Borderland between Anthropology, Medicine, and Psychiatry.* Comparative Studies of Health Systems and Medical Care, 3. Berkeley: University of California Press.

Kleinman, Arthur. 1988. *The Illness Narratives. Suffering, Healing, and the Human Condition.* New York: Basic Books.

Kleinman, Arthur, & Lilias H. Sung. 1979. Why Do Indigenous Practitioners Successfully Heal? *Social Science and Medicine* 13B: 7–26.

Kleinman, Arthur, & James M. Gale. 1982. Patients Treated by Physicians and Folk Healers: A Comparative Study in Taiwan. *Culture, Medicine and Psychiatry,* 6: 405–423.

Kleinman, Arthur, Joan Kleinman, & Sing Lee. 1999. Introduction to the Transformation of Social Experience in Chinese Society: Anthropological, Psychiatric, and Social Medicine Perspectives. *Culture, Medicine, and Psychiatry* 23: 1–6. Overview of special issue from 1996 conference.

Kleinman, Arthur, & Don Seeman. 2000. Personal Experience of Illness. In Albrecht et al. 2000, 230–242.

Kleinman, Arthur, et al. 2011. *Deep China. The Moral Life of the Person. What Anthropology and Psychiatry Tell Us about China Today.* Berkeley: University of California Press.

Kohn, Livia. 2000. *Daoism Handbook.* Handbook of Oriental Studies, section 4, vol. 14. Leiden: Brill.

Kohn, Livia, & Harold D. Roth, eds. 2002. *Daoist Identity: History, Lineage and Ritual.* Honolulu: University of Hawai'i Press.

Kotaki Tōru 小滝透. 1997. *Kamigami no mezame: kindai Nihon no shūkyō kakumei* 神々の目覚め: 近代日本の宗教革命 (Awakening of the gods: religious revolution in modern Japan). Tokyo: Shunjūsha, 1997.

Kovacs, Jürgen, & Paul U. Unschuld, translators. 1998. *Essential Subtleties on the Silver Sea. The Yin-hai jing-wei: A Chinese Classic on Opthalmology.* Comparative Studies of Health Systems and Medical Care, 38. Berkeley: University of California Press.

Kuhn, Dieter. 2009. *The Age of Confucian Rule. The Song Transformation of China.* History of Imperial China. Belknap Press of Harvard UP.

Lagerwey, John. 1987. *Taoist Ritual in Chinese Society and History.* New York: Macmillan.

Lagerwey, John. 2010. *China. A Religious State.* Hong Kong UP. Four lectures.

Lagerwey, John, & Lü Pengzhi, eds. 2010. *Early Chinese Religion. Part Two: The Period of Disunion (220–589 AD).* Handbook of Oriental Studies, section 4, vols. 21–22. Leiden: Brill.

Lai, Chi Tim [Li Zhitian 黎志添]. 1998. The Opposition of Celestial-master Taoism to Popular Cults during the Six Dynasties. *Asia Major* (Taipei), ser. 3, 11. 1: 1–20.

Lebra, William P., ed. 1976. *Culture-Bound Syndromes, Ethnopsychiatry, and Alternative Therapies.* Mental Health Research in Asia and the Pacific, 4. Honolulu: University Press of Hawaii.

Lee T'ao. 1940. Ten Celebrated Physicians and their Temple. *Chinese Medical Journal* 58: 267–274. On state cult and popular cults.

Legge, James. 1885/1968. *The Texts of Confucianism,* parts 3–4. *The Lî Kî.* Sacred Books of the East, 28. 2 vols. Oxford UP. Reprint, Delhi: Motilal Banarsidass, 1968.

Lerner, Barron H. 2006. *When Illness Goes Public. Celebrity Patients and How We Look at Medicine.* Baltimore: The Johns Hopkins UP.

Leung, Angela Ki Che. 2003. Medical Learning from the Song to the Ming. In Smith & von Glahn 2003, 374–398, 510–512.

Leung, Angela Ki Che. 2009. *Leprosy in China: A History.* Studies of the Weatherhead East Asian Institute. New York: Columbia UP.

Levine, Ari Daniel. 2009. The Reigns of Hui-tsung (1100–1126) and Ch'in-tsung (1126–1127) and the Fall of the Northern Sung. In *The Cambridge History of China.* Vol. 5, part 1. *The Sung Dynasty and its Precursors,* 556–643. Cambridge UP.

Lewis, I. M. 1971. *Ecstatic Religion. An Anthropological Study of Spirit Possession and Shamanism.* Harmondsworth: Penguin.

Leys, Simon, & Michael Nylan, translators. 2014. *Confucius. The Analects.* Norton Critical Editions. New York: W. W. Norton.

Li Fengmao 李豐楙. 1993. Daozang suo shou zao qi dao shu de wenyiguan 道藏所收早期道書的瘟疫觀 (Views of epidemics in early Daoist books in the Daoist Canon). *Bulletin of the Institute of Literature and Philosophy, Academia Sinica* 3: 1–38.

Li Feng-mao. 1994. Xing wen yu song wen. Daojiao yu minzhong wenyiguan de jiaoliu yu fenqi 行瘟與送瘟. 道教與民衆瘟疫觀的交流與分歧 (Parading the epidemic gods and sending them off. The interaction and divergence of Daoist and popular views of epidemics). In Anonymous 1994, 372–422.

Li Gang. 2012. Cao Cao and Taoism. In Mou Zhongjian 2012, 101–117.

Li Jianmin, ed. 2008. *Cong yiliao kan Zhongguo shi* 從醫療看中國史 (Medical Perspectives on Chinese History). Taipei: Academia Sinica, 2008.

Li Jingwei 李经纬. 1998. Shi lun Zhongguo gudai waike shoushu 试论中国古代之外科手术 (Essay on surgery in ancient China). In Li Jingwei 李经纬, *Zhongguo yixue zhi huihuang. Li Jingwei wen ji* 中国医学之辉煌. 李经纬文集 (The glory of Chinese medicine. Collected essays of Li Jingwei), 298–301. Beijing: Zhongguo Zhongyiyao Chubanshe.

Liang Jun 梁峻. 1995. *Zhongguo gudai yizheng shi lue* 中国古代医政史略 (Outline history of ancient Chinese medical administration). Hohhot: Neimenggu Renmin Chubanshe.

Liao Hsien-huei. 2007. Encountering Evil: Ghosts and Demonic Forces in the Lives of the Song Elite. *Journal of Song–Yuan Studies* 37: 89–134.

Lincoln, Bruce. 2001. Revisiting 'Magical Fright.' *American Ethnologist* 28. 4: 778–802.

Lindemann, Mary. 2010. *Health and Healing in Early Modern Europe.* Rev. ed. Cambridge UP.

Little, Stephen, & Shawn Eichmann. 2000. *Taoism and the Arts of China.* The Art Institute of Chicago. Catalogue of exhibition, Nov. 2000–Jan 2001, with essays by specialists.

Liu, James T. C. 1957. An Early Sung Reformer: Fan Chung-yen. In *Chinese Thought and Institutions,* ed. John K. Fairbank, 105–131. Comparative Studies of Cultures and Civilizations, 8. University of Chicago Press.

Liu, James T. C. 1959. *Reform in Song China. Wang An-shih (1021–1086) and his New Policies.* Harvard East Asian Studies, 3. Harvard UP.

Liu Shoushan 刘寿山, ed. in chief. 1963– . *Zhongyao yanjiu wenxian zhaiyao* 中药研究文献摘要 (Abstracts of research publications on Chinese drugs). Beijing: Kexue Chubanshe. Ongoing; the first volume covers research published between 1820 and 1961.

Liu Shufen 劉淑芬. 2008a. Tang Song shi sengren, guojia he yiliao de guanxi: Cong Yaofang dong dao Huimin ju 唐宋時僧人國家和醫療的關係: 從藥方洞到惠民局 (Buddhist monks, the state, and medical therapy in the Tang and Song periods. From Formulary Cave to the Bureau for Benefiting the People). In Li Jianmin 2008, 145–202.

Liu Shufen 刘淑芬. 2008b. *Zhonggu de fojiao yu shehui* 中古的佛教与社会 (Medieval Buddhism and Society). Shehui, jingji, guannian congshu 社会. 经济. 观念丛书. Shanghai Guji Chubanshe.

Liu Zhiwan 劉枝萬. 1967. *Taibei Songshan qi an jian jiao jidian* 臺北松山祈安建醮祭典 (Great propitiatory rites of petition for beneficence at Songshan, Taipei, Taiwan). Institute of Ethnology, Academia Sinica, Monographs, 14. Nankang: Academia Sinica.

Liu Zhiwan 劉枝萬. 1974a. *Zhongguo minjian xinyang lun ji* 中國民間信仰論集 (Essays on Chinese Folk Belief and Folk Cults). Institute of Ethnology, Academia Sinica, Monographs, 22. Nankang: Academia Sinica.

Liu Zhiwan. 1974b. Lüshan jiao zhi shou hun fa 閭山教之收魂法 (The method of retrieving the soul in the Lüshan sect). In Liu 1974a, 207–378.

Lloyd, G. E. R., & Nathan Sivin. 2002. *The Way and the Word. Science and Medicine in Early China and Greece.* New Haven: Yale UP.

Lock, Margaret. 2000. Accounting for Disease and Distress: Morals of the Normal and Abnormal. In Albrecht et al. 2000, 259–276.

Lock, Margaret. 2005. Symptom Reporting at the End of Menstruation: Biological Variation and Cultural Difference. In *Controversies in Science and Technologies: From Maize to Menopause,* ed. D.L. Kleinman, A.J. Kinchy, & J. Handelsman. Madison: University of Wisconsin Press, 236–253.

Lock, Margaret, & Nancy Scheper-Hughes. 1996. A Critical-Interpretive Approach in Medical Anthropology: Rituals and Routines of Discipline and Dissent. In Sargent & Johnson 1986, 41–70.

Loewe, Michael, ed. 1993. *Early Chinese Texts. A Bibliographical Guide.* Early China Special Monograph Series, 2. Berkeley: The Society for the Study of Early China & The Institute of East Asian Studies.

Lopez, Donald S., Jr. 1996. *Religions of China in Practice.* Princeton Readings in Religions. Princeton UP.

Ma Boying 马伯英. 1994/2010. *Zhongguo yixue wenhua shi* 中国医学文化史 (A history of medicine in Chinese culture). 2d ed. 2 vols. Shanghai Renmin Chubanshe.

Ma Jixing 馬繼興, ed. 1995. *Shennong bencao jing ji zhu* 神農本草經輯注 (Reconstituted and annotated *Divine Farmer's materia medica).* RW. A new text reconstructed from early primary sources, adding reconstructions of a 4-chapter ed. and Han and Wei commentaries, and 700 pp. of scholarly essays related to the reconstruction.

Ma Jixing 馬繼興 et al. 1998. *Dunhuang yiyao wenxian ji jiao* 敦煌醫藥文獻輯校 (Collected collations of the medical texts from Dunhuang). Dunhuang wenxian fen lei lu jiao congkan 敦煌文獻分類錄校叢刊. Nanjing: Jiangsu Guji Chubanshe.

MacDonald, Michael. 1981. *Medical Bedlam. Madness, Anxiety, and Healing in Seventeenth-century England.* Cambridge UP.

MacDonald, Michael. 1989. The Medicalization of Suicide in England: Laymen, Physicians, and Cultural Change, 1500–1870. *Milbank Quarterly* 67 (Suppl. 1), 69–91.

Matsumoto Kōichi 松本浩一. 2006. *Sōdai no dōkyō to minkan shingyō* 宋代の道教と民間信仰 (Daoism and folk belief in the Song period). Tokyo: Kyuko Shoin.

McFarland, H. Neill. 1967. *The Rush Hour of the Gods: A Study of New Religious Movements in Japan.* New York: Macmillan.

McGrath, Michael. 2009. The Reigns of Jen-tsung (1022–1063) and Ying-tsung (1063–1067). In *The Cambridge History of China.* Vol. 5, part 1. *The Sung Dynasty and its Precursors,* 279–346. Cambridge UP.

Megill, Allan, ed. 1994. *Rethinking Objectivity.* Durham: Duke UP.

Meng Yongliang 孟永亮 & Liang Yongxuan 梁永宣. 2014. Bei Song Jiaozheng Yishuju bian jiao yi ji gai shu 北宋校正医书局编校医籍概述 (An overview of the collation and editing of medical books by the Bureau for Revising Medical Books of the Northern Song dynasty). *Zhonghua yishi zazhi* 中华医史杂志 44. 4: 206–210.

Mitamura, Keiko. 2002. Daoist Hand Signs and Buddhist Mudras. In Kohn & Roth 2002, 235–255. On symbolic gestures.

Miyasita [Miyashita] Saburō. 1976. A Historical Study of Chinese Drugs for the Treatment of Jaundice. *American Journal of Chinese Medicine* 4. 3: 239–243.

Miyasita Saburō. 1977. A Historical Analysis of Chinese Formularies and Prescriptions: Three Examples. *Nihon ishigaku zasshi* 23. 2: 283–300.

Miyasita Saburō. 1979. Malaria *(yao)* [i.e. *nue* 瘧] in Chinese Medicine during the Chin and Yuan Periods. *Acta Asiatica* 36: 90–112.

Miyasita Saburō. 1980. An Historical Analysis of Chinese Drugs in the Treatment of Hormonal Diseases, Goitre, and Diabetes Mellitus. *American Journal of Chinese Medicine* 8. 1: 17–25.

Moerman, Daniel. 2000. Cultural Variations in the Placebo Effect: Ulcers, Anxiety, and Blood Pressure. *Medical Anthropology Quarterly* 14. 1: 1–22.

Moerman, Daniel. 2002. *Meaning, Medicine and the Placebo Effect.* Cambridge Studies in Medical Anthropology. Cambridge UP.

Mollier, Christine. 1990. *Une apocalypse taoïste du Ve siècle. Le livre des incantations divines des grottes abyssales.* Mémoires de l'Institut des Hautes Études Chinoises, 31. Paris: L'Institut.

Montaigne, Michel de. 1685/1711. *Essays of Michael Seigneur de Montaigne.* 4th ed., 3 vols. London: Daniel Brown et al.

Morris, David B. 1997. Placebo, Pain, and Belief: A Biocultural Model. In Harrington 1997, 187–207.

Mou Zhongjian, ed. 2012. *Taoism,* ed. and tr. Pan Junliang & Simone Normand, Religious Studies in Contemporary China Collection, 2. Boston: Brill, 2012. Surveys and research papers from Chinese scholars.

Mueggler, Erik. 2003. Review of Stephan Feuchtwang, *Popular Religion in China: The Imperial Metaphor* (Richmond, Surrey: Curzon Press, 2001). *American Anthropologist,* n.s., 105. 2: 410–411.

Munkhoff, Rachelle. 1999. Searchers of the Dead: Authority, Marginality, and the Interpretation of Plague in England, 1574–1665. *Gender and History* 11: 1–29.

Nakamura Jihei 中村治兵衛. 1978. KitaSōchō to fu 北宋朝と巫 (The Northern Song dynasty and wizards). *Chūo Daigaku Bungakubu kiyo. Shigaku ka* 中央大學文學部紀要. 史學科 23: 63–78.

Nakamura Jihei. 1982. Sōdai no fu no tokuchō 宋代の巫の特徵 (Special characteristics of wizards in the Song period). *Chūo Daigaku Bungakubu kiyo* 104: 51–75.

Naquin, Susan. 2012. Temples, Technology, and Material Culture in Shouzhou 壽州, Anhui. In Schäfer 2012, 184–207.

National Association of Chronic Disease Directors. 2007. *Public Health Advances through Chronic Disease Prevention: 1986–2006.* Atlanta: The Association.

National Institutes of Health. 2012. 'Attention Deficit Hyperactivity Disorder.' NIH Publication 12-3572. Http://www.nimh.nih.gov/health/publications/attention-deficit-hyperactivity-disorder/index.shtml (accessed 2015.3.2).

Needham, Joseph, et al. 1954– . *Science and Civilisation in China.* 24 vols. to date. Cambridge UP.

Needham, Joseph, et al. 1970. *Clerks and Craftsmen in China and the West. Lectures and Addresses on the History of Science and Technology.* Cambridge UP.

Nichter, Mark. 1980. The Layperson's Perception of Medicine as Perspective into the Utilization of Multiple Therapy Systems in the Indian Context. *Social Science and Medicine* 148: 225–233.

Nickerson, Peter. 1996. Abridged Codes of Master Lu for the Daoist Community. In Lopez 1996, 347–359.

Nickerson, Peter. 1997. The Great Petition for Sepulchral Plaints. In *Early Daoist Scriptures,* ed. Stephen R. Bokenkamp, 230–74. Berkeley: University of California Press.

Nickerson, Peter. 2000. The Southern Heavenly Masters. In Kohn 2000, 256–282.

Nickerson, Peter. 2006. 'Let Living and Dead Take Separate Paths.' Bureaucratisation and Textualisation in Early Chinese Mortuary Ritual. In Penny 2006, 10–40.

Obringer, Frédéric. 1997. *L'aconit et l'orpiment. Drogues et poisons en Chine ancienne et médiévale*. Penser la médecine, 4. Paris: Fayard.

Ogawa Takuji 小川琢治. 1935. Shina ni okeru honzōgaku no kigen to *Shinnō honzōkyō* 支那における本草學の起原と神農本草經 (The beginnings of materia medica in China and the *Divine Farmer's Materia Medica*). In Ogawa, *Shina rekishi chiri kenkyū* 支那歷史地理研究 (Studies in Chinese historical geography). 3d ed., Tokyo: Kōbundō Shobō 弘文堂書房.

Okanishi Tameto 岡西為人. 1958. *Song yiqian yiji kao* 宋以前醫籍考 (Studies of medical books of the Sung and earlier). B: RW.

Okanishi Tameto 岡西為人, editor. 1972. *Bencao jing jizhu* 本草經集注 (The Heavenly Farmer's canon of materia medica, with collected annotations). Osaka: Minami-Ōsaka Insatsu Sentaa.

Orzech, Charles D. 2002. *Fang yankou* and *Pudu:* Translation, Metaphor, and Religious Identity. In Kohn & Roth 2002, 213–234.

Payer, Lynn. 1988. *Medicine & Culture: Varieties of Treatment in the United States, England, West Germany, and France.* New York: Henry Holt.

Pellegrino, Edmund D. 1976. Prescribing and Drug Ingestion: Symbols and Substances. *Drug Intelligence and Clinical Pharmacy* 10: 624–630.

Pelling, Margaret. 1998. *The Common Lot: Sickness, Medical Occupations and the Urban Poor in Early Modern England.* London: Longman.

Penny, Benjamin, ed. 2006. *Daoism in History. Essays in Honour of Liu Ts'un-yan.* London: Routledge.

Poo, Mu-chou. 2010. Images and Ritual Treatment of Dangerous Spirits. In Lagerwey & Lü 2010, 2:1075–1094.

Porkert, Manfred. 1974. *The Theoretical Foundations of Chinese Medicine: Systems of Correspondence.* MIT East Asian Science Series, 3. Cambridge: The MIT Press.

Porter, Roy, ed. 1985. *Patients and Practitioners. Lay Perceptions of Medicine in Pre-industrial Society.* Cambridge History of Medicine, 9. Cambridge UP.

Porter, Roy. 1989. *Health for Sale. Quackery in England 1660–1850.* Manchester UP.

Potter, Jack M. 1974. Cantonese Shamanism. In Wolf 1974a, 207–231.

Pregadio, Fabrizio, ed. 2008. *The Encyclopedia Of Taoism*. 2 vols. New York: Routledge.

Price, Donald D., & Howard L. Fields. 1997. The Contribution of Desire and Expectation to Placebo Analgesia: Implications for New Research Strategies. In Harrington 1997, 116–137.

Ramsey, Matthew. 1988. *Professional and Popular Medicine in France, 1770–1830: The Social World of Medical Practice.* Cambridge history of medicine. Cambridge UP.

Rankin, Alisha. 2013. *Panaceia's Daughters: Noblewomen as Healers in Early Modern Germany.* Synthesis. University of Chicago Press.

Raz, Gil. 2007. Imperial Efficacy: Debates on Imperial Ritual in Early Medieval China and the Emergence of Daoist Ritual Schemata. In Reiter 2007b, 83–109.

Raz, Gil. 2012. *The Emergence of Daoism. Creation of Tradition.* Routledge Studies in Taoism. London: Routledge.

Reiter, Florian C., ed. 2007a. *Basic Conditions of Taoist Thunder Magic*. Abhandlungen für die Kunde des Morgenlandes, 61. Wiesbaden: Harrassowitz.

Reiter, Florian C., ed. 2007b. *Purposes, Means and Convictions in Daoism. A Berlin Symposium.* Humboldt Universiteit Asien- und Afrika-Studien, 29. Wiesbaden: Harrassowitz.

Ren Zongquan 任宗权. 2002. *Daojiao shouyin yanjiu* 道教手印研究 (Studies of Daoist symbolic gestures). Beijing: Daojiao Wenhua Chubanshe.

Robinet, Isabelle. 1984. *La revelation du Shangqing dans l'histoire du Taoisme.* 2 vols. Paris: Ècole Française d'Extrême-Orient.

Rosenberg, Charles E. 2003. What is Disease? In Memory of Owsei Temkin. *Bulletin of the History of Medicine* 77: 491–505.

Rubel, Arthur J., & Michael R. Haas. 1996. Ethnomedicine. In Sargent & Johnson 1996, 113–130.

Rubinstein, Robert A., & Ronald T. Brown. 1984. An Evaluation of the Validity of the Diagnostic Category of Attention Deficit Disorder. *American Journal of Orthopsychiatry* 543: 398–414.

Russell, Bertrand. 1945. *A History of Western Philosophy, and its Connection with Political and Social Circumstances from the Earliest Times to the Present Day.* New York: Simon and Schuster.

Salguero, C. Pierce. 2009. The Buddhist Medicine King in Literary Context: Reconsidering an Early Medieval Example of Indian Influence on Chinese Medicine and Surgery. *History of Religions* 48. 3: 183–210.

Salguero, C. Pierce. 2010. 'A Flock of Ghosts Bursting Forth and Scattering': Healing Narratives in a Sixth-century Chinese Buddhist Hagiography. EASTM 32: 89–120.

Salguero, C. Pierce. 2014. *Translating Buddhist Medicine in Medieval China.* Encounters with Asia. Philadelphia: University of Pennsylvania Press.

Salzman, Philip Carl. 2002. On Reflexivity. *American Anthropologist* 104. 3: 805–813. Fallacies connected with the concept.

Sargent, Carolyn F., & Thomas M. Johnson, eds. 1996. *Medical Anthropology: Contemporary Theory and Method.* Rev. ed. Westport, CT: Praeger.

Saunders, E. Dale. 1960. *Mudrā. A Study of Symbolic Gestures in Japanese Buddhist Sculpture.* Bollingen series, 58. New York: Pantheon Books.

Saunders, E. Dale. 1968. Notions of Medicine in Early Japan. In *Symposium on Chinese Studies Commemorating the Golden Jubilee of the University of Hong Kong,* 3:82–109.

Savill, Thomas Dixon. 1930. *A System of Clinical Medicine: Dealing with the Diagnosis, Prognosis, and Treatment of Disease: For Students and Practitioners.* 8th ed. New York: William Wood. First ed., 2 vols., London, 1903–1905.

Sawada Mizuho 澤田瑞穗. 1984. *Chūgoku no juhō* 中国の咒法 (Chinese incantations). Tokyo: Hirakawa Shuppansha.

Schafer, Edward H. 1977. *Pacing the Void. T'ang Approaches to the Stars.* Berkeley: University of California Press.

Schäfer, Dagmar, ed. 2012. *Cultures of Knowledge. Technology in Chinese History.* Sinica Leidensia, 103. Leiden: Brill.

Scheid, Volker. 2002. *Chinese Medicine in Contemporary China: Plurality and Synthesis*. Durham: Duke UP.

Scheid, Volker. 2007. *Currents of Tradition in Chinese Medicine. 1626–2006*. Seattle: Eastland Press.

Spindler, Kristofer M. 1975. *Concordance du Tao-tsang. Titres et ouvrages*. Publications, 102. Paris: École Française d'Extrême-orient.

Schipper, Kristofer M. 1982. *Le corps taoïste. Corps physique–corps social*. L'espace intérieur, 25. Paris.

Schipper, Kristofer M. 1985. Taoist Ritual and Local Cults of the Tang Dynasty. In Strickmann 1981–1985, 3:812–834.

Schipper, Kristofer. 1989. A study of Buxu: Taoist Liturgical Hymn and Dance. In *Studies of Taoist Rituals and Music of Today,* ed. Pen-yeh Tsao & Daniel P. L. Law, 110–120. Hong Kong: Society of Ethnomusicologica.

Schipper, Kristofer, & Franciscus Verellen, eds. 2004. *The Taoist Canon. A Historical Companion to the* Daozang. 3 vols. University of Chicago Press.

Seidel, Anna. 1983. Imperial Treasures and Taoist Sacraments. Taoist Roots in the Apocrypha. In Strickmann 1981–1985, 2:291–371.

Seidel, Anna K. 1969–1970. The Image of the Perfect Ruler in Early Taoist Messianism. Lao tzu and Li Hung. *History of Religions* 9: 216–247.

Seligman, Adam B., Robert P. Weller, Michael J. Puett, & Bennett Simon. 2008. *Ritual and its Consequences. An Essay on the Limits of Sincerity.* Oxford UP.

Seligman, Adam B. & Robert P. Weller. 2012. *Rethinking Pluralism: Ritual, Experience, and Ambiguity.* Oxford UP. Chapter 3 (pp. 93–145) is "Ritual and the Rhythms of Ambiguity."

Shahar, Meir, & Robert P. Weller, eds. 1996. *Unruly Gods. Divinity and Society in China.* Honolulu: University of Hawaii Press.

Shandong Zhongyi Xueyuan 山东中医学院 (Shandong Provincial College of Chinese Medicine) & Hebei Yixueyuan 河北医学院 (Hebei Provincial Hospital). 1982. *Huangdi neijing Su wen jiaoshi* 黄帝内经素问校释 (*Inner Canon of the Yellow Emperor, Basic Questions,* with critical and explanatory notes). RW.

Shapiro, Arthur K., & Elaine Shapiro. 1997. The Placebo: Is It Much Ado about Nothing? In Harrington 1997, 12–36. Medical reductionists' view.

Shinno, Reiko. 2007. Medical Schools and the Temples of the Three Progenitors in Yuan China: A Case of Cross-Cultural Interactions. *Harvard Journal of Asiatic Studies* 67. 1: 89–133.

Sivin, Nathan. 1968. *Chinese Alchemy: Preliminary Studies.* Harvard Monographs in the History of Science, 1. Harvard UP.

Sivin, Nathan. 1977. Social Relations of Curing in Traditional China: Preliminary Considerations. *Nihon ishigaku zasshi* 23: 505–532.

Sivin, Nathan. 1978. On the Word Taoism as a Source of Perplexity. With Special Reference to the Relations of Science and Religion in Traditional China. *History of Religions* 17: 303–330.

Sivin, Nathan. 1979. Report on the Third International Conference on Taoist Studies. *Bulletin,* Society for the Study of Chinese Religions 7: 1–23.

Sivin, Nathan. 1987. *Traditional Medicine in Contemporary China.* Science, Medicine, and Technology in East Asia, 2. Ann Arbor: Center for Chinese Studies, University of Michigan.

Sivin, Nathan. 1995a. *Medicine, Philosophy and Religion in Ancient China. Researches and Reflections.* Variorum Collected Studies Series. Aldershot, Hants: Variorum.

Sivin, Nathan. 1995b. Emotional Counter-therapy. In Sivin 1995a, chapter 2.

Sivin, Nathan. 1995c. Taoism and Science. In Sivin 1995a, chapter 7.

Sivin, Nathan. 1995d. Shen Kua (1031–1095). In *Science in Ancient China. Researches and Reflections,* chapter 3, 1–53. Variorum Collected Studies Series. Aldershot, Hants: Variorum.

Sivin, Nathan. 2010. Old and New Daoisms. *Religious Studies Review* 36. 1: 31–50.

Skar, Lowell. 2008. Lingbao dafa 靈寳大法. In Pregadio 2008, 671–672.

Skinner, G. William. 1985. Presidential Address: The Structure of Chinese History. *Journal of Asian Studies* 44. 2: 271–292.

Smith, Hilary. 2008. Foot Qi: History of a Chinese Medical Disorder. Ph.D. dissertation, History and Sociology of Science, University of Pennsylvania.

Smith, Paul Yakov. 2003. Problematizing the Song–Yuan–Ming Transition. In Smith & von Glahn 2003, 1–34.

Smith, Paul Yakov, & Richard von Glahn, eds. 2003. *The Song–Yuan–Ming Transition in Chinese History*. Harvard East Asian Monographs, 221. Harvard UP. On the period 1270–1550.

Snell, Bruno. 1953. *The Discovery of the Mind.* Oxford: Blackwell.

Spindler, George Dearborn, John Wesley, & Mayhew Whiting. 1978. *The Making of Psychological Anthropology.* Berkeley: University of California Press.

Spiro, Howard. 1986. *Doctors, Patients, and Placebos.* Yale UP.

Spiro, Howard. 1997. Clinical Reflections on the Placebo Phenomenon. In Harrington 1997, 37–55.

Spiro, Melford E. 1978. Culture and Human Nature. In Spindler 1978, 331–60.

Spiro, Melford E. 1986. Cultural Relativism and the Future of Anthropology. *Cultural Anthropology* 1. 3: 259–286.

Stein, Howard F. 1973. Ethanol and its Discontents: Paradoxes of Inebriation and Sobriety in American Culture. *Journal of Psychoanalytic Anthropology* 5. 4: 355–377.

Strickmann, Michel, ed. 1981–1985. *Tantric and Taoist Studies in Honour of R. A. Stein.* 3 vols. Brussels: Institut Belge des Hautes Études Chinoises.

Strickmann, Michel. 1993. The Seal of the Law: a Ritual Implement and the Origins of Printing. *Asia Major,* ser. 3, 6. 2: 1–83.

Strickmann, Michel. 2002. *Chinese Magical Medicine*, ed. Bernard Faure. Asian Religions and Cultures. Stanford UP. Posthumous.

Sue Takashi 須江隆. 1994. TōSōki ni okeru shibyo no byogaku hogo no kashi ni tsuite 唐宋期における祠廟の廟額封号の下賜について (On the conferral of temple plaques and ranks for spirits on temples in the Tang and Song periods). *Chūgoku shakai to bunka* 中国社会と文化 (Chinese society and culture) 9: 96–119.

Sun, Xiaochun 孫小淳. 2007. State and Science: Scientific Innovations in Northern Song China, 960–1127. Ph.D. dissertation, History and Sociology of Science, University of Pennsylvania.

Sun Xiaochun & Zeng Xiongsheng 曾雄生, eds. 2007. *Songdai guojia wenhua zhong de kexue* 宋代国家文化中的科学 (Science and the State in the Song Dynasty). Beijing: Zhongguo Kexue Jishu Chubanshe.

Swidler, Ann. 2001. *Talk of Love. How Culture Matters.* University of Chicago Press.

Szonyi, Michael. 1997. The Illusion of Standardizing the Gods. The Cult of Five Emperors in Late Imperial China. *Journal of Asian Studies* 56. 1: 113–135.

Tang Daijian 唐代劍. 2003. *Songdai daojiao guanli zhidu yanjiu* 宋代道教管理制度研究 (A study of regulation of the Daoist religion in the Song period). Beijing: Xianzhuang shuju.

Tao Yufeng 陶御风, Zhu Bangxian 朱邦贤, & Hung Pimo 洪丕漠. 1988. *Lidai biji yi shi bielu* 历代笔记医事别录 (Classified anthology of medical matters in the collected jottings of various periods). Tianjin: Tianjin Kexue Jishu Chubanshe. About 2000 jottings from the *biji* literature, arranged by topic; some censorship.

Taylor, Kim. 2004. Divergent Interests and Cultivated Misunderstandings: The Influence of the West on Modern Chinese Medicine. *Social History of Medicine* 17. 1: 93–111. On the origin of the term "Traditional Chinese Medicine."

Teiser, Stephen F. 1993. The Growth of Purgatory. In Ebrey & Gregory 1993, 115–145.

Teiser, Stephen F. 1995. Popular Religion. *Journal of Asian Studies* 54. 2: 378–395.

Topley, Marjorie. 1970. Chinese Traditional Ideas and the Treatment of Disease: Two Examples from Hong Kong. *Man,* n.s., 5: 421–437.

Topley, Marjorie. 1974. Cosmic Antagonisms: A Mother-Child Syndrome. In Wolf 1974a, 233–249.

Torrey, E. Fuller. 1974. Spiritualists and Shamans as Psychotherapists: An Account of Original Anthropological Sin. In *Religious Movements in Contemporary America,* ed. Irving I. Zaretsky & Mark P. Leone, 30–37. Princeton UP.

Tseng, Wen-shing. 1973. The Development of Psychiatric Concepts in Traditional Chinese Medicine. *Archives of General Psychiatry* 29: 569–575.

Tseng, Wen-shing. 1976. Folk Psychotherapy in Taiwan. In Lebra 1976, 164–178.

Tseng, Wen-shing. 2006. From Peculiar Psychiatric Disorders through Culture-bound Syndromes to Culture-related Specific Syndromes. *Transcultural Psychiatry* 43. 4: 554–576.

Ulrich, Laurel Thatcher. 1990. *A Midwife's Tale. The Life of Martha Ballard, Based on her Diary, 1785–1812.* New York: Alfred A. Knopf.

Unschuld, Paul Ulrich. 1989. *Forgotten Traditions in Ancient Chinese Medicine. The I-hsueh Yüan Liu Lun of 1757 by Hsü Ta-Ch'un.* Brookline, MA: Paradigm Publications.

Unschuld, Paul Ulrich. 2003. *Huang Di nei jing su wen. Nature, Knowledge, Imagery in an Ancient Chinese Medical Text.* Berkeley: University of California Press.

Unschuld, Paul U. 2010. The Berlin Collections of Chinese Medical Manuscripts: Rural Authors, Rural Contents. *Monumenta Serica* 58: 281–293.

Unschuld, Paul U., & Zheng Jinsheng. 2012. *Chinese Traditional Healing. The Berlin Collections of Manuscript Volumes from the Sixteenth through the Early Twentieth Century.* Sir Henry Wellcome Asian Series, 10. 3 vols. Leiden: Brill.

van der Loon, Piet. 1984. *Taoist Books in the Libraries of the Sung Period. A Critical Study and Index.* Oxford Oriental Institute Monographs, 7. London: Ithaca Press.

Waldram, James B. 2000. The Efficacy of Traditional Medicine: Current Theoretical and Methodological Issues. *Medical Anthropology Quarterly* 14. 4: 603–625.

Wang, Jing. 2001. Culture as Leisure and Culture as Capital. *Positions* 9. 1: 69–104.

Wang, Jing. 2005. Bourgeois Bohemians in China? Neo-Tribes and the Urban Imaginary. *The China Quarterly* 183: 532–548.

Wang Ming 王明. 1980. *Baopuzi neipian jiao shi* 抱朴子内篇校釋 (*The Inner Chapters of the Master who Embraces Simplicity,* with commentary). ZS.

Wang Zhenguo 王振国. 2006. *Zhongguo gudai yixue jiaoyu yu kaoshi zhidu yanjiu* 中国古代医学教育与考试制度研究 (A study of medical education and the examination system in ancient China). Jinan: Qi-Lu Shu She.

Ware, James R. 1966. *Alchemy, Medicine, and Religion in the China of A.D. 320. The Nei P'ien of Ko Hung.* Cambridge, Mass. Translation of *Baopuzi nei pian.*

Wear, Andrew, Johanna Geyer-Kordesch, & Roger French, eds. 1993. *Doctors and Ethics: The Earlier Historical Setting of Professional Ethics.* Wellcome Institute Series in the History of Medicine. Amsterdam: Rodopi.

Weerdt, Hilde de. 2006. Byways in the Imperial Chinese Information Order: The Dissemination and Commercial Publication of State Documents. *Harvard Journal of Asiatic Studies* 66. 1: 145–188.

Whyte, Susan Reynolds, Sjaak van der Geest, & Anita Harden. 2002. *Social Lives of Medicines.* Cambridge Studies in Medical Anthropology. Cambridge UP.

Wilkinson, Endymion. 2013. *Chinese History: A New Manual.* Third, revised printing. Cambridge: Harvard UP. This edition originally published 2012.

Wolf, Arthur P., ed. 1974a. *Religion and Ritual in Chinese Society.* Stanford UP. Essays on contemporary Hong Kong and Taiwan.

Wolf, Arthur P. 1974b. Gods, Ghosts, and Ancestors. In Wolf 1974a, 131–182.

Woods, Andrew H., M. D. 1929. The Nervous Diseases of the Chinese. *Archives of Neurology and Psychiatry* 2: 542–570.

Wu Yiyi. 1993. A Medical Line of Many Masters: A Prosopographical Study of Liu Wansu and his Disciples from the Jin to the Early Ming. *Chinese Science* 11: 36–65.

Wujastyk, Dominik. 1993. Indian medicine. In *Companion Encyclopedia of the History of Medicine*, ed. W. F. Bynum & Roy Porter, 755–778. London: Routledge.

Wujastyk, Dominik. 2001. *The Roots of Āyurveda: Selections from Sanskrit Medical Writings.* Penguin classics. New Delhi: Penguin Books.

Xu Fulin 徐复霖, Tian Weijun 田维君, & Wu Shijiu 吴仕九. 1985. *Gu jin jiu wu* 古今救誤 (The correction of medical errors in ancient and modern times). Changsha: Hunan Kexue Jishu Chubanshe. Anthology of therapeutic errors.

Xue Qinglu 薛清录 et al. 1991. *Quanguo Zhongyi tushu lianhe mulu* 全国中医图书聯合目录 (National union catalogue of primary sources for Chinese medicine). Beijing: Zhongyi Guji Chubanshe.

Yan Ruixue 閻瑞雪. 2009. Songdai yixue zhishi de kuosan 宋代医学知识的扩散 (Spread of Medical Knowledge in the Song Period). In Fang Xiaoyang 方晓阳 & Chen Tianjia 陈天嘉 2009, 63–85.

Yan Shiyun 严世芸. 1990–1994. *Zhongguo yi ji tong kao* 中国医籍通考 (General compendium on traditional Chinese medical books). 4 vols., 1 vol. index. Shanghai: Shanghai Zhongyi Xueyuan Chubanshe. Not a general compendium; merely reproduces prefaces to ca. 9000 books, extant and lost, with occasional notes on authors.

Yap, P. M. 1960. The Possession Syndrome: a Comparison of Hong Kong and French Findings. *Journal of Mental Science* 106: 114–137.

Yap, P. M. 1969. Classification of the Culture-bound Reactive Syndromes. *Far East Medical Journal* 7: 219–225.

Young, Allan. 1982. The Anthropologies of Illness and Sickness. *Annual Review of Anthropology* 11: 257–285.

Young, Allan. 1983. The Relevance of Traditional Medical Cultures to Modern Primary Health Care. *Social Science and Medicine* 17. 16: 1205–1211.

Yu, Anthony C. 2006. *State and Religion in China: Historical and Textual Perspectives.* Chicago: Open Court Books.

Yü, Chün-fang (Yu Junfang). 2001. *Kuan-yin. The Chinese Transformation of Avalokitesvara.* Institute for Advanced Studies of World Religions Books, 11. New York: Columbia UP.

Yu Gengzhe 于赓哲. 2011. *Tangdai jibing yiliao shi chu tan* 唐代疾病医疗史初探 (Preliminary historical studies of illness and therapy in the Tang period). Beijing: Zhongguo Shehui Kexue Chubanshe.

Zhang Haipeng 張海鵬. 2014. Cong Songren dui yizhe de jishu kan zhishi chuancheng moshi de zhuanbian 从宋人对医者的记述看医学知识传承模式的转变 (On changes in the model of medical knowledge in Song period depictions of physicians). *Zhonghua yishi zazhi* 中华医史杂志, 44. 6: 329-334.

Zhang, Yanhua. 2007. *Transforming Emotions with Chinese Medicine: An Ethnographic Account from Contemporary China.* Albany: State University of New York Press.

Zhang Zehong. 1999. *Daojiao zhaijiao keyi yanjiu* 道教斋醮科仪研究 (Studies in the liturgy of Daoist offering rituals). Ru Dao Shi boshi lunwen congshu 儒道释博士论文丛书. Chengdu: Ba-Shu Shushe.

Zhang Zuoji 张作记 & Zhang Ruixian 张瑞贤, eds. 1995. *Yaowang quan shu* 药王全书 (Collected books of the King of Medicine). Beijing: Huaxia Chubanshe. Collected works of Sun Simiao.

Zhong Jingwen 钟敬文, ed. in chief. 2008. *Zhongguo minsu shi (Song Liao Jin Yuan juan)* 中国民俗史 (宋辽金元卷) (The history of Chinese folklore: Song, Liao, Jin, and Yuan periods). Guojia sheke jijin chengguo wenku 国家社科基金成果文库. Beijing: Renmin Chubanshe.

Zhou Yimou 周一謀. 1983. *Lidai ming yi lun yide* 历代名医論医德 (Discussions of medical morality by famous doctors in successive dynasties). Changsha: Hunan Kexue Jishu Chubanshe. Anthology, from early classics to 1897.

Zhu Kewen 朱克文, Gao Sixian 高思显, & Gong Chun 龚纯. 1996. *Zhongguo junshi yixue shi* 中国军事医学史 (History of Chinese military medicine). Beijing: Renmin Junyi Chubanshe.

Zhuang Hongyi 莊宏誼. 1999. Songdai daojiao yiliao. Yi Hong Mai *Yijian zhi* wei zhu zhi yanjiu 宋代道教醫療－以洪邁夷堅志為主之研究 (Daoist therapy in the Song. A study based mainly on Hong Mai's *Records of the Listener). Furen zongjiao yanjiu* 輔仁宗教研究 12: 73–147.

Zimmerman, Francis. 1978. From Classic Texts to Learned Practice: Methodological Remarks on the Study of Indian Medicine. *Social Science and Medicine* 12: 97–103.

Zito, Angela. 1996. City Gods and their Magistrates. In Lopez 1996, 72–81.

Zong Li 宗力 & Liu Qun 刘群. 1987. *Zhongguo minjian zhu shen* 中国民間诸神 (Popular gods of China). Shijiazhuang: Hebei Renmin Chubanshe.

Index

© Springer International Publishing Switzerland 2015

N. Sivin, *Health Care in Eleventh-Century China*, Archimedes 43,
DOI 10.1007/978-3-319-20427-7

D

E

T

MIX
Papier aus verantwortungsvollen Quellen
Paper from responsible sources
FSC® C105338

If you have any concerns about our products,
you can contact us on
ProductSafety@springernature.com

In case Publisher is established outside the EU,
the EU authorized representative is:
Springer Nature Customer Service Center GmbH
Europaplatz 3, 69115 Heidelberg, Germany

Printed by Libri Plureos GmbH
in Hamburg, Germany